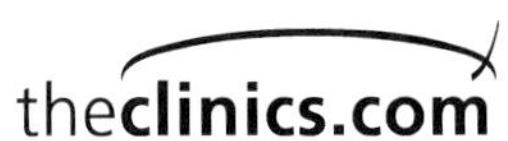

PHYSICAL MEDICINE AND REHABILITATION CLINICS OF NORTH AMERICA

Motor Neuron Disease

GUEST EDITORS
Michael D. Weiss, MD
Gregory T. Carter, MD, MS

CONSULTING EDITOR
George H. Kraft, MD, MS

August 2008 • Volume 19 • Number 3

SAUNDERS
An Imprint of Elsevier, Inc.
PHILADELPHIA LONDON TORONTO MONTREAL SYDNEY TOKYO

W.B. SAUNDERS COMPANY
A Division of Elsevier Inc.

1600 John F. Kennedy Blvd. • Suite 1800 • Philadelphia, Pennsylvania 19103

http://www.theclinics.com

PHYSICAL MEDICINE AND REHABILITATION CLINICS OF NORTH AMERICA
August 2008
Editor: Debora Dellapena

Volume 19, Number 3
ISSN 1047-9651
ISBN-10: 1-4160-6337-4
ISBN-13: 978-1-4160-6337-7

Physical Medicine and Rehabilitation Clinics of North America (ISSN 1047-9651) is published quarterly by Elsevier Inc., 360 Park Avenue South, New York, NY 10010-1710. Months of publication are February, May, August, and November. Business and Editorial Offices: 1600 John F. Kennedy Blvd., Suite 1800, Philadelphia, PA 19103-2899. Customer Service Office: 6277 Sea Harbor Drive, Orlando, FL 32887-4800. Periodicals postage paid at New York, NY and additional mailing offices. Subscription price per year is $197.00 (US individuals), $308.00 (US institutions), $99.00 (US students), $240.00 (Canadian individuals), $394.00 (Canadian institutions), $135.00 (Canadian students), $277.00 (foreign individuals), $394.00 (foreign institutions), and $135.00 (foreign students). Foreign air speed delivery is included in all *Clinics* subscription prices. All prices are subject to change without notice. POSTMASTER: Send address changes to *Physical Medicine and Rehabilitation Clinics of North America*, Elsevier Periodicals Customer Service, 6277 Sea Harbor Drive, Orlando, FL 32887-4800. **Customer Service: 1-800-654-2452 (US). From outside of the United States, call 1- 407-563-6020. Fax: 1-407-363-9661. E-mail: JournalsCustomerService-usa@elsevier.com.**

Physical Medicine and Rehabilitation Clinics of North America is indexed in *Excerpta Medica, MEDLINE/PubMed (Index Medicus), Cinahl,* and *Cumulative Index to Nursing and Allied Health Literature.*

Printed in the United States of America.

CONSULTING EDITOR

GEORGE H. KRAFT, MD, MS, Alvord Professor of Multiple Sclerosis Research; Professor, Rehabilitation Medicine; and Adjunct Professor, Neurology, University of Washington, School of Medicine, Seattle, Washington

GUEST EDITORS

MICHAEL D. WEISS, MD, Director, EMG Laboratory, Co-Director MDA/ALS Center, Associate Professor, Department of Neurology, University of Washington Medical Center, Seattle, Washington

GREGORY T. CARTER, MD, MS, Co-Director MDA/ALS Center, Clinical Professor, Department of Physical Medicine and Rehabilitation, University of Washington Medical Center, Seattle, Washington

CONTRIBUTORS

JOSHUA O. BENDITT, MD, Professor of Pulmonary and Critical Care Medicine, University of Washington Medical Center, Seattle, Washington

LOUIS BOITANO, MS, RRT, Respiratory Care Department, University of Washington Medical Center, Seattle, Washington

MARK B. BROMBERG, MD, PhD, Clinical Neurosciences Center, Department of Neurology, University of Utah Health Sciences Center, Salt Lake City, Utah

ALEXANDER A. BROWNELL, MS, Clinical Neurosciences Center, Department of Neurology, University of Utah Health Sciences Center, Salt Lake City, Utah

GREGORY T. CARTER, MD, MS, Co-Director MDA/ALS Center, Clinical Professor, Department of Physical Medicine and Rehabilitation, University of Washington Medical Center, Seattle, Washington

GREGORY A. CARY, BA, Department of Laboratory Medicine, University of Washington Medical Center; and Molecular & Cellular Biology Program, Department of Laboratory Medicine, University of Washington Medical Center, Seattle, Washington

AMY CHEN, MD, PhD, Post-Doctoral Fellow, Department of Neurology, Columbia University, New York, New York

B. JANE DISTAD, MD, Assistant Professor, Department of Neurology, University of Washington Medical Center, Seattle, Washington

AMY ELLIS, MPH, RD, CNSD, Department of Nutrition Science, University of Alabama at Birmingham, Birmingham, Alabama

JAY J. HAN, MD, Assistant Professor, Department of Physical Medicine and Rehabilitation, University of California–Davis, Sacramento, California

SUSAN T. IANNACCONE, MD, Professor of Neurology and Pediatrics, Southwestern Medical Center, University of Texas; Director of Pediatric Neurology, Children's Medical Center Dallas, Dallas, Texas

JONATHAN S. KATZ, MD, Forbes Norris MDA/ALS Research Center, California Pacific Medical Center, San Francisco, California

PETRA KAUFMANN, MD, MSc, Assistant Professor of Neurology, The Neurological Institute, Columbia University, New York, New York

LISA S. KRIVICKAS, MD, Harvard Medical School, Spaulding Rehabilitation Hospital, Boston, Massachusetts

ALBERT R. LA SPADA, MD, PhD, Director, Center for Neurogenetics & Neurotherapeutics, University of Washington; Associate Professor, Department of Laboratory Medicine, University of Washington Medical Center; Department of Neurology, University of Washington; Department of Medicine, University of Washington; Department of Pathology, University of Washington, Seattle, Washington

LEE L. LIOU, MD, PhD, Fellow, Department of Neurology, University of Washington Medical Center, Seattle, Washington

JAU-SHIN LOU, MD, PhD, Director, ALS Center of Oregon; Director, Oregon Health and Science University EMG Laboratory; and Associate Professor, Department of Neurology, Oregon Health and Science University, Portland, Oregon

ANGELI S. MAYADEV, MD, Assistant Professor, Department of Physical Medicine and Rehabilitation, University of Washington Medical Center, Seattle, Washington

CRAIG M. McDONALD, MD, Professor, Department of Physical Medicine and Rehabilitation, University of California–Davis, Sacramento, California

GREGG D. MEEKINS, MD, Assistant Professor, Department of Neurology, University of Washington Medical Center, Seattle, Washington

ROBERT G. MILLER, MD, California Pacific Medical Center, Forbes Norris MDA/ALS Research Center, San Francisco, California

HIROSHI MITSUMOTO, MD, DSc, Wesley J. Howe Professor of Neurology, College of Physicians and Surgeons, Columbia University; and Director, Neuromuscular Diseases Division, Eleanor & Lou Gehrig MDA/ALS Center, Columbia University, New York, New York

THOMAS MÖLLER, PhD, Department of Neurology, University of Washington, Seattle, Washington

JACQUELINE MONTES, PT, MA, NCS, Physical Therapist, SMA Clinical Research Center, Department of Neurology, Columbia University, New York, New York

ELSA RAIBON, PhD, Department of Neurology, University of Washington, Seattle, Washington

JOHN RAVITS, MD, FAAN, Staff Neurologist, Virginia Mason Medical Center; Research Associate Scientist, Benaroya Research Institute at Virginia Mason; and Clinical Professor, University of Washington School of Medicine, Seattle, Washington

JEFFREY ROSENFELD, PhD, MD, FAAN, Chief, Division of Neurology, University of California San Francisco-Fresno, Fresno, California

JEREMY M. SHEFNER, MD, PhD, Professor and Chair, Department of Neurology, State University of New York Upstate Medical University, Syracuse, New York

NAILAH SIDDIQUE, RN, MSN, Clinical Nurse Specialist, Neuromuscular Disorders Program, Northwestern University, Feinberg School of Medicine, Chicago, Illinois

TEEPU SIDDIQUE, MD, The Herbert C. Wenske/Les Turner ALS Foundation Professor, Neuromuscular Disorders Program, Northwestern University, Feinberg School of Medicine; Davee Department of Neurology and Clinical Neurosciences, Northwestern University, Feinberg School of Medicine, Chicago; Department of Cell and Molecular Biology, Northwestern University, Feinberg School of Medicine, Chicago, Illinois

LISA MARIE TODD, MD, Department of Rehabilitation Medicine, University of Washington, Seattle, Washington

BRYAN J. TRAYNOR, MD, Clinical Associate, Neurogenetics Branch, National Institute of Neurological Diseases and Stroke, National Institutes of Health, Bethesda, Maryland

MICHAEL D. WEISS, MD, Director, EMG Laboratory, Co-Director MDA/ALS Center, Associate Professor, Department of Neurology, University of Washington Medical Center, Seattle, Washington

SUSAN C. WOOLLEY, PhD, Forbes Norris MDA/ALS Research Center, California Pacific Medical Center, San Francisco, California

CONTENTS

FORTHCOMING ISSUES

November 2008

Dysphagia
Jeffrey B. Palmer, MD, *Guest Editor*

May 2009

Fatigue
Adrian Cristian, MD,
and Brian Greenwald, MD, *Guest Editors*

RECENT ISSUES

May 2008

The Child and Adolescent Athlete
Brian J. Krabak, MD, MBA, *Guest Editor*

February 2008

Neuromuscular Complications of Systemic Conditions
Kathryn A. Stolp, MD, *Guest Editor*

November 2007

Up-to-Date Advances in Rehabilitation: Review Issue
Seema R. Khurana, DO, *Guest Editor*

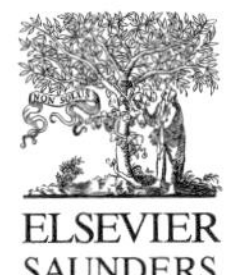

ELSEVIER
SAUNDERS

Phys Med Rehabil Clin N Am
19 (2008) xv–xvii

PHYSICAL MEDICINE
AND REHABILITATION
CLINICS OF
NORTH AMERICA

Foreword

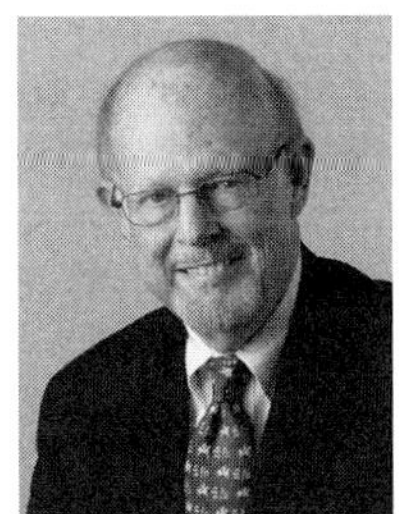

George H. Kraft, MD, MS
Consulting Editor

> *There is no other source of knowledge but the intellectual manipulation of carefully verified observations—in fact, what is called research...and no knowledge can be obtained from revelation, intuition, or inspiration.*
>
> —*Sigmund Freud (1856-1939)* [1]

Motor neuron diseases—amyotrophic lateral sclerosis (ALS) and related disorders—continue to be an enigma for the medical community. At the time of this writing (May 2008), only one drug has been approved by the Food and Drug Administration for the treatment of ALS. That drug, Rilutek, has only a modest effect. With high hopes, other drugs have been studied but have not cleared the bar of randomized, controlled trials.

It is clear that ALS is not just one disease: some ALS is sporadic and some is hereditary. There are some data that indicate there may be a "clustering" of the sporadic diseases, thus suggesting some communicable, environmental, or situational link. But the current state of knowledge is that the medical community has so far failed to identify the cause of sporadic ALS.

So what is known? It is known that one to two persons per 100,000 in the United States develops ALS in any given year. Males seem to be more likely to get it than females. The most common age of onset is between 40 and 60, although some of us in ALS clinics suspect that we may be seeing the disease even earlier. We know that the hereditary form of ALS accounts for 5% to 10% of all cases, and that some of these are linked to a mutation in copper/zinc dismutase, an enzyme responsible for scavenging free radicals. In

doi:10.1016/j.pmr.2008.05.005

addition, in three regions of the Pacific—most prominently in Guam—there is a very high prevalance of ALS.

Consequently, motor neuron disease continues to be both a puzzle and a challenge to the medical community. I am fortunate to be Co-Director, with Dr. Thomas Bird, of the University of Washington Muscular Dystrophy Association (MDA) Clinic. Within our MDA Clinic we have an ALS Center, directed by Drs. Gregory Carter and Michael Weiss, the Guest Editors of this issue. ALS is generally a rapidly progressing neuromuscular disease, producing progressive weakness of the skeletal muscles, including the muscles of respiration. The outcome is that after diagnosis, patients need a number of years of rehabilitative care.

As the Consulting Editor of the *Physical Medicine and Rehabilitation Clinics of North America*, I search out Guest Editors who can bring together outstanding physicians to present in a single issue the important clinical and research points necessary for a clinician to manage diseases. We strive for a relevant issue, but with the latest research underpinnings.

This issue has far, far surpassed my expectations. Drs. Michael Weiss and Gregory Carter, as Guest Editors, have taken a single issue of the *Clinics* to a new height. With their enthusiasm and contacts with the best ALS physicians and researchers available, they have filled this issue with 16 useful articles. The reader will note that this is probably the thickest issue of the *Clinics* that they have ever received. But there is tremendous sadness as well.

Tremendous sadness.

During the preparation of this issue, one of the article authors was diagnosed with ALS. She had been scheduled to write an article on EMG as well, but was unable to carry this out. Dr. Lisa Krivickas, an old friend of the Consulting and Guest Editors, has recently been diagnosed with a familial form of ALS.

This issue is dedicated to Dr. Lisa Krivickas, a remarkable physician, Harvard academician, role model, and mother. Drs. Weiss and Carter have more to say about Dr. Krivickas and her many contributions in their dedication.

Thank you, Lisa, for contributing so much, being such an outstanding physician, and for being a friend.

George H. Kraft, MD, MS
Alvord Professor of MS Research
Professor, Rehabilitation Medicine
Adjunct Professor, Neurology
University of Washington
Box 356490
1959 NE Pacific St.
Seattle, WA 98195-6490, USA

E-mail address: ghkraft@u.washington.edu

Reference

[1] Freud, S. New introductory lectures on psychoanalysis. 35;1933. In Pruner, HW. Freud: His Life and His Mind. New York: Grosset and Dunlapp; 1947. p. 13.

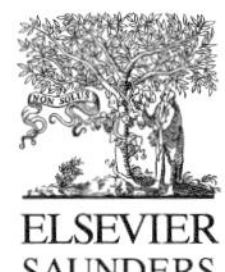
ELSEVIER
SAUNDERS

Phys Med Rehabil Clin N Am
19 (2008) xix–xx

PHYSICAL MEDICINE
AND REHABILITATION
CLINICS OF
NORTH AMERICA

Preface

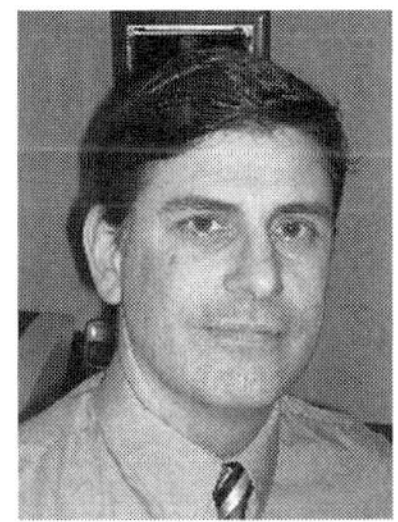
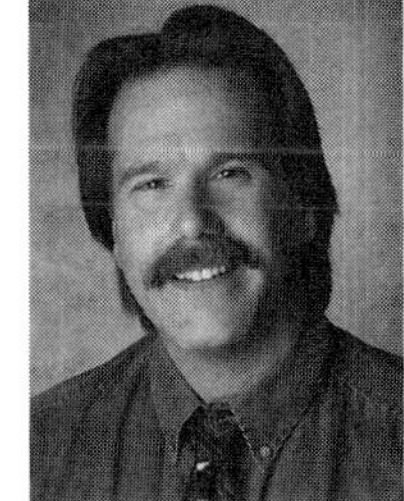

Michael D. Weiss, MD Gregory T. Carter, MD, MS
Guest Editors

We are very proud and honored to be the editors of this outstanding volume of the *Physical Medicine and Rehabilitation Clinics of North America* on motor neuron disease. Over the last few decades there have been tremendous advances in our understanding of the pathophysiology of many forms of motor neuron disease. Indeed, we now know the underlying molecular cause of most forms of spinal muscular atrophy. Our understanding of the genetic causes of familial amyotrophic lateral sclersosis (ALS) also has grown exponentially. The sporadic forms of ALS remain largely a pathophysiologic enigma, an entity that we all struggle to both study and treat, though well-designed and insightful studies continue to be published on the subject. In the context of all of this, we have assembled for this issue a group of nationally and internationally renowned researchers and clinicians to update you on the state of the science of all motor neuron diseases. While there are many articles on complex basic pathophysiology and molecular genetics, there are an equal number of articles discussing how to manage these patients, with an emphasis on improving quality of life and minimizing pain and physical disability: that is, taking optimal care of these patients.

We think this book will be of immense use to physicians and other clinicians who diagnose and treat people with motor neuron diseases. While we aimed for research at the cutting edge, we specifically chose the authors whose work we felt had potential clinical consequence, thus having an immediate impact on a clinician's practice, rather than a theoretical discussion

1047-9651/08/$ - see front matter
doi:10.1016/j.pmr.2008.05.006

of future research areas of interest. It is our hope that this issue will be most often found lying on a physician's desk, next to a stack of charts, with the pages open and a passage from an article highlighted.

Michael D. Weiss, MD
Director EMG Laboratory
Co-Director MDA/ALS Center
Associate Professor, Department of Neurology
University of Washington Medical Center
1959 NE Pacific Street
Room NN282A, Box 356115
Seattle, WA 98195, USA

E-mail address: mdweiss@u.washington.edu

Gregory T. Carter, MD, MS
Co-Director MDA/ALS Center
Clinical Professor, Department of Rehabilitation
University of Washington Medical Center
1800 Cooks Hill Road, Suite E
Centralia, WA 98531, USA

E-mail address: gtcarter@u.washington.edu

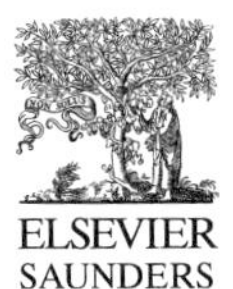
ELSEVIER
SAUNDERS

Phys Med Rehabil Clin N Am
19 (2008) xxi–xxii

PHYSICAL MEDICINE
AND REHABILITATION
CLINICS OF
NORTH AMERICA

Dedication

One sunny day last summer, Greg received an urgent call from a dear friend, colleague and fellow neuromuscular researcher, Dr. Lisa Krivickas. She proceeded to tell him that she had hereditary ALS attributed to an AV4 mutation in the superoxide dismutase 1 gene, which she had inherited from her mother. We had all known for years that Lisa's mother had died from ALS but had always assumed that her form was sporadic.

Greg has known Lisa for nearly 20 years, first meeting her when he was junior faculty at University of California, Davis. She had come out to do an acting internship with us and his first impression was that she was an absolute dynamo from Harvard Medical School whose numerical IQ was likely more than he could bench press. They tried hard to recruit her but she ultimately chose to train at Kessler in New Jersey. However, in that short time they became very good friends, initially because they both shared a headstrong determination to do research in neuromuscular disease, something not terribly common in our field of rehabilitation medicine. Over the years they began to do collaborative projects. When Michael came out to the University of Washington, Greg quickly introduced him to Lisa as well. Now the three of us have collaborated numerous times and co-authored many publications. We tried hard to recruit her to the University of Washington several years back, and she almost agreed but her husband Joe couldn't find a high tech job in the post Microsoft boom years.

Lisa's career has been marked by continuous production of top-notch, cutting-edge, basic science and clinical research. It is widely accepted that she is one of the brightest rising stars in our field of Rehabilitation Medicine. As the three of us have worked on so many projects over the years, we have always had the mind set that this would be the case our entire career. There would always be Lisa, our friend from Harvard, our colleague, co-author, fellow researcher and ALS clinician.

Now we struggle to even comprehend why or how this could even happen. Over the past few months, we have had many deep conversations, struggling with the age-old question of "Why do bad things happen to good people?" Indeed, that is one of the most difficult questions all of us struggle with as we see our ALS patients. Stop. Think. Have you ever seen a person with ALS who was mean or somehow deserved the disease? Personally, in almost 20 years of doing this, and God knows how many ALS patients,

1047-9651/08/$ - see front matter
doi:10.1016/j.pmr.2008.05.004

we have never seen one. In fact they uniformly seem to be the kindest, warmest souls.

Thus, it is with a mixture of joy and sadness, hope and love, compassion, and mostly a deep, heartfelt respect, that we dedicate this book to our dear friend and colleague, Dr. Lisa Krivickas.

Lisa, you continue to inspire us, and are now teaching us all not only how to diagnose and treat ALS, but how to live with it as well. Through your inspiration, it is our sincere hope that all of us will become kinder, more compassionate and caring physicians, enduring on to treat not only the body, but the heart and spirit of our ALS patients.

Respectfully,

Michael D. Weiss, MD
Director EMG Laboratory
Co-Director MDA/ALS Center
Associate Professor, Department of Neurology
University of Washington Medical Center
1959 NE Pacific Street
Room NN282A Box 356115
Seattle, WA 98195

E-mail address: mdweiss@u.washington.edu

Gregory T. Carter, MD, MS
Co-Director MDA/ALS Center
Clinical Professor, Department of Rehabilitation
University of Washington Medical Center
1800 Cooks Hill Road, Suite E
Centralia, WA 98531

E-mail address: gtcarter@u.washington.edu

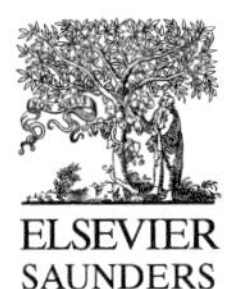
ELSEVIER
SAUNDERS

Phys Med Rehabil Clin N Am
19 (2008) 429–439

PHYSICAL MEDICINE
AND REHABILITATION
CLINICS OF
NORTH AMERICA

Genetics of Amyotrophic Lateral Sclerosis

Nailah Siddique, RN, MSN[a,b],
Teepu Siddique, MD[a,b,c,*]

[a]*Neuromuscular Disorders Program, Northwestern University, Feinberg School of Medicine, Tarry Building, Room13-715, 303 East Chicago Avenue, Chicago, IL 60611, USA*
[b]*Davee Department of Neurology and Clinical Neurosciences, Northwestern University, Feinberg School of Medicine,303 East Chicago Avenue, Chicago, IL 60611, USA*
[c]*Department of Cell and Molecular Biology, Northwestern University, Feinberg School of Medicine, 303 East Chicago Avenue, Chicago, IL 60611, USA*

Amyotrophic lateral sclerosis (ALS) was first described by Charcot in 1869 as what we would now call a sporadic disease—a disease believed to occur without a strong genetic influence. By 1880 Sir William Osler recognized that the Farr family of Vermont had a dominantly inherited progressive muscular atrophy, one phenotypic variation of ALS [1]. It took another 100 years to develop the tools of molecular biology that allowed examination of the clearly inherited forms of the disease. Only within the past 10 years has it been possible to fully explore genetic influence on disorders that seem to occur sporadically but are in fact quite complex—those that likely result from the convergence of multiple genetic and environmental factors. The roughly 90% of ALS that occurs in individuals who have no family history of ALS is called sporadic ALS (SALS), whereas the remaining 10% of ALS that occurs in at least two people in the same family is considered familial ALS (FALS) [1].

This article reviews the genetics of FALS and summarizes current investigations of genetic influence in SALS.

This work was supported by the National Institute of Neurologic Disorders and Stroke (NS40308, NS050641, NS046535), the National Institute of Environmental Health Science (ES014469), Les Turner ALS Foundation, Vena E. Schaff ALS Research Fund, Harold Post Research Professorship, Herbert and Florence C. Wenske Foundation, Ralph and Marian Falk Medical Research Trust, Abbott Labs Duane and Susan Burnham Professorship, David C. Asselin MD Memorial Fund.

* Corresponding author. Northwestern University, Feinberg School of Medicine, Tarry Building, Room 13-715, 303 East Chicago Avenue, Chicago, IL 60611.
E-mail address: t-siddique@northwestern.edu (T. Siddique).

1047-9651/08/$ - see front matter
doi:10.1016/j.pmr.2008.05.001

Familial amyotrophic lateral sclerosis

FALS can be transmitted as a dominant or a recessive trait, but is most commonly an adult-onset disorder of autosomal dominant transmission. Autosomal recessive inheritance is rare and seems to be limited to people who have juvenile-onset ALS or people who have a double dose of particular mutations in the SOD1 gene. We have reported a single family with X-linked dominantly inherited ALS, a rarely observed phenomenon in neurogenetics [2].

In 1991 positional cloning identified linkage of familial ALS to the SOD1 locus on chromosome 21q22 and demonstrated genetic locus heterogeneity in FALS [3]. Two years later mutations in SOD1 were linked to FALS, establishing SOD1 as the first causative gene for ALS (genetic nomenclature, ALS1) [4,5]. Subsequently, homozygosity mapping of highly consanguineous families identified the gene ALSIN causing autosomal recessive ALS2 [6] and the locus for ALS5 [7]. Since then five additional genetic loci for FALS and seven for related motor neuron degenerations have been identified (Tables 1 and 2), establishing a multi-etiologic basis for FALS [1].

SOD-ALS (ALS1)

The SOD1 gene is around 11 kilobases with five exons, four introns, and several alternatively spliced forms. More than 100 mutations, predominantly missense, have been reported in 68 of the 153 codons, spread over all five exons (http://alsod.iop.kcl.as.uk/index.aspx). The SOD1 protein is a 32 kd homodimeric protein consisting of 153 highly conserved amino acids. Each monomer has a Greek key β-barrel fold that binds to one copper and one zinc ion [8,9]. The dimer interface is stabilized by hydrophobic interactions, with dimerization doubling the dismutase activity of SOD1. An electrostatic guidance channel shepherds superoxide ions to the active Cu^{2+}-containing site [9]. In human SOD1 two cysteine residues are oxidized as a sulfhydryl bridge (C_{57}, C_{146}), which provides stability and increases melting temperature with the aid of the zinc ion. The dismutase reaction is likely limited only by substrate availability [9]. The size- and charge-selective access to the active site specifically allows in the negatively charged superoxide ion, while excluding larger and positively charged ions [9].

There are three superoxide dismutases (SOD1, 2, and 3), all three of which are isoenzymes that play major roles in reducing free radical–induced cellular damage. They scavenge superoxide free radicals that are byproducts of oxidative respiration and the cytochrome P450 system. SOD1, the only one of the three implicated in FALS, is primarily a cytosolic enzyme, but small amounts are also present in mitochondria and other organelles [8,9].

Human SOD-ALS (ALS1)

A typical presentation of FALS, particularly ALS1, is one of early monomelic weakness without significant loss of muscle bulk, which may persist

Table 1
Amyotrophic lateral sclerosis genes and loci

Frequency of cases	Genetic nomenclature	Inheritance pattern	Disease name	Gene	Locus	Protein product
20%	ALS1	AD	SOD-FALS	SOD1	21q22.1	Cu-Zn superoxide dismutase
Rare	ALS2	AR	Juvenile ALS type 3	ALS2	2q33	Alsin
Single family	ALS3	AD	FALS		18q21	Unknown
Rare	ALS5	AR	Juvenile ALS type 1		15q15.1–q21.1	Unknown
Three families	ALS6	AD	FALS		16q12	Unknown
Single family	ALS7	AD	FALS		20ptel	Unknown
Rare		AD	FALS and FALS/FTD	TDP-43	1p36	TAR DNA-binding protein
Single family	XALS	X- dominant	FALS		X	Unknown

Abbreviations: AD, autosomal dominant; AR, autosomal recessive; FTD, frontotemporal dementia; SMA, spinal muscular atrophy.

Data from Siddique T, Dellefave L. Amyotrophic lateral sclerosis. In: David Lynch, Jennifer Farmer, editors. Neurogenetics: scientific and clinical advances. New York and London: Taylor and Francis; 2006. p. 693–720.

Table 2
Amyotrophic lateral sclerosis–related motor neuron disorders with upper and lower motor neuron involvement

Frequency of cases	Genetic nomenclature	Inheritance pattern	Disease name	Gene	Locus	Protein product
Rare	ALS4[a]	AD	Distal hereditary motor neuronopathy with pyramidal features	SETX	9q34	Senataxin
Rare	ALS8[b]	AD	SMA IV, Finkel type SMA	VAPB	20q13	VAPB
Rare	ALS/FTD1	AD	ALS with FTD	Unknown	9q21–q22	Unknown
More common	ALS/FTD2	AD	ALS with FTD	Unknown	9p21	Unknown
Rare	FTDP17	AD	Disinhibition-dementia-parkinsonism-amyotrophy complex	Unknown	17q	Unknown
Uncommon	SPG17	AD	Silver syndrome	Unknown	11q12–q14	Unknown
Old order Amish	SPG20	AR	Troyer syndrome	SPG20	13q12.3	Spartin
Rare		AD	Inclusion body myopathy associated with Paget disease of bone and FTD	VCP	9p21.1–p12	Valosin-containing protein

Abbreviations: AD, autosomal dominant; AR, autosomal recessive; FTD, frontotemporal dementia.

[a] No bulbar involvement. Long, slow progression, distal wasting with pyramidal signs and sensory loss, previously called axonal Charcot Marie Tooth with pyramidal signs.

[b] This disorder seems to be proximal SMA IV (Finkel type) with some UMN findings.

Data from Siddique T, Dellefave L. Amyotrophic lateral sclerosis. In: David Lynch, Jennifer Farmer, editors. Neurogenetics: scientific and clinical advances. New York and London: Taylor and Francis; 2006. p. 693–720.

for many months before significant weakness or muscle wasting is noted at the site or elsewhere. In 2000, the Escorial Criteria were revised in recognition of this phenomenon. "Clinically definite familial ALS—laboratory supported" can be diagnosed if a pathogenic mutation has been identified in the presence of progressive upper or lower motor neuron signs in at least a single region in the absence of another cause for the abnormal neurologic signs [10]. In practice, however, lower motor neuron features predominate in ALS1 with the first sign frequently being mild weakness in calf muscles accompanied by loss of the S_1 glutamate-mediated monosynaptic Achilles reflex, calling in question the role of glutamate toxicity. (T. Siddique, unpublished observation, 1998).

Age of onset does not correlate with mutation, ranging from 15 to 81 years, with mean onset at age 47 $\pm$ 13 years. Extremity onset, particularly in the legs, is much more common than bulbar onset and both genders are equally affected. Disease duration or rate of disease progression does correlate with some mutations, however, with particularly the A4V mutation that causes about 50% of ALS1 in North American families being consistently associated with a rapid course of 1.0 $\pm$ 0.4 years from symptom onset until death [11]. A few other mutations confer a disease duration of 10 years or more, whereas some others exhibit extensive variability [1]. Penetrance of SOD1 mutations is variable and mutation specific, with the I113T and D90A mutations markedly reduced compared with the generally high A4V mutation [1].

The dosage of certain SOD1 mutations, particularly D90A, seems to affect age of disease onset also. Generally individuals of Scandinavian origin who are D90A heterozygotes do not develop ALS. More than 80 cases that had homozygous D90A mutations from 40 independent pedigrees originating in Northern Scandinavia developed ALS, however. A slowly progressive form, often presenting as SALS, has been identified in homozygotes of other populations. Dominant pedigrees have also been reported [1,12,13]. SOD1 enzyme activity is not associated with disease severity, with mutations that provide even marginally reduced activity producing disease [1].

Animal, biochemical, and cellular studies in SOD-ALS

The first mouse model overexpressing SOD1 was constructed in 1994 using the G93A mutation [14]. The model has since been replicated with other SOD1 mutations in both mouse and rat and extensively studied [1]. Transgenic mice or rats overexpressing mutant SOD1 develop an ALS-like phenotype, whereas those overexpressing wild-type SOD1 remain unaffected. SOD1 knockout mice show axonal damage; although their muscles show fiber-type grouping characteristic of denervation/reinnervation, they do not develop motor neuron degeneration or obvious clinical weakness. Despite the varied pathology described in animals that have ALS overexpressing mutant SOD1, the central lesson is that onset of disease correlates with levels of protein expression, which in turn is related to copy number of the transgene [1,15]. This correlation suggests that mutant SOD1 must reach a critical threshold in its expression, above which it causes disease by gain of a toxic property that triggers degeneration of motor neurons [1,15]. Two major hypotheses have been proposed. One is that although normal SOD1 activity serves as an antioxidant defense, the peroxidase, superoxide reductase, and superoxide generating properties of mutant SOD1 lead to the formation of toxic species, including peroxynitrite, superoxide, and decomposition products of hydrogen peroxide [16]. Removal of copper essential for these reactions with copper chaperone of SOD or copper chelators, however, did not ameliorate disease in mutant SOD1 transgenic mice [17], which makes it unlikely the basis for disease.

We propose that formation of aggregates of SOD1 identified in brain and spinal cord of both SOD1 transgenic mice and ALS1 patients, like the mutant prion aggregates of Creutzfeldt-Jakob disease, are the toxic mechanism in SOD-ALS. Investigations with double transgenic mice in our laboratory established that wild-type SOD1 is recruited in the presence of mutant SOD1, not only hastening disease onset in G93A and L126Z mutant mice but also converting the otherwise unaffected A4V mice into diseased mice. Analyses of spinal cord tissue of these double transgenic mice revealed this phenomenon is accompanied by conversion of both mutant and wild-type SOD1 from a soluble form to an aggregated and detergent-insoluble form. This conversion, observed in the mitochondrial fraction of the spinal cord, involved formation of insoluble SOD1 dimers and multimers that are cross-linked through intermolecular disulfide bonds. The dimers act as seeds in forming toxic intermediate species with possible membrane-disrupting properties. SOD1, normally an important protein in cellular defense against free radicals, is converted to an aggregated and apparently toxic species by redox processes, demonstrating direct links between oxidation, protein aggregation, mitochondrial damage, and SOD1-mediated ALS [18]. We have observed SOD1 protein levels are highest in spinal cord of G93A mutants, with lesser amounts in brain and liver and least in kidneys, and increased accumulation occurs with age (N. Cole and T. Siddique, unpublished observation, 1997). These studies, taken together, suggest that the spinal cord and brainstem are unable to effectively deal with the mutant protein load, leading to the region-specific pathology and dysfunction noted in ALS mice, and probably in humans. This finding is important because rational therapy based on these observations can now be developed and tested.

ALSIN-ALS (ALS2)

Mutations in the ALSIN gene, which encodes the protein alsin, produce either a recessive juvenile-onset primary lateral sclerosis (PLS) or a juvenile-onset upper motor neuron (UMN)–predominant ALS [6]. The alsin sequence contains three domains with homology to GTPases, proteins with roles in axonal outgrowth, signaling cascades, and vesicular trafficking [6]. ALSIN makes both a short and a long transcript by alternate splicing. We hypothesize a loss of normal function resulting in an ALS phenotype occurs from mutations that affect domains close to the N-terminal region of ALSIN, rendering both long and short transcripts nonfunctional. The milder PLS occurs from more distal mutations that leave the short transcript intact, so perhaps a short protein may allow preservation of some function [6]. ALSIN set the precedent that proteins related to the function of small GTPases and proteins involved in vesicular trafficking are determinants of motor neuron viability.

Knockout models of the ALSIN gene do not exhibit a robust phenotype of motor neuron degeneration, although special copper-silver staining demonstrates distal axonal degeneration in the corticospinal tracts of knockout mice [19]. Corticospinal tracts in rodents are small and lie behind the central cord, raising concern whether rodents are appropriate models of UMN disease and spinal cord injury. Cross-breeding experiments using G93A-SOD1 mice and ALSIN knockout mice did not alter the onset or survival of G93A mice, which may indicate that alsin-related UMN neurodegeneration uses a different pathway than SOD1-related neurodegeneration [19]. In vitro experiments suggest a protective role for alsin in SOD1-linked cell death [20].

TDP43-ALS

There has been much discussion recently over the relationship between ALS and frontotemporal dementia (FTD), with frontal temporal impairment being increasingly recognized as clinically associated with ALS [21]. A commonality between a subset of ALS cases and FTD cases is the presence of ubiquinated inclusions composed of the transactive response (TAR) DNA-binding protein with a molecular weight of 43 kd (TDP-43) [22,23]. Mutations in TDP-43 have recently been identified in several affected people in families who have FALS, both with and without FTD, and several patients who have apparently sporadic ALS [24–27].

Locus heterogeneity

With three ALS genes and five additional ALS loci identified, it is apparent that virtually identical clinical and pathologic phenotypes can arise from multiple causes (see Table 1). Related disorders involving motor neuron degeneration also have demonstrated locus heterogeneity, including ALS with frontotemporal dementia [28] (see Table 2). It is therefore crucial that additional ALS genes and loci be identified to further the understanding of the multiple pathways involved in the pathogenesis of ALS.

Sporadic amyotrophic lateral sclerosis

SALS is believed to be a multifactorial disease, likely produced by multiple genes interacting with multiple environmental factors, with its complex causes still undetermined. Identification of susceptibility genes may provide clues to pathogenesis and point to intersecting environmental factors. Some polymorphisms may not influence susceptibility but rather may affect onset, severity, and duration, thus influencing the phenotype. Successful gene mapping in complex diseases depends on many factors, including appropriate study design, adequate statistical power, extent of genetic heterogeneity, and appropriate mechanisms for verification of the susceptibility genes. Association studies using population-based case-control samples or family-based samples determine whether a specific allele of a given genetic marker is found with increased frequency in individuals who have disease compared with the frequency of the marker in individuals who do not have disease. Several association studies are highlighted.

The APOE gene polymorphisms, alleles 2, 3 and 4, have been the focus of at least five association studies with ALS, in which early reports of associations were not replicated with larger sample sizes. Our recent, larger study, which identified the E2 allele as protective against an early onset of ALS, was the first subclassification of the role of an APOE in ALS [29].

Three studies have looked at SMN2 copy number or deletions within the SMN1 gene and SALS, with one demonstrating deletions of SMN do not predispose one to ALS, another reporting modest differences in SMN2 copy numbers in patients who have SALS, and the third identifying homozygous deletion of SMN as a prognostic factor. None of the results has yet been replicated [1].

A case-control meta-analysis of three Belgian, Swedish, and British populations demonstrated an association with three polymorphisms known to affect vascular endothelial growth factor expression. No association was found in a different subset of the British population, a Dutch cohort, or our own North American cohort [1,30,31]. Interestingly, a single nucleotide polymorphism of the related protein angiogenin was associated with SALS in an Irish population [32].

Associations have been reported in polymorphisms of the heavy neurofilament subchain [33] and a frameshift mutation was identified in peripherin, a type III intermediate neurofilament protein expressed predominantly in the peripheral nervous system, in one individual who had ALS [34].

Members of the paraoxonase cluster, PONs1, 2, and 3, are enzymes involved in detoxification of organophosphate pesticides and chemical nerve agents. Our investigation of a large North American white family-based and case-control cohort (n = 2008) demonstrated significant evidence of association of variants in the PON cluster with SALS, indicating environmental toxicity in a susceptible host may precipitate ALS [35]. Importantly, these results have been replicated in Polish and Irish populations [36,37].

The first reported whole genome association study identified single nucleotide polymorphisms (SNPs) of interest, but none survived Bonferroni correction. The more than 300 million genotypes it produced have been made available on the Internet, which is the first time such data have been so easily accessible [38]. TGen's larger series identified 10 loci significantly associated with SALS in all three of their data sets, and 41 others that had significant association in two. Their most significant association was near the uncharacterized gene FLJ10986, which codes for a protein expressed in spinal cord and CSF of patients and controls [39]. The 19 SNPs that showed a trend toward association in a large British pathway-based, candidate gene, case-control association study were not associated with a moderately sized German replication group [40]. A three-armed European GWAS reported a variant in the inositol 1,4,5-triphosphate receptor 2 gene (ITPR2) is significantly associated with SALS, with combined analysis of all samples confirming this association. Additionally, ITPR2 expression was greater in the peripheral blood of 126 patients who had ALS compared with 126 healthy controls [41]. Recently, examination of publicly available data identified SNPs within guidance pathway genes as highly predictive of ALS susceptibility, survival free of ALS, age at onset of ALS, and overlap with genes associated with Parkinson disease, which may indicate they are involved more broadly in neurodegeneration [42]. As mentioned previously, mutations in TDP-43 have been recently identified in ten SALS patients [24,25].

Genetic study clearly offers the potential for identification of molecular targets that would allow development of rational therapies for various forms of ALS, but much work remains.

References

[1] Siddique T, Dellefave L. Amyotrophic lateral sclerosis. In: Lynch David, Farmer Jennifer, editors. Neurogenetics: scientific and clinical advances. New York and London: Taylor and Francis; 2006. p. 693–720.

[2] Hong SBB, Siddique T. X-linked dominant locus for late-onset familial amyotrophic lateral sclerosis. Abstr Soc Neurosci 1998;24:478.

[3] Siddique T, Figlewicz DA, Pericak-Vance MA, et al. Linkage of a gene causing familial amyotrophic lateral sclerosis to chromosome 21 and evidence of genetic-locus heterogeneity. N Engl J Med 1991;324(20):1381–4.

[4] Deng HX, Hentati A, Tainer JA, et al. Amyotrophic lateral sclerosis and structural defects in Cu, Zn superoxide dismutase. Science 1993;261(5124):1047–51.

[5] Rosen DR, Siddique T, Patterson D, et al. Mutations in Cu/Zn superoxide dismutase gene are associated with familial amyotrophic lateral sclerosis. Nature 1993;362(6415):59–62.

[6] Yang Y, Hentati A, Deng HX, et al. The gene encoding alsin, a protein with three guanine-nucleotide exchange factor domains, is mutated in a form of recessive amyotrophic lateral sclerosis. Nat Genet 2001;29(2):160–5.

[7] Hentati A, Ouahchi K, Pericak-Vance MA, et al. Linkage of a commoner form of recessive amyotrophic lateral sclerosis to chromosome 15q15-q22 markers. Neurogenetics 1998;2(1): 55–60.

[8] Getzoff ED, Tainer JA, Stempien MM, et al. Evolution of CuZn superoxide dismutase and the Greek key beta-barrel structural motif. Proteins 1989;5(4):322–36.

[9] Klug D, Rabani J, Fridovich I. A direct demonstration of the catalytic action of superoxide dismutase through the use of pulse radiolysis. J Biol Chem 1972;247(15):4839–42.

[10] Brooks BR, Miller RG, Swash M, et al. El Escorial revisited: revised criteria for the diagnosis of amyotrophic lateral sclerosis. Amyotroph Lateral Scler Other Motor Neuron Disord 2000;1(5):293–9.

[11] Juneja T, Pericak-Vance MA, Laing NG, et al. Prognosis in familial amyotrophic lateral sclerosis: progression and survival in patients with glu100gly and ala4val mutations in Cu, Zn superoxide dismutase. Neurology 1997;48(1):55–7.
[12] Cudkowicz ME, McKenna-Yasek D, Sapp PE, et al. Epidemiology of mutations in superoxide dismutase in amyotrophic lateral sclerosis. Ann Neurol 1997;41(2):210–21.
[13] Sjalander A, Beckman G, Deng HX, et al. The D90A mutation results in a polymorphism of Cu, Zn superoxide dismutase that is prevalent in northern Sweden and Finland. Hum Mol Genet 1995;4(6):1105–8.
[14] Gurney ME, Pu H, Chiu AY, et al. Motor neuron degeneration in mice that express a human Cu, Zn superoxide dismutase mutation. Science 1994;264(5166):1772–5.
[15] Dal Canto MC, Gurney ME. A low expressor line of transgenic mice carrying a mutant human Cu, Zn superoxide dismutase (SOD1) gene develops pathological changes that most closely resemble those in human amyotrophic lateral sclerosis. Acta Neuropathol 1997; 93(6):537–50.
[16] Liochev SI, Fridovich I. Copper- and zinc-containing superoxide dismutase can act as a superoxide reductase and a superoxide oxidase. J Biol Chem 2000;275(49):38482–5.
[17] Subramaniam JR, Lyons WE, Liu J, et al. Mutant SOD1 causes motor neuron disease independent of copper chaperone-mediated copper loading. Nat Neurosci 2002;5(4):301–7.
[18] Deng HX, Shi Y, Furukawa Y, et al. Conversion to the amyotrophic lateral sclerosis phenotype is associated with intermolecular linked insoluble aggregates of SOD1 in mitochondria. Proc Natl Acad Sci USA 2006;103(18):7142–7 [epub 2006 Apr 24].
[19] Deng H-X, Zhai H, Fu R, et al. Distal axonopathy in alsin-deficient mouse model. Hum Mol Genet 2007;16(23):2911–20.
[20] Kanekura K, Hashimoto Y, Niikura T, et al. Alsin, the product of ALS2 gene, suppresses SOD1 mutant neurotoxicity through RhoGEF domain by interacting with SOD1 mutants. J Biol Chem 2004;279(18):19247–56.
[21] Murphy JM, Henry RG, Langmore S, et al. Continuum of frontal lobe impairment in amyotrophic lateral sclerosis. Arch Neurol 2007;64(4):530–4.
[22] Forman M, Trojanowski JQ, Lee V. TDP-43: a novel neurodegenerative proteinopathy. Curr Opin Neurobiol 2007;17(5):548–55.
[23] Neumann M, Sampathu DM, Kwong LK, et al. Ubiquitinated TDP-43 in frontotemporal lobar degeneration and amyotrophic lateral sclerosis. Science 2006;314(5796):130–3.
[24] Gitcho MA, Baloh RH, Chakraverty S, et al. TDP-43 A315T mutation in familial motor neuron disease. Ann Neurol 2008;63(4):535–8.
[25] Sreedharan J, Blair IP, Tripathi VB, et al. TDP-43 mutations in familial and sporadic amyotrophic lateral sclerosis. Science 2008;319(5870):1668–72 [epub 2008 Feb 28].
[26] Kabashi E, Valdmanis PN, Dion P, et al. TARDBP mutations in individuals with sporadic and familial amyotrophic lateral sclerosis. Nat Genet 2008 Mar 30 [epub ahead of print].
[27] Van Deerlin VM, Leverenz JB, Bekris LM, et al. TARDBP mutations in amyotrophic lateral sclerosis with TDP-43 neuropathology: a genetic and histopathological analysis. Lancet Neurol 2008;7(5):409–16 [epub 2008 Apr 7].
[28] Morita M, Al-Chalabi A, Andersen PM, et al. A locus on chromosome 9p confers susceptibility to ALS and frontotemporal dementia. Neurology 2006;6(6):839–44.
[29] Li Y, Pericak-Vance M, Haines J, et al. Age at onset modulates the effect of apolipoprotein E in amyotrophic lateral sclerosis. Neurogenetics 2004;5(4):209–13 [epub 2004 Oct].
[30] Van Vught PW, Sutedja NA, Veldink JH, et al. Lack of association between VEGF polymorphisms and ALS in a Dutch population. Neurology 2005;65(10):1643–5.
[31] Chen W, Saeed M, Mao H, et al. Lack of association of VEGF promoter polymorphisms with sporadic ALS. Neurology 2006;67(3):508–10.
[32] Greenway MJ, Alexander MD, Ennis S, et al. A novel candidate region for ALS on chromosome 14q11.2. Neurology 2004;63(10):1936–8.
[33] Julien J-P. Neurofilament function in health and disease. Curr Opin Neurobiol 1999;9(5): 554–60.

[34] Gros-Louis F, Lariviere R, Gowing G, et al. A frameshift deletion in peripherin gene associated with amyotrophic lateral sclerosis. J Biol Chem 2004;279(44):45951–6.
[35] Saeed M, Siddique N, Hung WY, et al. Paraoxonase cluster polymorphisms are associated with sporadic ALS. Neurology 2006;67(5):771–6 [epub 2006 Jul 5].
[36] Slowik A, Tomik B, Wolkow PP, et al. Paraoxonase promoter and intronic variants modify risk of sporadic amyotrophic lateral sclerosis. J Neurol Neurosurg Psychiatry 2007;78(9): 984–6.
[37] Cronin S, Greenway MJ, Prehn JH, et al. Paraoxonase promoter and intronic variants modify risk of sporadic amyotrophic lateral sclerosis. J Neurol Neurosurg Psychiatry 2007;78(9): 984–6.
[38] Schymick JC, Scholz SW, Fung HC, et al. Genome-wide genotyping in amyotrophic lateral sclerosis and neurologically normal controls: first stage analysis and public release of data. Lancet Neurol 2007;6(4):322–8.
[39] Dunckley T, Huentelman MJ, Craig DW, et al. Whole-genome analysis of sporadic amyotrophic lateral sclerosis. N Engl J Med 2007;357(8):775–88 [epub 2007 Aug 1].
[40] Kasperaviciute D, Weale ME, Shianna KV, et al. Large-scale pathways-based association study in amyotrophic lateral sclerosis. Brain 2007;130(Pt 9):2292–301 [epub 2007 Apr 17].
[41] van Es MA, Van Vught PW, Blauw HM, et al. ITPR2 as a susceptibility gene in sporadic amyotrophic lateral sclerosis: a genome-wide association study. Lancet Neurol 2007;6(10): 869–77.
[42] Lesnick TG, Sorenson EJ, Ahlskog JE, et al. Beyond Parkinson disease: amyotrophic lateral sclerosis and the axon guidance pathway. PLoS ONE. 2008;3(1):e1449.

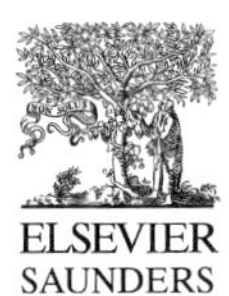
ELSEVIER
SAUNDERS

Phys Med Rehabil Clin N Am
19 (2008) 441–459

PHYSICAL MEDICINE
AND REHABILITATION
CLINICS OF
NORTH AMERICA

Glial Cells in ALS: The Missing Link?

Elsa Raibon, PhD[a], Lisa Marie Todd, MD[b], Thomas Möller, PhD[a,*]

[a]*Department of Neurology, University of Washington, Box 356465, 1959 NE Pacific Street, Seattle, WA 98195, USA*

[b]*Department of Rehabilitation Medicine, University of Washington, Box 356490, 1959 NE Pacific Street, Seattle, WA 98195, USA*

Amyotrophic lateral sclerosis

Amyotrophic lateral sclerosis (ALS), initially known as *Charcot's sclerosis*, was named after the French neurobiologist and physician Jean-Martin Charcot who first described this type of muscular atrophy in the early nineteenth century [1]. In the United States, ALS became widely known as *Lou Gehrig's disease* after the famous baseball player who succumbed to the disease in the late 1930s. Currently, ALS is the most common motor neuron disease, with a worldwide incidence of 8 cases per 100,000 population per year [2–4]. Familial forms constitute approximately 5% to 10% of all cases. Onset increases with age, with a peak in the seventh decade and a slight preponderance among men compared with women. Rapid progression of motor neuron loss leads to death an average of 3 to 5 years after symptom onset [2–4]. The cause of ALS remains unknown and there is still no curative therapy.

The term *amyotrophy* refers to peripheral denervation producing lower motor neuron signs of weakness, muscular atrophy, and fasciculations. Upper motor neuron signs of spasticity and hyperreflexia are appreciated as the disease advances, because of sclerosis of the lateral corticospinal tracts. Symptom onset is typically characterized by weakness or clumsiness in an upper extremity with or without fasciculations. In a subset of cases, presenting weakness in the bulbar musculature leads to progressive dysphagia and dysarthria. Bulbar onset infers a rapidly poor prognosis with life expectancy 1 to 2 years after the onset of symptoms.

As the disease progresses, widespread limb and trunk weakness leads to a rapid decline in physical function. Regardless of the initial site of disease

* Corresponding author.
E-mail address: moeller@u.washington.edu (T. Möller).

doi:10.1016/j.pmr.2008.04.003 **pmr.theclinics.com**

manifestation, weakness in the bulbar and respiratory muscles places patients at risk for aspiration pneumonia, which is often the eventual cause of death.

Although the events leading to neuronal toxicity are not clearly understood, ALS is now widely accepted to most likely be a multifactorial disease. Many factors, not necessarily related, have been shown to participate in motor neuron cell death in ALS, including glutamate toxicity, oxidative stress, neurofilament accumulation and neuroinflammation [3,5–9]. These pathways are not mutually exclusive and may act individually or in unison to cause motor neuron disease [10,11].

Diverse neurologic disorders such as Alzheimer's disease, Parkinson's disease, HIV-associated dementia, and other neurodegenerative diseases share common pathologic themes. Understanding these commonalities may help in developing new neuroprotective strategies [12]. One common feature is neuroinflammation.

Key players in neuroinflammation

Microglia

The primary mediators of neuroinflammation are microglia cells, the resident macrophage-like population of the central nervous system (CNS) [13,14]. Studies in the past 2 decades have shown involvement of microglia in many acute and chronic neurologic diseases, such as stroke, trauma, Alzheimer's disease, and multiple sclerosis [13,15–17].

In the unperturbed, healthy CNS, the microglia phenotype is called *resting microglia*, characterized by a small cell body with fine, ramified processes and minimal surface-antigen expression. On injury to the CNS, microglia are swiftly activated and participate in the pathogenesis of neurologic disorders. It now is widely accepted that substances released from damaged cells trigger microglial activation, leading to acute responses and long-term reorganization of the cell phenotype [13,14,18,19].

Once activated, microglia exert their effects on neurons and macroglia (astrocytes and oligodendrocytes) through the release of cytotoxic substances such as oxygen radicals, nitric oxide, glutamate, proteases, neurotoxic cytokines, and cytoprotective agents such as growth factors, plasminogen, plasminogen activator, and neuroprotective cytokines [13,15,20]. The effects of microglia are themselves modulated by astrocytes and neurons through cytokines and neurotransmitters, producing complex interactions among microglia, neurons, and astrocytes [21].

Astrocytes

Astrocytes are the most numerous glial cells. They constitute 50% to 60% of CNS cells and share a common lineage with neurons and oligodendrocytes. Although initially regarded as mere "in-between" neurons (*glia* is the Greek word for *glue*), astrocytes are now known to come in as many shapes and with as many functions as neurons.

Astrocytes provide crucial metabolic support to neurons [22], regulate local blood flow depending on neuronal activity [23], and shape and modulate synaptic strength [24,25]. They actively maintain the blood–brain barrier [23] and are the key players in removing excess glutamate from the CNS [26]. Together with microglia cells they resemble the innate immune response "squat" [27,28], and feedback loops between astrocytes and microglia regulate the expression of pro- and anti-inflammatory cytokines in many neuropathologic conditions [29,30].

Neuroinflammation in amyotrophic lateral sclerosis

Although microglia and neuroinflammation are implicated in nearly all disorders of the CNS, the role of microglial cells in ALS recently came into focus. In histopathologic studies of human ALS tissue, strong activation and proliferation of microglia have been described in the primary motor cortex, brainstem motor nuclei, and ventral horns of the spinal cord: all areas with motor neuron loss [31,32]. Activated microglia were seen in areas with not only severe motor neuron death but also mild neuronal death [31,33]. Furthermore, a recent positron emission tomographic (PET) scan study showed that microglial activation strongly correlated with clinical signs of upper motor neuron loss in sporadic ALS [34].

Evidence implicating activation of microglia in motor neuron disease was also seen in studies on mutant SOD1 (mtSOD1) transgenic mice, the predominant animal model of ALS. These studies showed that microglial activation occurred in the earliest stages of motor neuron degeneration, even before symptoms of weakness [35,36]. Several groups reported expression of proinflammatory mediators, such as interleukin (IL)-1β, IL-6, cyclooxygenase-2 (COX-2), inducible nitric oxide synthase (iNOS), or tumor necrosis factor (TNF)-α, even preceding the development of clinical signs [37–44]. The expression profile of these inflammatory molecules was microglia/macrophage-like.

Elevated levels of MCP-1 and IL-6, for example, were also reported in patients who had ALS [45,46]. Motor neurons are exquisitely sensitive to neuroinflammation. Several studies have shown that mediators associated with neuroinflammation, such as TNF-α, IL-1β, or FAS ligand (FasL), can readily trigger motor neuron apoptosis [47–49].

In ALS, in contrast to other neurodegenerative diseases such as multiple sclerosis or Alzheimer's disease, influx of peripheral immune cells such as lymphocytes or neutrophils is rare and mainly associated with end-stage disease [3,32,35,50]. However, recent progress in understanding T-cell subsets has led to experts to question whether a neuroprotective T-cell response is initially mounted in ALS but fails because of unknown reasons [51]. Therefore, in ALS, neuroinflammation is solely sustained by the interactions of microglia, neurons, and macroglia.

Growth factors are a group of proteins promoting the growth and survival of cells. Important neurotrophic growth factors include neural growth factor, brain-derived neurotrophic factor, insulin-like growth factor I, and vascular endothelial growth factor (VEGF) [52].

Dysregulation of several growth factors have been implicated in ALS [3,53]. For example, deletions in the VEGF promoter caused ALS-like symptoms in mice [54], and patients who have ALS show reduced VEGF levels in cerebrospinal fluid. In the CNS, astrocytes and microglia—the main mediators of neuroinflammation—are also the main sources of neurotrophic factors [27,53,55]. Neuroinflammation leads not only to an increase in inflammatory products but also is usually accompanied by the down-regulation of neurotrophic factors [27,53,55]. This withdrawal of trophic support could add insult to injury and finally drive damaged motor neurons into apoptosis [52,53].

The increased expression of inflammatory factors or down-regulation of growth factors could also explain how damage to lower motor neurons (spinal cord) could propagate to upper motor neurons (cortex). Proapoptotic inflammatory signals (eg, TNF-α, FasL) in the spinal cord could be detected by the axonal projections of upper motor neurons and trigger apoptosis in these cells. Likewise, the down-regulation of VEGF, for example, in the target area of an upper motor neuron could lead to apoptosis of this cell from failure of trophic support (Fig. 1) [56,57].

The (mis)conception of cell autonomous effects

Motor neuron cell loss was long seen from a neurocentric viewpoint as a "disease from within the motor neuron." Recently, it became clear that cell–cell interactions must be considered part of the cascade leading to cell death. Therefore, motor neuron degeneration occurring from intrinsic dysfunction and was called *cell autonomous*, even though *motor neuron–autonomous* seems to be the more correct term. When surrounding cells contribute to the event leading to motor neuron loss, the effect would be called *non–cell autonomous*. Clearly, neuroinflammation would be a non–cell autonomous effect from the motor neuron viewpoint.

Compelling evidence from the mtSOD1 transgenic animal models of ALS showed the involvement of non–cell autonomous effects in the pathogenesis of motor neuron disease. In wild-type/mtSOD1 chimeric mice, wild-type motor neurons surrounded by mtSOD1 glia were damaged, whereas mtSOD1 neurons surrounded by wild-type glia were healthier [58]. This finding strongly indicates a non–cell autonomous disease mechanism and the critical involvement of cell types other than neurons.

Very recently, using an elegant approach, mtSOD1 was selectively removed from microglial cells and macrophages through a CD11b-driven Cre/LoxP system. These animals showed a dramatically slowed disease progression. Removing mtSOD1 from motor neurons, however, delayed the

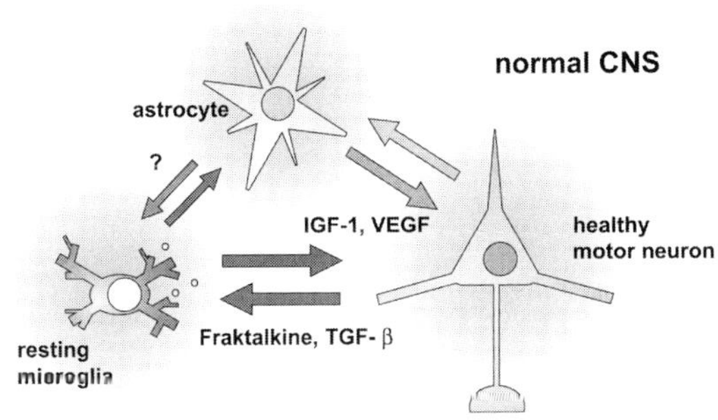

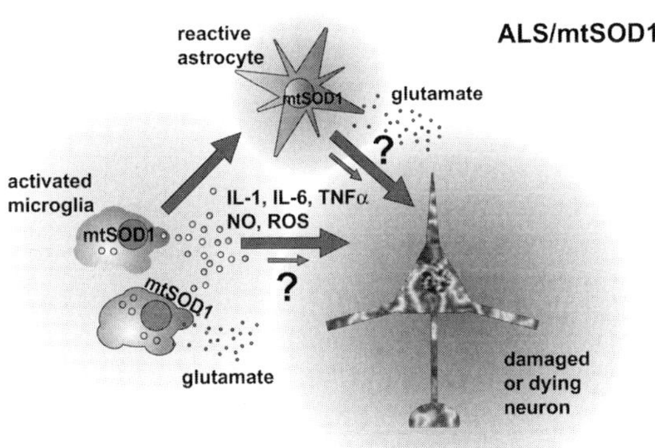

Fig. 1. Neuroinflammatory view of glia–motor neuron interactions in the normal and ALS/mtSOD1 CNS. In the unperturbed CNS, microglia, astrocytes, and motor neurons interact through the release of soluble messengers, such as growth factors, cytokines, and cell–cell contacts. The cells are in a quiescent state. The expression of mtSOD1 or, in the case of sporadic ALS, an unknown trigger leads to activation of glial cells. Activated microglia produce proinflammatory cytokines and glutamate and down-regulate growth factor expression, the SOD1 mutation critically alters this expression profile. Astrocytes, by virtue of mtSOD1 expression and in response to the inflamed tissue, also down-regulate growth factor expression and release inflammatory mediators. Furthermore, they lose their capacity to buffer glutamate. The prolonged exposure of motor neurons to the inflammatory and excitotoxic microenvironment leads to degeneration through apoptosis. *Green arrows*, trophic support; *red arrows*, inflammatory mediators. All named factors are prominent examples only.

onset of disease but had little influence on disease progression [59]. Although some open questions remain about these data pertaining to limited recombination efficiency, the results clearly indicate a role for mtSOD1 within microglial cells in the disease process.

Similar data were obtained through crossing the mtSOD1 into the PU.1 knockout strain, which are unable to develop myeloid and lymphoid cells without bone marrow transplantation. Disease in mtSOD1/PU.1$^{-/-}$ animals receiving wild-type bone marrow progressed considerably slower compared with mtSOD1 bone marrow controls [60]. This article and an earlier report showed that the expression of mtSOD1 in microglial cells leads to an increase in their cytotoxic potential, because they release increased amounts of superoxide, nitrate, and TNF-α in vitro [60–62].

Clearly, microglial intracellular mtSOD1 leads to unidentified changes in microglial phenotype with relevance to disease progression. In contrast, the activation of microglial cells by extracellular mtSOD1 was recently shown [63]. The authors showed that chaperone-associated mtSOD1 secreted from neuronal cells triggered microglial activation and in turn led to motor neuron death in vitro. Taken together, both pathways, intracellular and extracellular mtSOD1, could trigger a vicious neuroinflammatory circle with microglia at center stage.

Astrocytes have recently reappeared on the center stage of ALS [64–66]. They have been implicated early on as key players in the glutamate toxicity hypothesis because their transport capacity seems hampered in ALS [67,68]. However, recent data showed that mtSOD1 within astrocytes changes their properties and that they secrete an unknown factor leading to motor neuron degeneration [69].

Using their mtSOD1 CreLloxP system, the Cleveland group used a GFAP-Cre mouse to excise mtSOD1 from astrocytes. In contrast to the CD11b/microglial Cre model, the recombination efficiency was very high. Although genetic ablation of mtSOD1 in astrocytes did not affect the onset of disease, it significantly slowed its progression. The removal of mtSOD1 from astrocytes reduced the activation of microglial cells, as assessed using MAC-2 and iNOS staining. These indirect effects on microglia also show the close relationship of the two arms of the CNS' immune system.

Non–cell autonomous has been used to define the involvement of other cells contributing to motor neuron death. Both microglia and astrocytes seem to play crucial roles in the motor neuron's demise in ALS, although this may imply that mtSOD1 has a cell autonomous effect on glial cells. How microglia or astrocytes actually transmit these effects to motor neurons and induce their loss remains to be shown. The fact cannot be excluded that the mtSOD1 protein accumulation in microglia or astrocytes could also induce intrinsic loss of properties, such as a diminished neuroprotective function, which may be one mechanism contributing to the loss of motor neurons. Nevertheless, the inflammatory cascade doubtlessly plays a important role in ALS, lending credibility to the idea that therapeutic modulation of inflammation may help treat this currently incurable disease (Table 1).

Current therapy in amyotrophic lateral sclerosis: neuroprotective, anti-inflammatory, or both?

Although a sizable number of medications have been tested in ALS, there is currently only one FDA-approved drug, riluzole, available for therapy [70–73]. Riluzole, believed to exert its effect through presynaptic reduction of glutamate release, prolongs survival by a mere 3 months and does not clearly improve quality of life or functional parameters in patients who have ALS [74].

Although most studies indicate that riluzole works on neurons, some argue that microglia could be a target of the drug. Microglia can release high levels of glutamate, creating the possibility that riluzole could also slow down disease progression through an anti-inflammatory effect on microglia [75].

The advent of ALS animal models has prompted a surge in preclinical studies. The predictability of disease onset and progression makes these animals useful for pharmacologic trials [3,76,77]. Although some concern has been expressed about the inherent limitations of mtSOD1 models (eg, they resemble only a small population of patients who have ALS, several pharmacologic results from these models do not hold true in humans [73,78]), these animals are the only models currently available and have already greatly advanced understanding of ALS [3,72,77,79].

The current list of compounds in preclinical and clinical studies is long and includes targets for all suspected causes (eg, glutamate toxicity, oxidative stress) [3,73,80,81]. Most relevant for this article, however, are the group of drugs that are believed to exert their effects through an anti-inflammatory mode of action.

Celecoxib

Cyclooxygenase-2 (COX-2) is an enzyme central to the production of prostaglandins (PG), a family of powerful lipid mediators of inflammation [82,83]. COX-2 has been shown to be involved in many inflammatory diseases, including rheumatoid arthritis, inflammatory bowel disease, and multiple sclerosis [82,83]. In the CNS, COX-2 is constitutively expressed in a subset of neurons in vitro and in vivo [84,85], but can be readily induced through injury in most neurons and astrocytes [85,86].

Activated microglia also express COX-2 and produce considerable amounts of PGE2, which has been shown to be detrimental to neuronal survival [85,87,88]. Both COX-2 and PGE2 are elevated in the CNS of patients who have ALS [42,85,89–92].

Celecoxib is a COX-2 inhibitor that was introduced as an improved therapy for rheumatoid arthritis. It is currently being pursued as a therapeutic approach in neurodegenerative disease [85,93–95]. In mtSOD1 mice, celecoxib prolonged survival and reduced microglial activation as assessed through immunohistochemistry [93,95]. Unfortunately, clinical studies in humans have not shown efficacy, and celecoxib, although safe and well tolerated, did not improve muscle strength nor reduce motor neuron loss during 12 months of treatment [96].

Minocycline

Minocycline, known as a semisynthetic second-generation tetracycline antibiotic, is also an inhibitor of microglial activation [97,98]. It has been

Table 1
Therapeutics with known or proposed anti-inflammatory properties: trials and effects on patients who have amyotrophic lateral sclerosis and animal models

Pharmaceutical class	Drug name	Animal model trials	Clinical trials (n of patients enrolled)	Comments	References
Antioxidant	Coenzyme Q(10) (ubiquinone)	SOD^{G93Aa}		No effect on survival and possible gender effect on neurologic scores, which were improved for men only; effect on weight loss	ALS Therapy Development Institute (TDI) [119]
Anti-inflammatory molecules	Prednisolone	SOD^{G93A}		No effect on survival and onset of symptoms; possible weight loss from treatment	ALS TDI [120]
		Immunosuppressive treatment		No effect	Werdelin et al, [121]
	Minocycline	SOD^{G93A}		Delayed disease onset and prolonged survival in a dose-dependant manner; contradictory results; slight or no effect of minocycline Additive neuroprotective effect when coupled with creatine	Kriz et al, [103] Van Den Bosch et al, [104] ALS TDI [122] Diguet et al, [123] Zhang et al, [124]
			Multicenter, randomized, placebo-controlled phase III (412)	Harmful side effect on patients who have ALS	Gordon et al, [125]

	Thalidomide	SOD^{G93A}		Various doses tested, gender differences, and slight increase of survival	ALS TDI [126]
				Reduce production of proinflammatory molecules (TNF)	Kiaei et al, [118]
			Pilot study (40, ongoing) Phase II (24, ongoing)	Cotreatment with riluzole	Charite University Hospital (Thomas Meyer), Dartmouth Hitchcock Medical Center
	Celebrex/ celecoxib	SOD^{G93A}		Cox-2 inhibitor treatment delayed onset of symptoms and prolonged survival	Drachman et al, [93]
				Celebrex treatment results are inconclusive but not confirmatory; problem in validity of doses used	ALS TDI [127]
			Double-blind, placebo-controlled study (300)	No biologic effect in patients	Cudkowicz et al, [96]
Growth factors	CNTF		Phase II/III randomized, placebo-controlled, double-blind study (730)	Adverse side effects of rHCNTF (weight loss, anorexia, and cough) resulting from withdrawal of treatment; no beneficial effect?	ALS CNTF Treatment Study Group [128]

(*continued on next page*)

Table 1
(continued)

Pharmaceutical class	Drug name	Animal model trials	Clinical trials (n of patients enrolled)	Comments	References
			Phase I study ex vivo gene therapy [6]	Continuous delivery presented no limiting side effects	Aebischer et al, [129]
	GDNF	SOD^{G93A} (rat)		Prevent motor neuron loss but fail to maintain functional neuromuscular function	Suzuki et al, [130]
		SOD^{G93A}		Retrograde transport (GDNF in muscle) slowed down disease progression whereas GDNF overexpressed in astrocytes had no effect	Li et al, [131]
	VEGF	SOD^{G93A}		Prolonged survival and delayed onset	Azzouz et al, [132]
				Reduced astrogliosis and increased number of neuromuscular junctions	Zheng et al, [133]
		SOD^{G93A} (rat)		Delayed onset and prolonged survival; particularly effective for most severe forms of ALS	Storkebaum et al, [134]

Immunosuppressors	Cyclosporin A	SOD^{G93A}		12% extension survival; difference of effect between gender	Karlsson et al, [135] Kirkinezos et al, [136]
			Double-blind study (74)	Beneficial only in men on early onset	Appel et al, [137]
	FK 506	SOD^{G93A}		No beneficial effect on survival and symptoms	Anneser et al, [138]
HDAC inhibitors	Sodium phenyl butyrate	SOD^{G93A}		Extends survival	Ryu et al, [110]
	Sodium valproate	SOD^{G93A}		Increases survival and delay onset	ALS TDI [139]
			Double-blind, randomized study (173, ongoing)		UMC Utrecht [140]
	Trichostatin A	SOD^{G93A}		No effect on survival and symptoms	ALS TDI [141]

[a] Mouse model unless specified

Abbreviations: ALS, amyotrophic lateral sclerosis; CNTF, ciliary neurotrophic factor; GDNF, glial cell line–derived neurotrophic factor; rHCTNF, recombinant human ciliary neurotrophic factor; UMC, University Medical Center; VEGF, vascular endothelial growth factor.

shown to be neuroprotective in models of ischemia, Parkinson's disease, and spinal cord injury. Its function is most likely through inhibition of microglial activation [99–102]. In mtSOD1 mice, minocycline significantly slowed disease onset and progression and reduced microglial activation [103–105]. Based on these data, phase I/II trials are currently underway for the use of minocycline in ALS [106,107]. Despite these encouraging results, the molecular mechanisms underlying these effects are still unclear. Proposed actions of minocycline are p38 mitogen-activated protein kinase inhibition [100] and inhibition of mitochondrial cytochrome c-release [105].

Histone deacetylases inhibitors

Transcriptional dysregulation has recently been recognized as a important factor in neurodegeneration [108,109] and there is good indication that it also plays an important role in ALS [110,111]. Inhibitors of histone deacetylases (HDAC), the central regulators of transcriptional activity, have received increasing attention as potential tools to interfere with transcriptional dysregulation [108,109]. HDAC inhibitors were first developed as antitumoral agents, but they also seem to have strong anti-inflammatory properties [112–114].

Treatment with different HDAC inhibitors improved the survival and delayed motor neuron impairment in mtSOD1 mice [110]. A phase II clinical trial involving 40 patients who have ALS is currently underway to establish human safety for one type of HDAC inhibitor [73]. Suberoylanilide hydroxamic acid, a third-generation HDAC inhibitor, was shown to suppress cytokine expression in macrophage and mononuclear cells [115], supporting the hypothesis that HDAC inhibitors might exert their effects on macrophage/microglia activation.

Thalidomide

Thalidomide, originally introduced as a sedative and withdrawn from the market because of its devastating teratogenic effects, has recently received renewed interest as an anti-inflammatory drug [116,117]. Thalidomide inhibits the expression of cytokines such as TNF-α, which are linked to neuroinflammation in many neurodegenerative diseases, including ALS. In the mouse ALS model, thalidomide significantly increased survival [118]; however, the molecular mechanisms of this effect remain unknown.

Taken together, these reports stress the attractiveness of anti-inflammatory therapy as a therapeutic option in ALS [9,80]. Different classes of drugs, such as minocycline, celecoxib, thalidomide, and HDAC inhibitors may act through a shared anti-inflammatory mechanism. To provide a more tailored (and hopefully more successful) anti-inflammatory therapy, the shared and specific effects of each drug must be understood in the context of ALS-associated neuroinflammation. Once better understood, targeted interference with neuroinflammatory processes could be a tool to develop new therapeutic approaches.

References

[1] Rowland LP. How amyotrophic lateral sclerosis got its name: the clinical-pathologic genius of Jean-Martin Charcot. Arch Neurol 2001;58(3):512–5.

[2] Brown RH, Meininger V, Swash M. Amyotrophic lateral sclerosis. In: Brown RH, Meininger V, Swash M, editors. Amyotrophic lateral sclerosis. London: Martin Dunitz; 2000. p. 3–31.

[3] Bruijn LI, Miller TM, Cleveland DW. Unraveling the mechanisms involved in motor neuron degeneration in ALS. Annu Rev Neurosci 2004;27:723–49.

[4] Strong M, Rosenfeld J. Amyotrophic lateral sclerosis: a review of current concepts. Amyotroph Lateral Scler Other Motor Neuron Disord 2003;4(3):136–43.

[5] Cleveland DW, Rothstein JD. From Charcot to Lou Gehrig: deciphering selective motor neuron death in ALS. Nat Rev Neurosci 2001;2(11):806–19.

[6] Ludolph AC, Meyer T, Riepe MW. The role of excitotoxicity in ALS—what is the evidence? J Neurol 2000;247(Suppl 1):I7–16.

[7] Robberecht W. Oxidative stress in amyotrophic lateral sclerosis. J Neurol 2000; 247(Suppl 1):I1–6.

[8] Shaw PJ, Eggett CJ. Molecular factors underlying selective vulnerability of motor neurons to neurodegeneration in amyotrophic lateral sclerosis. J Neurol 2000;247(Suppl 1):I17–27.

[9] Weydt P, Möller T. Neuroinflammation in the pathogenesis of amyotrophic lateral sclerosis. Neuroreport 2005;16(6):527–31.

[10] Eisen AA. Amyotrophic lateral sclerosis is a multifactorial disease. Muscle Nerve 1995; 18(7):741–52.

[11] Strong MJ, Kesavapany S, Pant HC. The pathobiology of amyotrophic lateral sclerosis: a proteinopathy? J Neuropathol Exp Neurol 2005;64(8):649–64.

[12] Dhib-Jalbut S, Arnold DL, Cleveland DW, et al. Neurodegeneration and neuroprotection in multiple sclerosis and other neurodegenerative diseases. J Neuroimmunol 2006;176(1–2): 198–215.

[13] Kreutzberg GW. Microglia: a sensor for pathological events in the CNS. Trends Neurosci 1996;19(8):312–8.

[14] Streit WJ. Microglial senescence: does the brain's immune system have an expiration date? Trends Neurosci 2006;29(9):506–10.

[15] Streit WJ, Walter SA, Pennell NA. Reactive microgliosis. Prog Neurobiol 1999;57(6):563–81.

[16] McGeer EG, McGeer PL. Brain inflammation in Alzheimer disease and the therapeutic implications. Curr Pharm Des 1999;5(10):821–36.

[17] Hanisch UK, Kohsaka S, Möller T, editors. Special Issue Microglia. Glia 2002 ;40(2):131–3.

[18] Streit WJ. Microglia as neuroprotective, immunocompetent cells of the CNS. Glia 2002; 40(2):133–9.

[19] Nimmerjahn A, Kirchhoff F, Helmchen F. Resting microglial cells are highly dynamic surveillants of brain parenchyma in vivo. Science 2005;308(5726):1314–8.

[20] Hanisch UK. Microglia as a source and target of cytokines activities in the brain. In: Streit WJ, editor. Microglia in the degenerating and regenerating CNS. New York: Springer Verlag; 2001. p. 79–125.

[21] Wyss-Coray T, Mucke L. Inflammation in neurodegenerative disease—a double-edged sword. Neuron 2002;35(5):419–32.

[22] Brown AM, Ransom BR. Astrocyte glycogen and brain energy metabolism. Glia 2007; 55(12):1263–71.

[23] Abbott NJ, Ronnback L, Hansson E. Astrocyte-endothelial interactions at the blood-brain barrier. Nat Rev Neurosci 2006;7(1):41–53.

[24] Haydon PG, Carmignoto G. Astrocyte control of synaptic transmission and neurovascular coupling. Physiol Rev 2006;86(3):1009–31.
[25] Montana V, Malarkey EB, Verderio C, et al. Vesicular transmitter release from astrocytes. Glia 2006;54(7):700–15.
[26] Sattler R, Rothstein JD. Regulation and dysregulation of glutamate transporters. Handb Exp Pharmacol 2006;175:277–303.
[27] Dong Y, Benveniste EN. Immune function of astrocytes. Glia 2001;36(2):180–90.
[28] Farina C, Aloisi F, Meinl E. Astrocytes are active players in cerebral innate immunity. Trends Immunol 2007;28(3):138–45.
[29] Tilleux S, Hermans E. Neuroinflammation and regulation of glial glutamate uptake in neurological disorders. J Neurosci Res 2007;85(10):2059–70.
[30] de Haas AH, van Weering HR, de Jong EK, et al. Neuronal chemokines: versatile messengers in central nervous system cell interaction. Mol Neurobiol 2007;36(2):137–51.
[31] Ince PG, Shaw PJ, Slade JY, et al. Familial amyotrophic lateral sclerosis with a mutation in exon 4 of the Cu/Zn superoxide dismutase gene: pathological and immunocytochemical changes. Acta Neuropathol (Berl) 1996;92(4):395–403.
[32] Kawamata T, Akiyama H, Yamada T, et al. Immunologic reactions in amyotrophic lateral sclerosis brain and spinal cord tissue. Am J Pathol 1992;140(3):691–707.
[33] Ince PG. Neuropathology of ALS. In: Brown RH, Meininger V, Swash M, editors. Amyotrophic lateral sclerosis. London: Martin Dunitz; 2000. p. 83–112.
[34] Turner MR, Cagnin A, Turkheimer FE, et al. Evidence of widespread cerebral microglial activation in amyotrophic lateral sclerosis: an [11C](R)-PK11195 positron emission tomography study. Neurobiol Dis 2004;15(3):601–9.
[35] Alexianu ME, Kozovska M, Appel SH. Immune reactivity in a mouse model of familial ALS correlates with disease progression. Neurology 2001;57(7):1282–9.
[36] Hall ED, Oostveen JA, Gurney ME. Relationship of microglial and astrocytic activation to disease onset and progression in a transgenic model of familial ALS. Glia 1998;23(3): 249–56.
[37] Olsen MK, Roberds SL, Ellerbrock BR, et al. Disease mechanisms revealed by transcription profiling in SOD1-G93A transgenic mouse spinal cord. Ann Neurol 2001; 50(6):730–40.
[38] Yoshihara T, Ishigaki S, Yamamoto M, et al. Differential expression of inflammation- and apoptosis-related genes in spinal cords of a mutant SOD1 transgenic mouse model of familial amyotrophic lateral sclerosis. J Neurochem 2002;80(1):158–67.
[39] Elliott JL. Cytokine upregulation in a murine model of familial amyotrophic lateral sclerosis. Brain Res Mol Brain Res 2001;95(1–2):172–8.
[40] Nguyen MD, Julien JP, Rivest S. Induction of proinflammatory molecules in mice with amyotrophic lateral sclerosis: no requirement for proapoptotic interleukin-1beta in neurodegeneration. Ann Neurol 2001;50(5):630–9.
[41] Hensley K, Floyd RA, Gordon B, et al. Temporal patterns of cytokine and apoptosis-related gene expression in spinal cords of the G93A-SOD1 mouse model of amyotrophic lateral sclerosis. J Neurochem 2002;82(2):365–74.
[42] Almer G, Guegan C, Teismann P, et al. Increased expression of the pro-inflammatory enzyme cyclooxygenase-2 in amyotrophic lateral sclerosis. Ann Neurol 2001;49:176–85.
[43] Chen LC, Smith A, Ben Y, et al. Temporal gene expression patterns in G93A/SOD1 mouse. Amyotroph Lateral Scler Other Motor Neuron Disord 2004;5(3):164–71.
[44] Xie Y, Weydt P, Howland DS, et al. Expression of neuroinflammatory mediators and growth factors in the spinal cord of the G93A SOD1 transgenic rats. Neuroreport 2004; 15(16):2513–6.
[45] Moreau C, Devos D, Brunaud-Danel V, et al. Elevated IL-6 and TNF-alpha levels in patients with ALS: inflammation or hypoxia? Neurology 2005;65(12):1958–60.
[46] Dengler R, von Neuhoff N, Bufler J, et al. Amyotrophic lateral sclerosis: new developments in diagnostic markers. Neurodegener Dis 2005;2(3–4):177–84.

[47] Raoul C, Estevez AG, Nishimune H, et al. Motoneuron death triggered by a specific pathway downstream of Fas. potentiation by ALS-linked SOD1 mutations. Neuron 2002;35(6):1067–83.
[48] Figlewicz DA, Dong L, Mlodzienski M, et al. Culture models of neurodegenerative disease. Ann N Y Acad Sci 2000;919:106–18.
[49] Wen W, Sanelli T, Ge W, et al. Activated microglial supernatant induced motor neuron cytotoxicity is associated with upregulation of the TNFR1 receptor. Neurosci Res 2006; 55(1):87–95.
[50] Engelhardt JI, Tajti J, Appel SH. Lymphocytic infiltrates in the spinal cord in amyotrophic lateral sclerosis. Arch Neurol 1993;50(1):30–6.
[51] Holmoy T. T cells in amyotrophic lateral sclerosis. Eur J Neurol 2008;15(4):360–6.
[52] Villoslada P, Genain CP. Role of nerve growth factor and other trophic factors in brain inflammation. Prog Brain Res 2004;146:403.
[53] Beck M, Karch C, Wiese S, et al. Motoneuron cell death and neurotrophic factors: basic models for development of new therapeutic strategies in ALS. Amyotroph Lateral Scler Other Motor Neuron Disord 2001;2(Suppl 1):S55–68.
[54] Oosthuyse B, Moons L, Storkebaum E, et al. Deletion of the hypoxia-response element in the vascular endothelial growth factor promoter causes motor neuron degeneration. Nat Genet 2001;28(2):131–8.
[55] Markus A, Patel TD, Snider WD. Neurotrophic factors and axonal growth. Curr Opin Neurobiol 2002;12(5):523–31.
[56] Lambrechts D, Storkebaum E, Carmeliet P. VEGF: necessary to prevent motoneuron degeneration, sufficient to treat ALS? Trends Mol Med 2004;10(6):275–82.
[57] Greenberg DA, Jin K. VEGF and ALS: the luckiest growth factor? Trends Mol Med 2004; 10(1):1–3.
[58] Clement AM, Nguyen MD, Roberts EA, et al. Wild-type nonneuronal cells extend survival of SOD1 mutant motor neurons in ALS mice. Science 2003;302(5642):113–7.
[59] Boillee S, Yamanaka K, Lobsiger CS, et al. Onset and progression in inherited ALS determined by motor neurons and microglia. Science 2006;312(5778):1389–92.
[60] Beers DR, Henkel JS, Xiao Q, et al. Wild-type microglia extend survival in PU.1 knockout mice with familial amyotrophic lateral sclerosis. Proc Natl Acad Sci U S A 2006;103(43): 16021–6.
[61] Weydt P, Yuen EC, Ransom BR, et al. Increased cytotoxic potential of microglia from ALS-transgenic mice. Glia 2004;48(2):179–82.
[62] Xiao Q, Zhao W, Beers DR, et al. Mutant SOD1(G93A) microglia are more neurotoxic relative to wild-type microglia. J Neurochem 2007;102(6):2008–19.
[63] Urushitani M, Sik A, Sakurai T, et al. Chromogranin-mediated secretion of mutant superoxide dismutase proteins linked to amyotrophic lateral sclerosis. Nat Neurosci 2006;9(1): 108–18.
[64] Knott AB, Bossy-Wetzel E. ALS: astrocytes take center stage, but must they share the spotlight? Cell Death Differ 2007;14(12):1985–8.
[65] Holden C. Neuroscience. Astrocytes secrete substance that kills motor neurons in ALS. Science 2007;316(5823):353.
[66] Julien JP. ALS: astrocytes move in as deadly neighbors. Nat Neurosci 2007;10(5):535–7.
[67] Rothstein JD. Excitotoxicity and neurodegeneration in amyotrophic lateral sclerosis. Clin Neurosci 1995;3(6):348–59.
[68] Van Den Bosch L, Van Damme P, Bogaert E, et al. The role of excitotoxicity in the pathogenesis of amyotrophic lateral sclerosis. Biochim Biophys Acta 2006;1762(11–12): 1068–82.
[69] Nagai M, Re DB, Nagata T, et al. Astrocytes expressing ALS-linked mutated SOD1 release factors selectively toxic to motor neurons. Nat Neurosci 2007;10(5):615–22.
[70] Als-Tdf. Treatment master list. Available at: http://www.als.net/research/treatments/treatmentList.asp. Accessed 2006.

[71] Turner MR, Parton MJ, Leigh PN. Clinical trials in ALS: an overview. Semin Neurol 2001; 21(2):167–75.
[72] Carri MT, Grignaschi G, Bendotti C. Targets in ALS: designing multidrug therapies. Trends Pharmacol Sci 2006;27(5):267–73.
[73] Traynor BJ, Bruijn L, Conwit R, et al. Neuroprotective agents for clinical trials in ALS: a systematic assessment. Neurology 2006;67(1):20–7.
[74] Miller RG, Mitchell JD, Lyon M, et al. Riluzole for amyotrophic lateral sclerosis (ALS)/motor neuron disease (MND). Amyotroph Lateral Scler Other Motor Neuron Disord 2003;4(3):191–206.
[75] McGeer PL, McGeer EG. Inflammatory processes in amyotrophic lateral sclerosis. Muscle Nerve 2002;26(4):459–70.
[76] Jankowsky JL, Savonenko A, Schilling G, et al. Transgenic mouse models of neurodegenerative disease: opportunities for therapeutic development. Curr Neurol Neurosci Rep 2002;2(5):457–64.
[77] Julien JP, Kriz J. Transgenic mouse models of amyotrophic lateral sclerosis. Biochim Biophys Acta 2006;1762(11–12):1013–24.
[78] Benatar M. Lost in translation: treatment trials in the SOD1 mouse and in human ALS. Neurobiol Dis 2007;26:1.
[79] Rothstein JD. Of mice and men: reconciling preclinical ALS mouse studies and human clinical trials. Ann Neurol 2003;53(4):423–6.
[80] Weydt P, Weiss MD, Moller T, et al. Neuro-inflammation as a therapeutic target in amyotrophic lateral sclerosis. Curr Opin Investig Drugs 2002;3(12):1720–4.
[81] Dimayuga FO, Wang C, Clark JM, et al. SOD1 overexpression alters ROS production and reduces neurotoxic inflammatory signaling in microglial cells. J Neuroimmunol 2007; 182(1–2):89–99.
[82] Rocca B, FitzGerald GA. Cyclooxygenases and prostaglandins: shaping up the immune response. Int Immunopharmacol 2002;2(5):603–30.
[83] FitzGerald GA. COX-2 and beyond: approaches to prostaglandin inhibition in human disease. Nat Rev Drug Discov 2003;2(11):879–90.
[84] Kaufmann WE, Worley PF, Pegg J, et al. COX-2, a synaptically induced enzyme, is expressed by excitatory neurons at postsynaptic sites in rat cerebral cortex. Proc Natl Acad Sci U S A 1996;93(6):2317–21.
[85] Consilvio C, Vincent AM, Feldman EL. Neuroinflammation, COX-2, and ALS—a dual role? Exp Neurol 2004;187(1):1–10.
[86] Engblom D, Ek M, Saha S, et al. Prostaglandins as inflammatory messengers across the blood-brain barrier. J Mol Med 2002;80(1):5–15.
[87] Takadera T, Yumoto H, Tozuka Y, et al. Prostaglandin E(2) induces caspase-dependent apoptosis in rat cortical cells. Neurosci Lett 2002;317(2):61–4.
[88] Wang T, Qin L, Liu B, et al. Role of reactive oxygen species in LPS-induced production of prostaglandin E2 in microglia. J Neurochem 2004;88(4):939–47.
[89] Ilzecka J. Prostaglandin E2 is increased in amyotrophic lateral sclerosis patients. Acta Neurol Scand 2003;108(2):125–9.
[90] Almer G, Teismann P, Stevic Z, et al. Increased levels of the pro-inflammatory prostaglandin PGE2 in CSF from ALS patients. Neurology 2002;58(8):1277–9.
[91] Yokota O, Terada S, Ishizu H, et al. Increased expression of neuronal cyclooxygenase-2 in the hippocampus in amyotrophic lateral sclerosis both with and without dementia. Acta Neuropathol 2004;107(5):399–405.
[92] Yasojima K, Tourtellotte WW, McGeer EG, et al. Marked increase in cyclooxygenase-2 in ALS spinal cord: implications for therapy. Neurology 2001;57(6):952–6.
[93] Drachman DB, Frank K, Dykes-Hoberg M, et al. Cyclooxygenase 2 inhibition protects motor neurons and prolongs survival in a transgenic mouse model of ALS. Ann Neurol 2002;52(6):771–8.

[94] Pompl PN, Ho L, Bianchi M, et al. A therapeutic role for cyclooxygenase-2 inhibitors in a transgenic mouse model of amyotrophic lateral sclerosis. FASEB J 2003;17(6):725–7.
[95] Klivenyi P, Gardian G, Calingasan NY, et al. Additive neuroprotective effects of creatine and a cyclooxygenase 2 inhibitor against dopamine depletion in the 1-methyl-4-phenyl-1,2,3,6-tetrahydropyridine (MPTP) mouse model of Parkinson's disease. J Mol Neurosci 2003;21(3):191–8.
[96] Cudkowicz ME, Shefner JM, Schoenfeld DA, et al. Trial of celecoxib in amyotrophic lateral sclerosis. Ann Neurol 2006;60(1):22–31.
[97] Yrjanheikki J, Keinanen R, Pellikka M, et al. Tetracyclines inhibit microglial activation and are neuroprotective in global brain ischemia. Proc Natl Acad Sci U S A 1998;95(26): 15769–74.
[98] Yrjanheikki J, Tikka T, Keinanen R, et al. A tetracycline derivative, minocycline, reduces inflammation and protects against focal cerebral ischemia with a wide therapeutic window. Proc Natl Acad Sci U S A 1999;96(23):13496–500.
[99] Teng YD, Choi H, Onario RC, et al. Minocycline inhibits contusion-triggered mitochondrial cytochrome c release and mitigates functional deficits after spinal cord injury. Proc Natl Acad Sci U S A 2004;101(9):3071–6.
[100] Tikka T, Fiebich BL, Goldsteins G, et al. Minocycline, a tetracycline derivative, is neuroprotective against excitotoxicity by inhibiting activation and proliferation of microglia. J Neurosci 2001;21(8):2580–8.
[101] Tikka TM, Koistinaho JE. Minocycline provides neuroprotection against N-methyl-D-aspartate neurotoxicity by inhibiting microglia. J Immunol 2001;166(12):7527–33.
[102] Wu DC, Jackson-Lewis V, Vila M, et al. Blockade of microglial activation is neuroprotective in the 1-methyl-4-phenyl-1,2,3,6-tetrahydropyridine mouse model of Parkinson disease. J Neurosci 2002;22(5):1763–71.
[103] Kriz J, Nguyen MD, Julien JP. Minocycline slows disease progression in a mouse model of amyotrophic lateral sclerosis. Neurobiol Dis 2002;10(3):268–78.
[104] Van Den Bosch L, Tilkin P, Lemmens G, et al. Minocycline delays disease onset and mortality in a transgenic model of ALS. Neuroreport 2002;13(8):1067–70.
[105] Zhu S, Stavrovskaya IG, Drozda M, et al. Minocycline inhibits cytochrome c release and delays progression of amyotrophic lateral sclerosis in mice. Nature 2002;417(6884):74–8.
[106] Gordon PH, Moore DH, Gelinas DF, et al. Placebo-controlled phase I/II studies of minocycline in amyotrophic lateral sclerosis. Neurology 2004;62(10):1845–7.
[107] Pontieri FE, Ricci A, Pellicano C, et al. Minocycline in amyotrophic lateral sclerosis: a pilot study. Neurol Sci 2005;26(4):285–7.
[108] Butler R, Bates GP. Histone deacetylase inhibitors as therapeutics for polyglutamine disorders. Nat Rev Neurosci 2006;7(10):784–96.
[109] Saha RN, Pahan K. HATs and HDACs in neurodegeneration: a tale of disconcerted acetylation homeostasis. Cell Death Differ 2006;13(4):539–50.
[110] Ryu H, Smith K, Camelo SI, et al. Sodium phenylbutyrate prolongs survival and regulates expression of anti-apoptotic genes in transgenic amyotrophic lateral sclerosis mice. J Neurochem 2005;93(5):1087–98.
[111] Tremolizzo L, Rodriguez-Menendez V, Sala G, et al. Valproate and HDAC inhibition: a new epigenetic strategy to mitigate phenotypic severity in ALS? Amyotroph Lateral Scler Other Motor Neuron Disord 2005;6(3):185–6.
[112] Blanchard F, Chipoy C. Histone deacetylase inhibitors: new drugs for the treatment of inflammatory diseases? Drug Discov Today 2005;10(3):197–204.
[113] Kelly WK, O'Connor OA, Krug LM, et al. Phase I study of an oral histone deacetylase inhibitor, suberoylanilide hydroxamic acid, in patients with advanced cancer. J Clin Oncol 2005;23(17):3923–31.
[114] Adcock IM. Histone deacetylase inhibitors as novel anti-inflammatory agents. Curr Opin Investig Drugs 2006;7(11):966–73.

[115] Leoni F, Zaliani A, Bertolini G, et al. The antitumor histone deacetylase inhibitor suberoylanilide hydroxamic acid exhibits antiinflammatory properties via suppression of cytokines. Proc Natl Acad Sci U S A 2002;99(5):2995–3000.
[116] Franks ME, Macpherson GR, Figg WD. Thalidomide. Lancet 2004;363(9423):1802–11.
[117] Teo SK, Stirling DI, Zeldis JB. Thalidomide as a novel therapeutic agent: new uses for an old product. Drug Discov Today 2005;10(2):107–14.
[118] Kiaei M, Petri S, Kipiani K, et al. Thalidomide and Lenalidomide extend survival in a transgenic mouse model of amyotrophic lateral sclerosis. J Neurosci 2006;26(9):2467–73.
[119] ALS-TDI. ALS TDI Animal Studies: CoQ10 I. 2003. Available at: http://www.als.net/research/studies/animalStudyDetail.asp?studyType = internal&studyID = 44.
[120] ALS-TDI. ALS TDI Animals studies: Prednisolone I. 2003. Available at: http://www.als.net/research/studies/animalStudyDetail.asp?studyType = internal&studyID = 170.
[121] Werdelin L, Boysen G, Jensen TS, et al. Immunosuppressive treatment of patients with amyotrophic lateral sclerosis. Acta Neurol Scand 1990;82:132.
[122] ALS-TDI. ALS TDI Animals studies: Minocycline I II III. 2003. Available at: http://www.als.net/research/treatments/treatmentDetail.asp?studyType = all&treatmentId = 459.
[123] Diguet E, Gross CE, Tison F, et al. Rise and fall of minocycline in neuroprotection: need to promote publication of negative results. Exp Neurol 2004;189:1.
[124] Zhang W, Narayanan M, Friedlander RM. Additive neuroprotective effects of minocycline with creatine in a mouse model of ALS. Ann Neurol 2003;53:267.
[125] Gordon PH, Moore DH, Miller RG, et al. Efficacy of minocycline in patients with amyotrophic lateral sclerosis: a phase III randomised trial. Lancet Neurol 2007;6:1045.
[126] ALS-TDI. ALS TDI Animals studies: Thalidomide I–IV. 2001–2005. Available at: http://www.als.net/research/treatments/treatmentDetail.asp?studyType = internal&treatmentId = 707.
[127] ALS-TDI. ALS TDI Animal Studies: Celebrex I–III. 2001–2005. Available at: http://www.als.net/research/treatments/treatmentDetail.asp?studyType = internal&treatmentId = 137.
[128] A double-blind placebo-controlled clinical trial of subcutaneous recombinant human ciliary neurotrophic factor (rHCNTF) in amyotrophic lateral sclerosis. ALS CNTF Treatment Study Group. Neurology 1996;46:1244.
[129] Aebischer P, Schluep M, Deglon N, et al. Intrathecal delivery of CNTF using encapsulated genetically modified xenogeneic cells in amyotrophic lateral sclerosis patients. Nat Med 1996;2:696.
[130] Suzuki M, McHugh J, Tork C, et al. GDNF secreting human neural progenitor cells protect dying motor neurons, but not their projection to muscle, in a rat model of familial ALS. PLoS ONE 2007;2:e689.
[131] Li W, Brakefield D, Pan Y, et al. Muscle-derived but not centrally derived transgene GDNF is neuroprotective in G93A-SOD1 mouse model of ALS. Exp Neurol 2007;203:457.
[132] Azzouz M, Ralph GS, Storkebaum E, et al. VEGF delivery with retrogradely transported lentivector prolongs survival in a mouse ALS model. Nature 2004;429:413.
[133] Zheng C, Skold MK, Li J, et al. VEGF reduces astrogliosis and preserves neuromuscular junctions in ALS transgenic mice. Biochem Biophys Res Commun 2007;363:989.
[134] Storkebaum E, Lambrechts D, Dewerchin M, et al. Treatment of motoneuron degeneration by intracerebroventricular delivery of VEGF in a rat model of ALS. Nat Neurosci 2005;8:85.
[135] Karlsson J, Fong KS, Hansson MJ, et al. Life span extension and reduced neuronal death after weekly intraventricular cyclosporin injections in the G93A transgenic mouse model of amyotrophic lateral sclerosis. J Neurosurg 2004;101:128.
[136] Kirkinezos IG, Hernandez D, Bradley WG, et al. An ALS mouse model with a permeable blood-brain barrier benefits from systemic cyclosporine A treatment. J Neurochem 2004;88:821.
[137] Appel SH, Stewart SS, Appel V, et al. A double-blind study of the effectiveness of cyclosporine in amyotrophic lateral sclerosis. Arch Neurol 1988;45:381.

[138] Anneser JM, Gmerek A, Gerkrath J, et al. Immunosuppressant FK506 does not exert beneficial effects in symptomatic G93A superoxide dismutase-1 transgenic mice. Neuroreport 2001;12:2663.

[139] ALS-TDI. ALS TDI Animals studies: Sodium Valproate I. 2001. Available at: http://www.als.net/research/studies/animalStudyDetail.asp?studyType = internal&studyID = 215.

[140] UMC Utrecht Clinical Trials Phase III. Sodium Valproate. 2005. Available at: http://www.als.net/research/studies/currentClinicalTrialDetail.asp?studyID = 18.

[141] ALS-TDI. ALS TDI Animals studies: Trichostatin A I. 2002. Available at: http://www.als.net/research/studies/animalStudyDetail.asp?studyType = internal&studyID = 238.

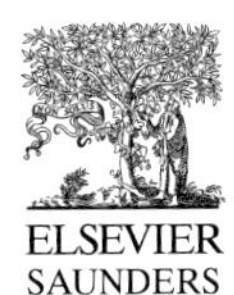

ELSEVIER
SAUNDERS

Phys Med Rehabil Clin N Am
19 (2008) 461–477

PHYSICAL MEDICINE
AND REHABILITATION
CLINICS OF
NORTH AMERICA

Current and Future Directions in Genomics of Amyotrophic Lateral Sclerosis

John Ravits, MD, FAAN[a,b,c,*], Bryan J. Traynor, MD[d]

[a]*Virginia Mason Medical Center, 1100 Ninth Avenue, Seattle, WA 98101, USA*
[b]*Benaroya Research Institute at Virginia Mason, 1201 Ninth Avenue, Seattle, WA 98101, USA*
[c]*Department of Neurology, University of Washington School of Medicine, 1959 NE Pacific Street, Seattle, WA 98195, USA*
[d]*Neurogenetics Branch, National Institute of Neurological Diseases and Stroke, National Institutes of Health, Building 35, Room 1A/110, 35 Convent Drive, Bethesda, MD 20892-3720, USA*

Mendelian and complex genetics of familial and sporadic amyotrophic lateral sclerosis

Advances in science in the past decade have accelerated the pace of discovery in amyotrophic lateral sclerosis (ALS), especially its genomics. This article discusses the Human Genome Project, the International HapMap, and emerging microarray and microdissection technologies, which have set the stage for several studies seeking fundamental insights into mechanisms of diseases and targets for therapy. Directly understanding the 90% to 95% of ALS that is sporadic (SALS) as opposed to the 5% to 10% that is familial (FALS) [1,2] now seems possible.

FALS follows simple Mendelian autosomal dominant inheritance; 20% are caused by mutations in the gene encoding superoxide dismutase 1 (SOD1) at chromosome 21q22.1 [3] and the remaining 80% by unknown mutations. SALS, by contrast, is widely believed to be a complex genetic

Dr. Traynor's work was supported by the intramural programmes of the National Institute on Aging (NIA) and the National Institute on Neurological Disorders and Stroke (NINDS).

Dr. Ravits' work was supported by the National Institute of Health (R21 NS051738-01A1), Department of Defense (USAMRMC Proposal #06054001), the Moyer Foundation, the Juniper Foundation, the Benaroya Foundation, and private philanthropists.

* Corresponding author. Benaroya Research Institute at Virginia Mason, 1201 Ninth Avenue, Seattle, WA 98101.

E-mail address: jravits@benaroyaresearch.org (J. Ravits).

doi:10.1016/j.pmr.2008.04.001

disease [2,4], which means genetic factors are important, but how much genetic factors contribute and the interplay of genetic and environmental factors are unknown. This article summarizes recent developments in genomics and efforts to apply them to understanding ALS, and highlights possible future directions of genomic research.

The Human Genome Project

The Human Genome Project was completed in 2001 and was the culmination of major advances in science, technology, and diplomacy. It was an international collaboration to sequence the 3.5 billion nucleotides in the human genome (http://www.ncbi.nlm.nih.gov/sites/entrez?db=nucleotide).

The human genome's nucleotide sequence can be divided into genic and intergenic regions. The genic regions are a minority of the code, coding for approximately 25,000 different genes. These genes are composed of promoter regions, which regulate its downstream gene; exons, which code for protein; and introns, which separate one exon from another. An average gene is 27,000 base pairs in length and consists of nine exons. In a complex assembly process in the nucleus, genes are transcribed into messenger RNA (mRNA), introns are removed, and exons are spliced together. The new assembly is then transported to the cytoplasm where protein is synthesized. The exact sequence in which exons are spliced together generates *exon splice variants*, which produce greater variations of proteins than code alone could provide, and likely plays an important role in pathogenesis of some diseases [5].

The intergenic regions, accounting for 99% of the human genome, once dismissed as "junk," are now recognized as having critical regulatory functions [6].

The International HapMap Project

The International HapMap Project was the natural successor to the Human Genome Project [7]. It was also conducted by an international collaboration that officially began in 2002. The motivating force was to provide a practical navigation map for exploring the human genome [8]. This map is possible because interspersed throughout the genome are 11 or more million sites of predictable variation called *single nucleotide polymorphisms* (SNPs). Variations that appear at one SNP are often parallel or "linked" to those that appear at others, a phenomenon called *linkage disequilibrium* [9]. The HapMap project catalogued approximately 3.5 million SNPs across the four main ethnic groups of the human species, namely north European Caucasians, Yorubans from Nigeria, Han Chinese, and Japanese. Exact numerical measurements of linkage disequilibrium between SNPs were included. Since SNPs with high linkage disequilibrium to each other could serve as proxies for each other, a representative selection of a few hundred thousand

SNPs (called *tagging SNPs*) could adequately represent SNP variation in the entire genome [10]. These could then be used to search the genome.

Microarray technology

Simultaneous with the Human Genome and International HapMap Projects was the emergence of microarray technologies. These technologies simultaneously profile hundreds of thousands of DNA or RNA sequences through microchip and microbead technologies.

In this technology, a small nucleotide probe of known sequence is synthesized and attached using laser technology to a microchip at specific *x*- and *y*-coordinate locations. The resolution of the coordinates is in the range of 3 to 10 μm and millions of probes can be placed on one microchip, which can thus represent the entire genome systematically. A labeled biologic test sample, derived from DNA or RNA, is applied to the microchip and, if sequences in the biologic test sample are complementary to those on the microchip, hybridization occurs. Signal recognition software registers what sequences hybridized and the degree of the hybridization. A digital file is then generated that profiles the biologic test sample.

Many microarray platforms exist, depending on what is being sought. The most common platforms are (1) SNP arrays, which have probes designed to detect single nucleotide polymorphisms; (2) expression arrays, which have probes designed to detect genes; (3) exon arrays, which have probes designed to detect the exons that comprise genes; and (4) tiling arrays, which have probes that detect short sequences systematically throughout the genome.

Microarray technology has engendered a new investigational paradigm that is referred to as *exploration* or *discovery* because does not depend on candidate biology or prior hypotheses. Instead, a specific test condition, such as SALS, is defined and comprehensively profiled and significant patterns and hypotheses are sought [11,12]. This paradigm generates enormous data, creating major challenges to computational biology for data mining (ie, methods for searching data for meaning) and has created a new field called *bioinformatics* [13]. One major challenge is the huge numbers of false leads that are generated. For example, if one microarray platform measures 550,000 items and the statistical analysis defines significance as the top 2% ($P < .02$), up to 11,000 findings are potentially false.

Several complex methods are emerging to better refine statistical analysis for multiple testing. One common test is the *Bonferroni correction*, which posits that the P value of true significance is the usual P value (ie, $P = .02$) divided by the number of hypotheses being tested (Fig. 1).

Whole genome association studies

With the International HapMap and the ability to represent the genetic variation through tagging SNPs, and the advances of the high throughput

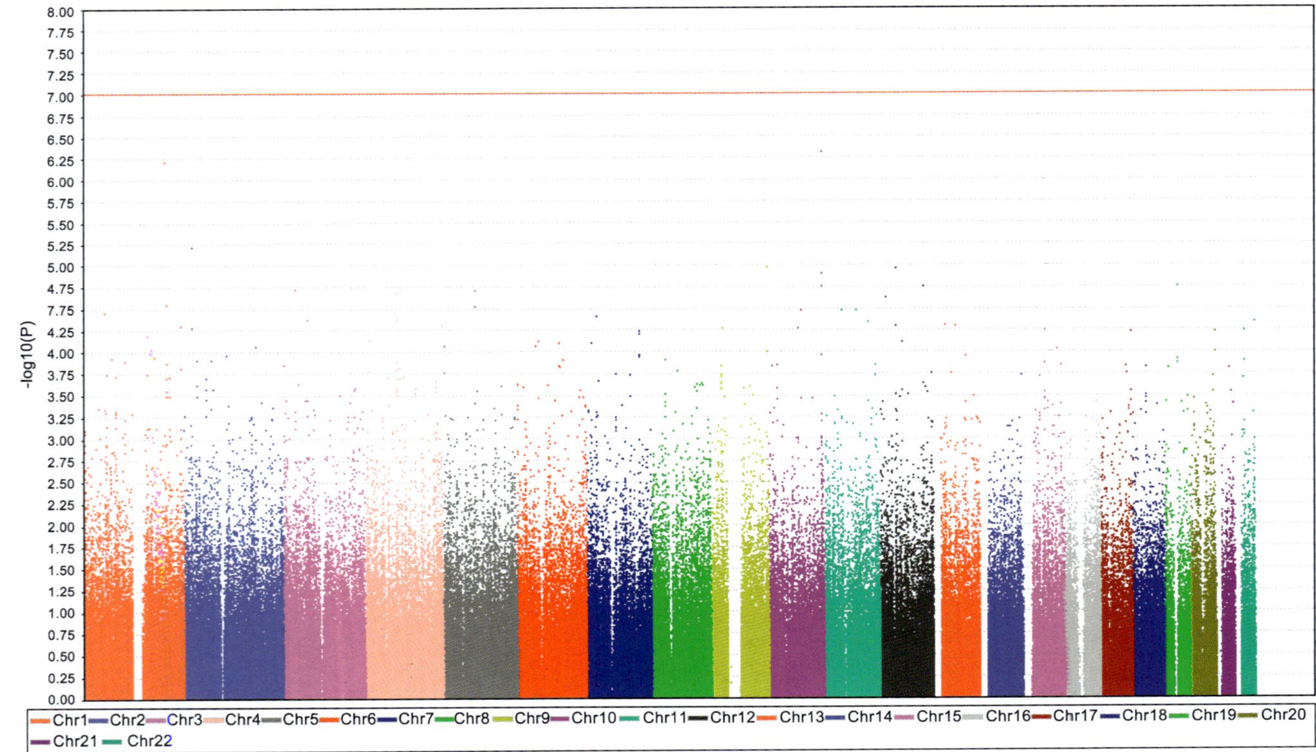

Fig. 1. Whole genome SNP association study. The plot displays the degree of association of particular SNPs with SALS: the *x*-axis displays SNPs chromosomal position and the *y*-axis shows −log10(*P* value obtained by allelic association test). The red line represents threshold for significance after Bonferroni correction for multiple testing. (*Data from* Schymick J, Scholz SW, Fung H-C et al. Genome-wide genotyping in amyotrophic lateral sclerosis and neurologically normal controls. Lancet Neurol 2007;6(4):322–8.)

microarray technologies, one microchip became able to adequately profile genetic variation across the genome. Suddenly, studies for disease association could be genome-wide through comparing cases with a disease to controls without (*case-control studies*) [14].

The manner in which whole genome association (WGA) studies ascertain association is as follows. The frequencies of alleles or genotypes (combination of alleles) of each tagging SNP are ascertained in disease and nondisease populations and then statistically compared [15]. A wide variety of statistical tests to assess for association have been described. The so-called "Cochrane Armitage trend test" is a favorite because of its (1) robustness to cryptic relatedness, wherein two samples are related to each other without the knowledge of the investigator (eg, second-degree cousins); (2) deviations from Hardy-Weinberg equilibrium, which are deviations from the frequency with which an allele is in a population when steady-state is established; and (3) ability to factor risk for disease in an additive fashion, accounting for the possibility that a causative allele may have either dominant or recessive actions.

The premise of WGA studies is that disease-predisposing alleles exist with relatively high frequency. This hypothesis is often referred to as the *common disease/common variant hypothesis* [16]. The recent explosion in the number of published whole genome studies has also made it clear that causative genetic variants typically confer only minor to moderate risk for disease. Many associations are finding odds ratios between 1.1 and 1.4, meaning that an individual's risk for disease is increased by 10% to 40%, which seems minor for rare diseases.

Not all diseases are yielding clear results, either because of low association to disease susceptibility or because the complexity of the association, if even genetic, is created through many alleles of such low frequency that they elude detection, a hypothesis referred to as *multiple rare variants hypothesis* [17–19].

Whole genome association studies of sporadic amyotrophic lateral sclerosis

Four WGA studies have been published for SALS [20–23]. The first study consisted of a cohort of 276 American patients who had SALS and 275 neurologically normal American control samples [20]. Although this study identified several loci that may be important in the pathogenesis of motor neuron degeneration, none exceeded Bonferroni correction (see Fig. 1).

The second WGA study used a technique that pooled DNA to analyze a cohort of 386 patients who had SALS and 542 neurologically normal controls [21]. This study implicated the FLJ10986 gene on chromosome 1 as being associated with increased risk for ALS (P value in replication series = 3.0×10^{-4}; odds ratio = 1.35).

The third study, involving 461 Dutch patients who had SALS and 450 controls, identified several SNPs of interest (including one on the ITPR2 gene on chromosome 12), although none met Bonferroni threshold [22]. However, a separate but related study from this same group identified dipeptidylpeptidase 6 (DPP6) on chromosome 7 as a risk allele (P value = 3.28×10^{-6} and 5.04×10^{-8}) [24].

A fourth study involving 221 Irish patients who had ALS and 211 Irish controls identified several loci of possible importance, but none exceeded Bonferroni threshold. However, pooled analysis also identified DPP6 (combined P value = 2.53×10^{-6}), which seems to increase risk for ALS by 37% [23].

Limitations

The WGA studies have two main problems [25]. First, with the possible exception of DPP6, no loci identified in individual studies have replicated each other. Second, the observed associations seem modest. Large cohorts of several thousand cases and controls are required to have sufficient power to discriminate moderate-effect alleles, and therefore each study was underpowered in the size of the initial cohorts [26]. Efforts are underway to pool data from the various WGA studies; this combined cohort of several thousand cases and controls may have sufficient power to identify moderate effect alleles.

Whole genome expression profiling

Expression and expression arrays

In contrast to genetic association studies, which examine sites in DNA for genetic associations to disease, gene expression studies explore transcribed mRNA for gene expression in disease. These studies are therefore more rooted in biology than genetics and are sometimes referred to as *functional genomics*.

The basis of these studies is expression microarray technology [27]. Expression microarrays capitalize on the fact that the 3′ tail of the 3′ exon is polyadenylated, and therefore can serve as a tag with which to identify expressed genes. Molecular techniques are used that prime with poly-dT sequences complementary to the poly-dA tails and are thus able to separate mRNA from non-mRNA (only 1%–3% of total RNA is mRNA), amplify the mRNA, and label it [28–30].

These studies use two kinds of microarray platforms. In one, called *cDNA* or *spotted microarrays*, the probes for detecting genes are maintained from in vivo stock and spotted onto the array. In the other, called *oligonucleotide microarrays*, the probes are computer designed and synthesized using laser technology. This platform has the advantage of being whole genome.

Interpreting expression data is complex. Statistical methods define genes that are differentially expressed and which can then be analyzed for biologic meaning (Fig. 2) [31]. Newer methods seek enrichment of biologic processes [32–34]. Rather than differential levels of expression of any one gene, these methods seek differential expression of sets or networks of genes that work together (Fig. 3). One challenge to data interpretation is that gene function annotation is at a relatively early stage of development and is skewed in the direction of current greatest research.

Cell-specific gene expression

Microarray technologies can be used with laser microdissection, a computer-assisted microscopic technique that microdissects tissue to isolate specific cells for molecular analysis [35,36]. Through microdissecting and pooling a single-cell population, mRNA from the relevant cells residing in tissues with complex architecture, such as the nervous system, can be isolated and pooled [37,38].

This technique is especially useful for overcoming some main difficulties in investigating sporadic neurodegenerative diseases, such as the selectivity of the pathologic process; the variable location of pathology along the neuraxis; the reduction caused by the disease; and the low pathogenic-to-non-pathogenic signal-to-noise ratio.

ALS lends itself to study with this technique. Clinically, ALS motor neuron degeneration begins in a discrete region of the motor system and propagates outward and summates over space and time until it appears to be diffuse [39]. The outward propagation of the disease from a focus creates a gradient of neurodegeneration around the site of onset, which, because of the direct involvement of respiration, is usually still active and present at death [40]. This finding can be exploited, especially when applied to regions in early stages of degeneration with relatively early molecular events [41].

Limitations

This technique has problems and cautions. Expression profiling depends on the quality of the input, underscoring the critical importance of upstream tissue processing. Expression profiles may be incomplete and only represent 75% of a cell's expressed genes, therefore causing false-negatives (ie, mistakenly thinking that a gene that is expressed is not) [42,43]. The genes identified represent the summation of the captured neurons; even though the neuronal population is homogeneous, the cells are at various stages of development or disease and the gene expression profile is a summation of this. As with all research such as this, molecular discoveries do not differentiate between primary and secondary changes. Even if primary gene expression changes can be defined, the initial causative factors initiating this expression remain to be defined. Furthermore, the relationship between genomics and proteomics is unknown; what occurs at the gene level may not accurately reflect what is happening at the protein level [44,45].

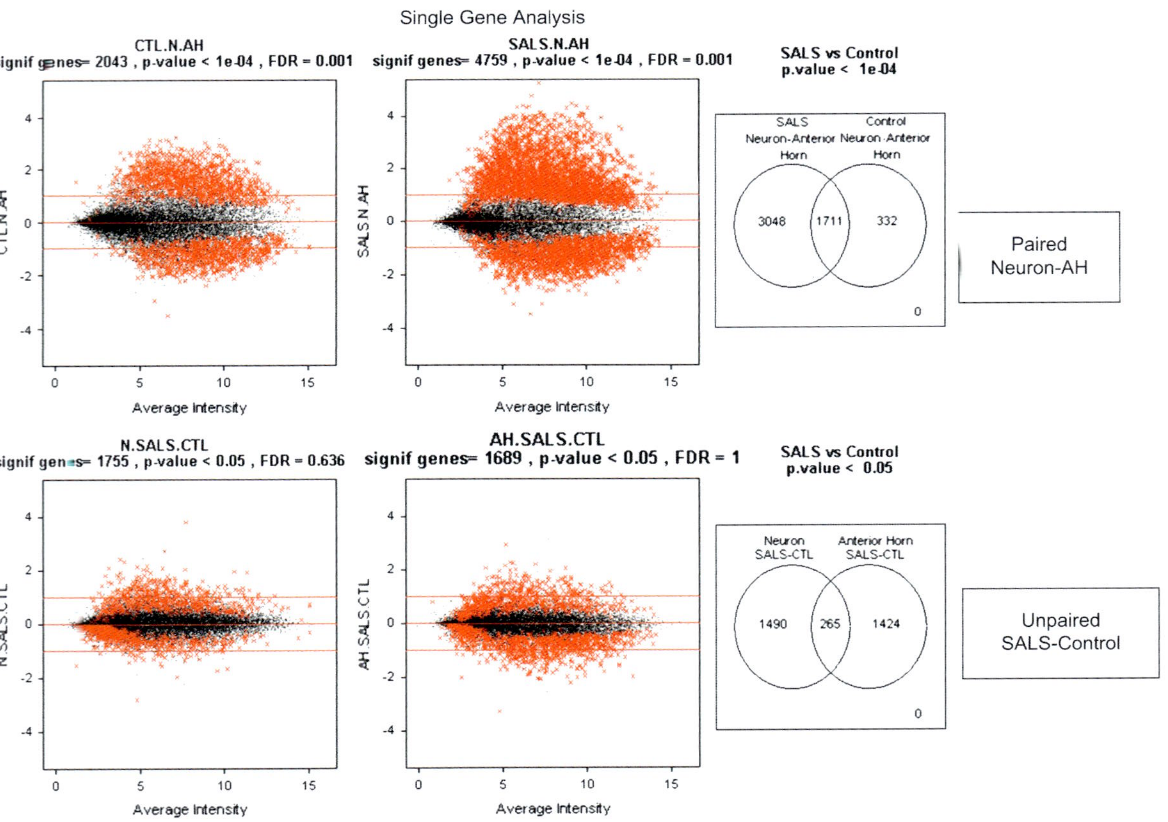
Single Gene Analysis
CTL.N.AH
signif genes= 2043 , p-value < 1e-04 , FDR = 0.001
CTL.N.AH
Average Intensity
SALS.N.AH
signif genes= 4759 , p-value < 1e-04 , FDR = 0.001
SALS.N.AH
Average Intensity
SALS vs Control
p.value < 1e-04
SALS
Neuron-Anterior
Horn
Control
Neuron-Anterior
Horn
3048
1711
332
0
Paired
Neuron-AH
N.SALS.CTL
signif genes= 1755 , p-value < 0.05 , FDR = 0.636
N.SALS.CTL
Average Intensity
AH.SALS.CTL
signif genes= 1689 , p-value < 0.05 , FDR = 1
AH.SALS.CTL
Average Intensity
SALS vs Control
p.value < 0.05
Neuron
SALS-CTL
Anterior Horn
SALS-CTL
1490
265
1424
0
Unpaired
SALS-Control

Expression studies in amyotrophic lateral sclerosis

Several investigations have used either tissue microdissection [46,47] or microarray technologies [48–53] for ALS, but only one has combined them in human SALS [54], and three have combined them in transgenic models (Tables 1 and 2) [55–57].

Jiang and colleagues [54] were the first to use microdissection to isolate motor neurons from postmortem frozen lumbar spinal cords of patients who had SALS, and used cDNA microarrays containing 4845 genes. They found that 3% of genes were down-regulated and were associated with cytoskeleton and axonal transport, transcription, and cell surface antigens and receptors; 1% of genes were up-regulated and included promoters for cell death pathways.

Based on these data, they further pursued expression in several genes using molecular pathology, including dynactin 1 (DCTN1), which is related to cytoskeleton/axonal transport and down-regulated; early growth response 3 (EGR3), which is related to transcription and down-regulated; death receptor 5 (DR5), which is related to cell death and up-regulated; cyclin C (CCNC), which is related to cell death and up-regulated; and acetyl-CoA transporter (ACATN), which is related to cell death and up-regulated [58]. One key finding was that DCTN1 seems to be one of the earliest changes in motor neurons, preceding other known markers such as accumulation of phosphorylated neurofilament or ubiquitinated proteins.

Perrin and colleagues [55] were the first to report studies of transgenic mice. They studied the G93A SOD1 genotype at 60, 90, and 120 days. At the early presymptomatic time (60 days), 17 genes were up-regulated and 11 genes were down-regulated; approximately half the genes that were differentially expressed at the early presymptomatic time remained differentially expressed throughout the disease. The differentially expressed genes functioned in areas such as intermediate filaments, protein catabolism, cell communication, and regulation of cell growth, but no induction of apoptotic pathways was apparent. One gene that was particularly important because it was also identified in other models of select motor neuron degeneration was the neurofilament protein vimentin, which was up-regulated early and remained up-regulated throughout the course. When studied with immunohistochemistry, it was deposited within the cytoplasm of motor neurons in disease.

Fig. 2. Differential gene expression. The plots show gene expression in motor neurons and anterior horns in lumbar spinal cords of SALS. The motor neurons were isolated from the surrounding anterior horn using a technique called *laser capture microdissection*, which allows histologic sections to be dissected with a specialized microscope. Gene expressions were performed using a technology called *whole genome oligonucleotide microarray*, which measure expression of each gene. The top plots compare anterior horns to motor neurons in control (*left*) and SALS (*right*); the bottom plots compare SALS to control in the neurons (*left*) and anterior horn (*right*.) (*Data from* John Ravits, MD, unpublished.)

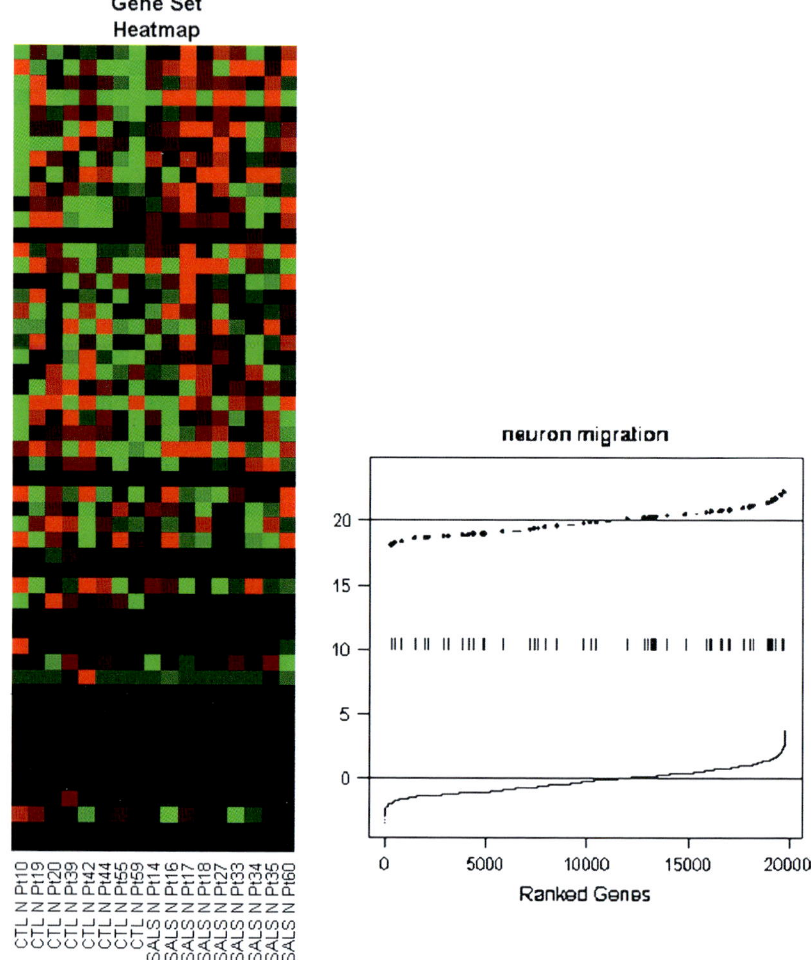

Fig. 3. Differential gene set expression. The plots show the neuron migration pathway of 54 genes that seems to be up-regulated in SALS motor neurons. The left plot shows what is called a *heat map*, which is a way of visualizing patterns. In the example, the groups of interest are in columns (control on the left and SALS on the right) and the genes in the pathway of interest are in rows (the top rows are the most differentiated between the groups). The right had plot shows the overall up-regulation (shift to the right) in the expression levels of these genes. (*Data from* John Ravits, MD, unpublished.)

Lobsiger and colleagues [56] studied SOD1 transgenic mouse and rat models and compared a model that had active SOD1 activity (SOD1 G37R) with one that had inactive activity (SOD1 G85R) at early time points. Both models showed early induction of components of the classic complement system and the regenerative/injury response; in addition, the model that was SOD1-active also showed early dysregulation of the D/L-serine biosynthetic pathway.

Table 1
Published genome wide association studies in amyotrophic lateral sclerosis

Population	Cases	Controls	Method	Gene described (P value)	Reference
US	276	271	HumanHap550K (Illumina)	No clearly associated gene	Schymick et al [20]
US	386	542	Human Mapping 500K (Affymetrix) + HumanHap300 (Illumina)	FLJ10986 (pooled $P = 3.0 \times 10^{-4}$)	Dunckley et al [21]
Dutch	461	450	HumanHap300K (Illumina)	ITPR2 (3.5×10^{-6}); DPP6 (pooled $P = 5.0 \times 10^{-8}$)	van Es et al [22,24]
Irish	222	217	HumanHap550k (Illumina)	No clearly associated gene; DPP6 (pooled $P = 2.53 \times 10^{-6}$)	Cronin et al [23]

DNA samples were pooled and then results between SNP typing platforms were pooled.

Ferraiuolo and colleagues [57] also studied G93A SOD1 transgenic mouse model at 60, 90, and 120 days. At the early presymptomatic time (60 days), an increase was seen in transcriptional and translational functions, lipid and carbohydrate metabolism, mitochondrial preprotein translocation, and respiratory chain function. Later in the course (90 days), up-regulation of genes involved in carbohydrate metabolism still occurred, but genes involved in transcription and mRNA processing genes begin to show down-regulation. Late in the disease course (120 days), repression of transcription and metabolic functions and up-regulation of complement system components and cyclins involved in cell-cycle regulation occurred.

Exon profiling

Variation in how exons are spliced together vastly expands the repertoire of proteins, and alterations of this phenomenon likely participate in disease pathogenesis [5]. Genome-wide profiling of exon splicing is now possible using a new microarray technology called *exon arrays* (Fig. 4) [59,60]. This technology capitalizes on the fact that much of the coding sequences within exons are conserved, and therefore probes to these sequences will query their individual expression, which can then be analyzed for increase or decrease.

These studies rely on a complicated scheme of random priming of mRNA to perform isolation, amplification, and labeling that differs from the expression profiles that use 3′-based mRNA amplification and array platforms. Important technical, biologic, and bioinformatics issues must be addressed for this to succeed, and there is little practical experience, especially in neurologic diseases [61]. Because significant portions of SNPS identified in the WGA studies reside in introns, which if pathogenic would likely exert their effect through exon splicing, and because the nuclear factor TDP-43, a primary ubiquitinated and mislocalized protein in SALS [62,63], is

Table 2
Microarray studies of microdissected motor neurons

Tissue	Microarray	Time points	Controls	Method of analysis	Major findings	
SALS	cDNA microarray of 4845 selected genes	NA	Non-SALS	Differential gene expression (O3-fold change)	Up-regulated promoters for cell death pathways; down-regulated cytoskeleton and axonal transport, transcription, and cell surface antigens and receptors	Jiang et al [54]
SOD1 G93A Tg mice	Whole genome oligonucleotide microarray	60, 90, and 120 days	G93A non-Tg littermates	Differential gene expression (O1.5-fold change)	Early and persistent dysregulation of intermediate filaments, protein catabolism, cell communication, and regulation of cell growth	Perrin et al [55]
SOD1 G37R and G85R Tg mice; G93A Tg rats	Whole genome oligonucleotide microarray	8 and 15 weeks	SOD1 WT Tg mice and rats	Differential gene expression (R1.5-fold change)	Early dysregulation of the D/L-serine biosynthetic pathway, induction of components of the classic complement system and of the regenerative/injury response	Lobsiger et al [56]
SOD1 G93A Tg mice	Whole genome oligonucleotide microarray	60, 90, and 120 days	G93A non-Tg littermates; SOD1 WT Tg mice; and wild-type SOD1 transgenic mice littermates	Differential gene expression (O2.0-fold change)	Early dysregulation in transcriptional and translational functions, lipid, and carbohydrate metabolism, mitochondrial preprotein translocation, and respiratory chain function	Ferraiuolo et al [57]

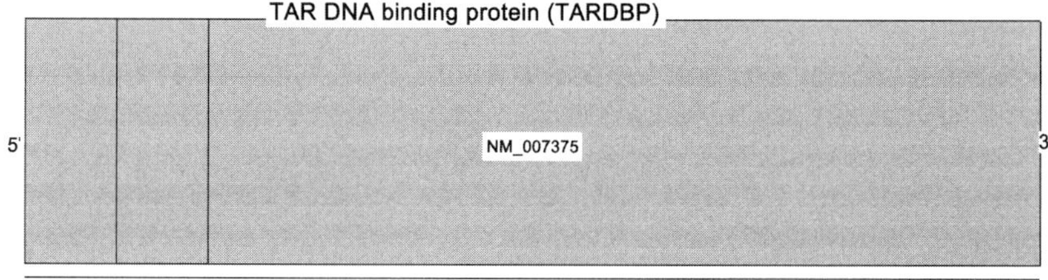

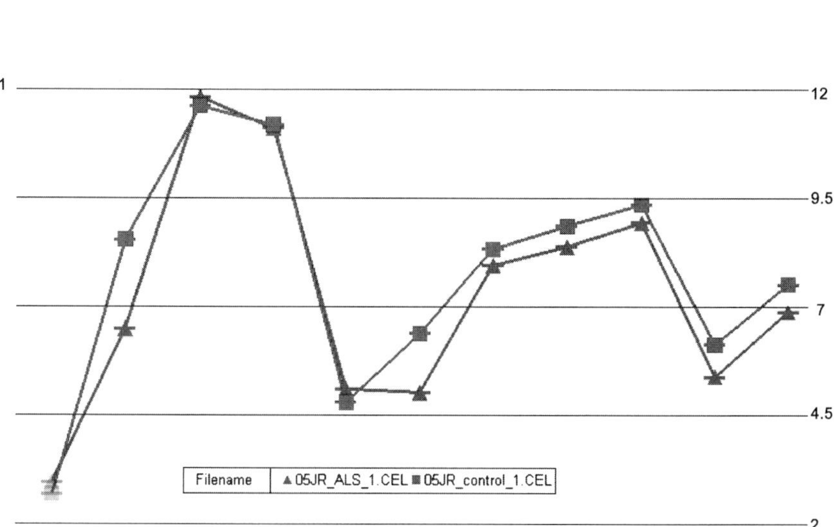

Fig. 4. Exon profiling and splicing. The plots show the expression levels of the exons comprising the *TARDBP* gene, here chosen to illustrate what is possible. They are taken from a technology called *whole genome exon microarrays*, which are able to measure each exon of each gene throughout the genome. The data is then processed by specialized computer software. The samples are obtained from motor neurons that were isolated by laser capture microdissection. The red graph is SALS and the blue graph is control. *TARDBP* is the gene coding for a protein called TDP-43, which is mislocalized in SALS. One of its functions is exon splicing. (*Data from* Stuart Rabin, PhD and John Ravits, MD, unpublished.)

a regulator of alternative splicing of exons [64], exon splice variants in SALS are important to examine.

Dark matter of the genome, noncoding RNA, and epigenetics

Vast portions of the genome code RNA transcripts that do not then code for protein (so-called "noncoding RNA") [6]. These transcripts include microRNA, which are transcribed in nucleus and transported to cytoplasm to knock-down gene expression [65,66]; small nucleolar RNA, which reside in the nucleolus to modify genes; and small nuclear RNA, which reside in the nucleus to alter pre-mRNA splicing. Noncoding RNA are believed to be particularly important as regulators of genome function and are particularly important in the nervous system [67,68].

Various new array technologies perform high-throughput profiling of genetic codes [69–71]. These allow systematic high-density profiling of the entire genome using 25-mer probes tiled at an average of 35 base pair probe spacing, thus leaving gaps of 10 base pair. With this platform, genic (exonic and intronic) and intergenic regions can be profiled. Current limitations to this technology include amplification strategies that select sense (+) strands; the large quantities of RNA needed for the seven microarrays containing approximately 45 million oligonucleotide probes that interrogate the whole human genome; and complex bioinformatics. Soon, direct whole genome sequencing will be available. The combined efforts of computational and direct biology is critical to exploring this area [72–75].

Epigenetics is the study of gene expression and regulation that occur separate from change in DNA sequence [76,77]. One important area is DNA methylation, which mutes gene expression through adding a methyl group to the 5-position of the cytosine ring. New technologies are emerging for high-throughput profiling of methylation changes, thus profiling the so-called "methylome," and this could reveal fundamental aspects of ALS pathogenesis [69,70].

Summary

High-resolution exploration of the genome is now possible and can be applied to understanding SALS biology, including exploration of the DNA, which might provide clues to SALS susceptibility, and of the RNA, which might provide clues of the SALS gene expression and molecular pathogenesis. Both genic regions, including introns and exons and their splicing, and nongenic regions, including structural, regulatory, and other elements, can be explored. Micro- and nanotechnologies, informatics, and computational biology could potentially lead to a deep understanding of molecular pathogenesis and identify targets for therapy.

References

[1] Figlewicz DA, Orrell RW. The genetics of motor neuron disease. Amyotroph Lateral Scler Other Motor Neuron Disord 2003;4:225–31.

[2] Valdmanis PN, Rouleau GA. Genetics of familial amyotrophic lateral sclerosis. Neurology 2008;70:144–52.

[3] Andersen PM. Amyotrophic lateral sclerosis associated with mutations in the Cu Zn superoxide dismutase gene. Curr Neurol Neuroscie Rep 2006;6:37–46.

[4] Simpson CL, Al-Chalabi A. Amyotrophic lateral sclerosis as a complex genetic disease. Biochim Biophys Acta 2006;1762:973–85.

[5] Novoyatleva T, Tang Y, Rafalska I, et al. Pre-mRNA missplicing as a cause of human disease. Prog Mol Subcell Biol 2006;44:27–46.
[6] Johnson JM, Edwards S, Shoemaker D, et al. Dark matter in the genome: evidence of widespread transcription detected by microarray tiling experiments. Trends Genet 2005;21(2): 93–102.
[7] The International HapMap Consortium. A haplotype of the human genome. Nature 2005; 437:1299–320.
[8] Barnes MR. Navigating the HapMap. Brief Bioinform 2006;7:211–24.
[9] Hartyl DL, Clark AG. Principles of population genetics. 4th edition. Sunderland (MA): Sinauer Associates, Inc.; 2007. p. 652.
[10] Abecasis GR, Ghosh D, Nichols TE. Linkage disequilibrium: ancient history drives the new genetics. Hum Hered 2005;59:118–24.
[11] Brown PO, Botstein D. Exploring the new world of the genome with DNA microarrays. Nat Genet 1999;21(1 Suppl):33–7.
[12] Goodman L. Hypothesis-limited research. Genome Res 1999;9:673–4.
[13] Barnes MR, editor. Bioinformatics for geneticists. A bioinformatics primer for the analysis of genetic data. 2nd edition. West Sussex (England): Wiley and Sons; 2007. p. 554.
[14] Hirschhorn JM, Daly MJ. Genome-wide association studies for complex diseases and complex traits. Nat Rev Genet 2005;6:95–108.
[15] Balding DJ. A tutorial on statistical methods for population association studies. Nat Rev Genet 2006;7:781–91.
[16] Reich DE, Lander ES. On the allelic spectrum of human disease. Trends Genet 2001;17:502–10.
[17] Pritchard JK. Are rare variants responsible for susceptibility to complex diseases? Am J Hum Genet 2001;69:124–37.
[18] Terwilliger JD, Hiekkalinna T. An utter refutation of the fundamental theorem of the HapMap. Eur J Hum Genet 2006;14:426–37.
[19] Wright AF, Hastie ND. Complex genetic diseases: controversy over the Croesus code. Genome Biol 2001;2(8):[comment/2007].
[20] Schymick J, Scholz SW, Fung H-C, et al. Genome-wide genotyping in amyotrophic lateral sclerosis and neurologically normal controls. Lancet Neurol 2007;6(4):322–8.
[21] Dunckley T, Huentelman MJ, Craig DW, et al. Whole-genome analysis of sporadic amyotrophic lateral sclerosis. NEJM 2007;357:1–14.
[22] van Es MA, van Vught PW, Blauw HW, et al. ITPR2 as a susceptibility gene in sporadic amyotrophic lateral sclerosis: a genome-wide association study. Lancet Neurol 2007;6(10): 869–77.
[23] Cronin S, Berger S, Ding J, et al. A genome-wide association study of sporadic ALS in a homogenous Irish population. Hum Mol Genet 2008;17:768–74.
[24] van Es MA, van Vught PW, Blauw HM, et al. Genetic variation in DPP6 is associated with susceptibility to amyotrophic lateral sclerosis. Nat Genet 2008;40(1):29–31.
[25] Garber K. The elusive ALS genes. Science 2008;319(5859):20.
[26] Skol AD, Scott LJ, Abecasis GR, et al. Joint analysis is more efficient than replication-based analysis for two-stage genome-wide association studies. Nat Genet 2006;38:209–13. Available at: http://www.sph.umich.edu/csg/abecasis/CaTS/index.html.
[27] Kirby J, Heath PR, Shaw PJ, et al. Gene expression assays. Adv Clin Chem 2007;44:247–92.
[28] Li J, Schwartz SM, Bumgarner RE. RNA amplification, fidelity and reproducibility of expression profiling. Comptes Rendus Biol 2003;326:1021–30.
[29] Ginsberg SD, Che S. RNA amplification in brain tissues. Neurochem Res 2002;27: 981–92.
[30] Kelz MB, Dent GW, Therlanos S, et al. Single-cell antisense RNA amplification and microarray analysis as a tool for studying neurological degeneration and restoration. Sci Aging Knowledge Environ 2002;1:1–10.
[31] Speed T, editor. Statistical analysis of gene expression microarray data. Boca Raton (FL): Chapman and Hall/CRC Press LLC; 2003. p. 1–222.

[32] Subramanian A, Tamayo P, Mootha V, et al. Gene set enrichment analysis: a knowledge-based approach for interpreting genome-wide expression profiles. Proc Natl Acad Sci U S A 2005;102:15545–50.
[33] Bild A, Febbo PG. Application of a priori established gene sets to discover biologically important differential expression in microarray data. Proc Natl Acad Sci U S A 2005; 1073:15278–9.
[34] Efron B, Tibshirani R. On testing the significance of sets of genes. Available at: http://www-stat.stanford.edu/~tibs/ftp/GSA.pdf.
[35] Emmert-Buck MR, Bonner RF, Smith PD, et al. Laser capture microdissection. Science 1996;274:998–1001.
[36] Bonner RF, Emmert-Buck M, Cole K, et al. Laser capture microdissection: molecular analysis of tissue. Science 1997;278:1481–3.
[37] Nisenbaum LK. The ultimate chip shot: can microarray technology deliver for neuroscience? Genes Brain Behav 2002;1:27–34.
[38] Mills JC, Roth KA, Cagan RL, et al. DNA microarrays and beyond: completing the journey from tissue to cell. Nat Cell Biol 2001;3:E175–8.
[39] Ravits J, Paul P, Jorg C. Focality of upper and lower motor neuron degeneration at the clinical onset of ALS. Neurology 2007;68:1571–5.
[40] Ravits J, Laurie P, Fan Y, et al. Implications of ALS focality: rostral-caudal distribution of lower motor neuron loss postmortem. Neurology 2007;68:1576–82.
[41] Ravits J, Laurie P, Stone B. Amyotrophic lateral sclerosis microgenomics. Phys Med Rehabil Clin N Am 2005;16(4):909–24.
[42] Kacharmina JE, Crino PB, Eberwine J. Preparation of cDNA from single cells and sub cellular regions. Methods Enzymol 1999;303:3–18.
[43] Crino PB, Trojanowski JQ, Dichter MA, et al. Embryonic neuronal markers in tuberous sclerosis: single-cell molecular pathology. Proc Natl Acad Sci USA 1996;93:14152–7.
[44] Humphery-Smith I, Cordwell SJ, Blackstock WP. Proteome research: complementarity and limitations with respect to the RNA and DNA worlds. Electrophoresis 1997;18:1217–42.
[45] Greenbaum D, Colangelo C, Williams K, et al. Comparing protein abundance and mRNA expression levels on a genomic scale. Genome Biol 2003;4(9):117.
[46] Heath PR, Tomkins J, Ince PG, et al. Quantitative assessment of AMPA receptor mRNA in human spinal motor neurons isolated by laser capture microdissection. Neuroreport 2002; 13(14):1753–7.
[47] Mawrin C, Kirches E, Dietzmann K. Single-cell analysis of mtDNA in amyotrophic lateral sclerosis: towards the characterization of individual neurons in neurodegenerative disorders. Pathol Res Pract 2003;199:415–8.
[48] Malaspina A, Kaushik N, de Belleroche J. Differential expression of 14 genes in amyotrophic lateral sclerosis spinal cord detected using gridded cDNA arrays. J Neurochem 2001;77: 132–45.
[49] Ishigaki S, Niwa J, Ando Y, et al. Differentially expressed genes in sporadic amyotrophic lateral sclerosis spinal cords–screening by molecular indexing and subsequent cDNA microarray analysis. FEBS Lett 2002;531:354–8.
[50] Dangond F, Hwang D, Camelo S, et al. Molecular signature of late-stage human ALS revealed by expression profiling of postmortem spinal cord gray matter. Physiol Genomics 2004;16:229–39.
[51] Olsen MK, Roberds SL, Ellerbrock BR, et al. Disease mechanisms revealed by transcription profiling in SOD1-G93A transgenic mouse spinal cord. Ann Neurol 2001;50:730–40.
[52] Yoshihara T, Ishigaki S, Yamamoto M, et al. Differential expression of inflammation- and apoptosis-related genes in spinal cords of a mutant SOD1 transgenic mouse model of familial amyotrophic lateral sclerosis. J Neurochem 2002;80:158–67.
[53] Hensley K, Floyd RA, Gordon B, et al. Temporal patterns of cytokine and apoptosis-related gene expression in spinal cords of the G93A-SOD1 mouse model of amyotrophic lateral sclerosis. J Neurochem 2002;82:365–74.

[54] Jiang Y-M, Yamamoto M, Koyayashi Y, et al. Gene expression profile of spinal motor neurons in sporadic amyotrophic lateral sclerosis. Ann Neurol 2005;57:236–51.
[55] Perrin F, Boisset G, Docquier M, et al. No widespread induction of cell death genes occurs in pure motoneurons in an amyotrophic lateral sclerosis mouse model. Hum Mol Genet 2005; 14:3309–20.
[56] Lobsiger CS, Boillee S, Cleveland DW. Toxicity from different SOD1 mutants dysregulates the complement system and the neuronal regenerative response in ALS motor neurons. Proc Natl Acad Sci U S A 2007;104:7319–26.
[57] Ferraiuolo L, Heath PR, Holden H, et al. Microarray analysis of the cellular pathways involved in the adaptation to and progression of motor neuron injury in the SOD1 G93A mouse model of familial ALS. J Neurosci 2007;27:9201–19.
[58] Jiang YM, Yamamoto M, Tanaka F, et al. Gene expression specifically detected in motor neurons (dynactin 1, early growth response 3, acetyl-CoA transporter, death receptor 5, and cyclin C) differentially correlate to pathologic markers in sporadic amyotrophic lateral sclerosis. J Neuropthol Exp Neurol 2007;66:617–27.
[59] Cuperlovic-Culf M, Belacel N, Culf AS, et al. Microarray analysis of alternative splicing. OMICS 2006;10(3):344–57.
[60] Clark TA, Schweitzer AC, Chen TX, et al. Discovery of tissue-specific exons using comprehensive human exon microarrays. Genome Biol 2007;8(4):R64, 1–16.
[61] Heinzen EL, Yoon W, Weale ME, et al. Alternative ion channel splicing in mesial temporal lobe epilepsy and Alzheimer's disease. Genome Biol 2007;8(3):R32, 1–18.
[62] Newmann M, Sampathu DM, Kwong LK, et al. Ubiquitinated TDP-43 in frontotemporal lobar degeneration and amyotrophic lateral sclerosis. Science 2006;314(5796):130–3.
[63] Arai T, Hasegawa LM, Akiyama H, et al. TDP-43 is a component of ubiquitin-positive tau-negative inclusions in frontotemporal lobar degeneration and amyotrophic lateral sclerosis. Biochem Biophys Res Commun 2006;351:602–11.
[64] Buratti E, Dork T, Zuccato E, et al. Nuclear factor TDP-43 and SR proteins promote in vitro and in vivo CFTR exon 9 skipping. EMBO J 2001;20(7):1774–84.
[65] Krichevsky AM. MicroRNA profiling: from dark matter to white matter, or identifying new players in neurobiology. ScientificWorldJournal 2007;7(S2):155–66.
[66] Kim VN, Nam J-W. Genomics of microRNA. Trends Genet 2005;22:165–73.
[67] Mehler MF, Mattick JS. Non-coding RNAs in the nervous system. J Physiol 2006;575: 333–41.
[68] Nelson PT, Keller JN. RNA in brain disease: no longer just "the messenger in the middle". J Neuropathol Exp Neurol 2007;66:461–8.
[69] Mockler TC, Ecker JR. Applications of DNA tiling arrays for whole-genome analysis. Genomics 2005;85:1–15.
[70] Hoheisel J. Microarray technology: beyond transcript profiling and genotype analysis. Nat Rev Genet 2006;7:200–10.
[71] Cowell JK, Hawthorn L. The application of microarray technology to the analysis of the cancer genome. Curr Mol Med 2007;7:103–20.
[72] Chaudhuri K, Chatterjee R. MicroRNA detection and target prediction: integration of computational and experimental approaches. DNA Cell Biol 2007;26:321–37
[73] Berezikow E, Cuppen E, Plasterek RH. Approaches to microRNA discovery. Nat Genet 2006;38:52–7.
[74] Zhang B, Pan X, Wang Q, et al. Computational identification of microRNAs and their targets. Comput Biol Chem 2006;30:395–407.
[75] Huang JC, Morris QD, Frey BJ. Bayesian inference of microRNA targets from sequence and expression data. J Comput Biol 2007;14:550–63.
[76] Saetrom P, Snøve O Jr, Rossi JJ. Epigenetics and microRNA. Pediatr Res 2007;61:17R–23R.
[77] Chuang JC, Jones PA. Epigenetics and microRNA. Pediatr Res 2007;61:24R–9R.

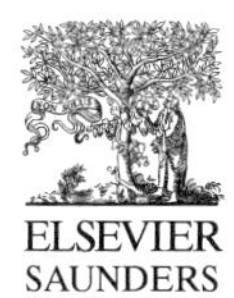
ELSEVIER
SAUNDERS

Phys Med Rehabil Clin N Am
19 (2008) 479–494

PHYSICAL MEDICINE
AND REHABILITATION
CLINICS OF
NORTH AMERICA

Androgen Receptor Function in Motor Neuron Survival and Degeneration

Gregory A. Cary, BA[a,b],
Albert R. La Spada, MD, PhD[a,c,d,e,f,*]

[a]*Department of Laboratory Medicine, University of Washington Medical Center, Box 357110, Room NW 120, Seattle, WA 98195-7110, USA*
[b]*Molecular & Cellular Biology Program, Department of Laboratory Medicine, University of Washington Medical Center, Box 357110, Room NW 120, Seattle, WA 98195-7110, USA*
[c]*Department of Neurology, University of Washington, Seattle, WA, USA*
[d]*Department of Medicine, University of Washington, Seattle, WA, USA*
[e]*Department of Pathology, University of Washington, Seattle, WA, USA*
[f]*Center for Neurogenetics & Neurotherapeutics, University of Washington, Seattle, WA, USA*

The androgen receptor (AR) is a nuclear hormone receptor of approximately 110 kd that is responsible for the biological actions of androgens, including testosterone and its metabolite dihydrotestosterone (DHT). Androgens regulate a wide range of developmental and physiologic processes including the growth of muscle and bone, spermatogenesis, and the development of secondary sexual characteristics [1]. The AR mediates these effects primarily by influencing the expression of androgen responsive genes. The AR affects transcription in a ligand-dependent manner by nuclear translocation, dimerization, DNA binding, and association with various co-activators/co-repressors and other components of the transcriptional machinery [2]. The functional domains of the AR – an N-terminal transcriptional activation domain, a DNA-binding domain (DBD) and a C-terminal ligand-binding domain (Fig. 1) – reflect these processes involved in androgen signaling. Both gain-of-function and loss-of-function mutations have been identified in the AR, and these alterations respectively give rise to distinct pathologies. These conditions include the various forms of androgen insensitivity syndromes (AIS): ranging from testicular feminization

Motor neuron disease research in the La Spada laboratory is supported by the NIH (NS41648) and the Muscular Dystrophy Association.

* Corresponding author. Department of Laboratory Medicine, University of Washington Medical Center, Box 357110, Room NW 120, Seattle, WA 98195-7110.
E-mail address: laspada@u.washington.edu (A.R. La Spada).

doi:10.1016/j.pmr.2008.03.002

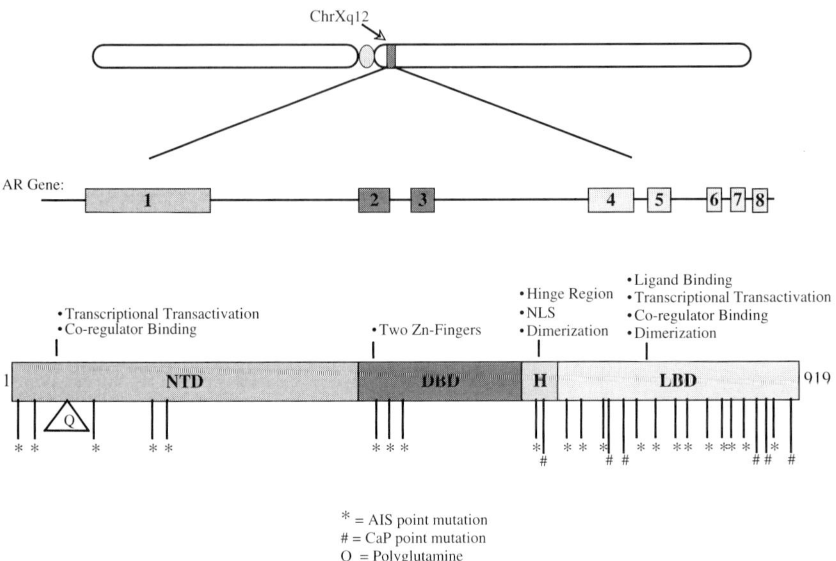

Fig. 1. Schematic illustration of the androgen receptor. The location of the androgen receptor locus on the long arm of the X chromosome at q12 (gray bar) and an expanded map of the androgen receptor gene, depicting the relative sizes and distribution of its eight exons, are shown. The colors of the exons reflect the different functional domains of the translated protein that are encoded by the various exons, including the amino-terminal domain (NTD; blue), the DNA-binding domain (DBD; red) and the ligand-binding domain (LBD; yellow). An illustration of the final protein product is shown below, highlighting these functional domains, along with the short hinge region (H). Representative disease-causing mutations have been identified and mapped onto the protein, including mutations that cause androgen insensitivity syndrome (AIS; *), mutations that are associated with prostate cancer (CaP; #), and the polyglutamine tract that is expanded in SBMA (Q).

(Tfm) and partial androgen insensitivity syndrome (PAIS) to male infertility, prostate cancer (CaP), breast cancer susceptibility, and X-linked spinal and bulbar muscular atrophy (SBMA), which is also known as Kennedy's disease [3]. SBMA is of particular interest because it exhibits characteristics of both loss-of-function and gain-of-function mutations in the AR.

SBMA is a heritable, adult onset disease that causes preferential degeneration of lower motor neurons leading to weakness and atrophy of bulbar, facial, and limb muscles [4,5]. It is clinically similar to amyotrophic lateral sclerosis (ALS), another form of motor neuron disease (MND). The main clinical distinction between the two diseases is that ALS involves degeneration of both upper and lower motor neurons, whereas the affected cell type in SBMA is lower motor neurons. Another interesting difference is that Onuf's nucleus, an androgen-sensitive spinal cord motor neuron nucleus, is spared in ALS, although it degenerates in SBMA [6,7]. Degeneration of sensory neurons of the dorsal root ganglia is also a typical sign associated with SBMA, often preceding the onset of motor dysfunction [8,9]. In addition to the neurologic phenotype, SBMA patients display some of the characteristic signs of androgen insensitivity syndromes including testicular atrophy, decreased fertility, gynecomastia, and elevated androgen levels [10,11]. This mild androgen insensitivity, along with the X-linked pattern of inheritance, caused the AR to be considered as a candidate gene for SBMA. This association was further supported by linkage mapping of the SBMA gene to a locus on the X chromosome that includes the AR gene [12]. Ultimately, the work to identify the gene responsible for SBMA led to the discovery of a novel mutation, the expansion of a trinucleotide CAG repeat, in the first exon of the AR gene [13]. This CAG repeat encodes a stretch of glutamine residues within the N-terminal transcriptional activation domain of the AR. Unaffected individuals have a polyglutamine repeat size that ranges between 5 and 35 glutamines, while symptomatic individuals always have a polyglutamine stretch of at least 37 glutamines [13]. This absolute association indicates that the polyglutamine expansion in the AR is the source of the pathology in SBMA. SBMA is a member of a family of nine dominantly inherited neurodegenerative diseases caused by polyglutamine (polyQ) repeat expansions in specific proteins. Other polyQ diseases include Hungtington's disease (HD), dentatorubral-pallidoluysian atrophy, and six forms of spinocerebellar ataxia. Interestingly, though each of the polyQ diseases has a CAG repeat expansion in a different gene, and each disease seems to specifically affect different subsets of neuronal populations, SBMA is the only polyQ repeat expansion disease known to cause selective degeneration of motor neurons [14]. This observation implies that there is something unique about AR biology that is important for motor neuron function.

Studies of other polyQ expansion diseases, as well as research specifically investigating SBMA, indicate that the pathology associated with polyQ-expanded proteins is due to a toxic gain of function of the mutant protein [14–16]. The polyQ expansion of the AR in SBMA, like all polyQ repeat expansion diseases, is a dominantly inherited mutation; numerous lines of investigation, including ascertainment of homozygous females with CAG repeat expansions [17] and androgen ablation experiments in SBMA transgenic mouse models [18], have shown that SBMA disease pathogenesis requires AR activation by ligand binding. Heterozygous female carriers are thus spared the neurodegenerative SBMA phenotype due to a significantly reduced concentration of available ligands for the AR. Although considerable work in the polyQ research field has emphasized the polyQ protein misfolding gain-of-function toxicity as the principal mechanism for molecular pathology, gain-of-function and loss-of-function are not mutually exclusive explanations for the etiology of the disease. Indeed, numerous studies have implicated loss of polyQ protein normal function in the pathogenesis of each disease [19–25]. In the case of SBMA, one of the primary indicators of a loss of normal AR function is the mild androgen insensitivity phenotype that is seen in affected patients. This insensitivity reflects the fact that polyQ-expanded AR is not competent to fully stimulate androgen-dependent physiologic pathways or to fully maintain male secondary sexual characteristics. Consequently, in a motor neuron-like cell culture model of SBMA, cells transfected with polyQ-expanded AR differentially express genes in response to androgens when compared with cells expressing a non-pathologic form of AR [26], confirming that polyQ-expanded AR is not functionally interchangeable with unexpanded AR. In a highly representative SBMA transgenic mouse model, the authors' lab has further demonstrated that endogenous mouse AR partially compensates for, and thus retards, motor neuron loss, as SBMA mice develop a more severe motor neuron phenotype when the endogenous AR is absent [18]. These observations indicate that normal AR might be playing a role in supporting motor neurons and protecting them from degeneration. Hence, polyQ-expanded AR is dysfunctional in this protective capacity, an effect that agonizes the process of motor neuron degeneration in SBMA. This article examines the evidence supporting the idea that normal AR has a protective, trophic role in motor neuron biology, first by examining the trophic requirements of motor neurons in general, and then by delineating the trophic properties of the AR in the central nervous system.

Trophic requirements of motor neurons

The neuronal requirements for trophic factor support are well established and have been investigated for over 50 years. Nerve growth factor (NGF) was the first target-derived neuronal growth factor identified. Since its discovery in 1951, a whole family of similar trophic factors, called neurotrophins, have been recognized [27–29]. Neurotrophins are small peptide growth hormones that promote neuronal differentiation, synaptic plasticity, regeneration, and survival [27–29]. The family includes molecules such as neurotrophin-3 (NT-3), brain-derived neurotrophic factor (BDNF), ciliary neurotrophic factor (CNTF), and glial cell line-derived neurotrophic factor (GDNF) [27–29]. Neurotrophin signals are transduced in a variety of ways, but most involve the activation of receptor tyrosine kinases. NGF, BDNF, and NT-3 involve signaling through the Trk receptors (ie, TrkA, TrkB, and TrkC) and also through the $p75^{NTR}$ (neurotrophin receptor). GDNF signals through the RET family of receptor tyrosine kinases and CNTF signals through a receptor that is structurally very similar to the IL-6 receptor.

Of all of these neurotrophic factors, GDNF, BDNF, and CNTF display the greatest growth promotion and neuroprotective effects on motor neuron populations. GDNF is produced by glial cells of the CNS; is a very potent neuroprotective agent; and exerts its effects on both astrocytes and motor neurons. Mutations in murine GDNF are associated with a loss of 20%–30% of motor neurons [30], whereas GDNF over-expression prevents the developmental programmed cell death of motor neurons [31] and axotomy-induced motor neuron cell death [32]. Muscle from patients who have SBMA and ALS demonstrates decreased expression of GDNF [33]. BDNF is target-derived and retrogradely transported by motor neurons from muscle [34,35]. BDNF can also protect motor neurons from axotomy-induced cell death [36–38], as well as prevent toxic neuronal nitric oxide synthase production [39] and glutamate excitotoxicity [40,41]. Despite these protective effects, BDNF has shown little promise in the treatment of several MNDs, including ALS [42], though it did ameliorate the disease phenotype in the Wobbler mouse [43]. CNTF is a peptide growth factor that is produced predominantly by glial cells postnatally, but, unlike the other neurotrophins, does not contain a signal sequence, indicating that it is not normally secreted [44]. This has led some to hypothesize that CNTF release occurs in response to nerve injury [28]. Despite some conflicting reports [45,46], CNTF appears to rescue axotomized neurons from cell death [47]. In addition, both homozygous null CNTF mice [48] and mice deficient in the CNTFα receptor [49] develop motor neuron loss.

Beyond these classical neurotrophic factors, there are several other growth factors that display motor neuron specific trophism, including vascular endothelial growth factor (VEGF) and insulin-like growth factor 1 (IGF-1). VEGF is a cytokine that is typically associated with angiogenesis and can support motor neurons by increasing local blood supply, but also exhibits many direct neuroprotective effects on motor neurons [50–52]. VEGF is able to promote the survival of motor neurons in vitro [53], and increase neurogenesis after axotomy [54]. Decreased VEGF levels have been correlated with various forms of MND including ALS, both in patients [55] and in mouse models, including the authors' transgenic mouse model of SBMA [56]. Intriguingly, deletion of a hypoxia-responsive element within the promoter of VEGF leads to the degeneration of motor neurons [57] and a correlation between VEGF promoter haplotypes and ALS has been observed [58]. In addition, VEGF treatment has been beneficial in a variety of models of MND [50–52,59].

IGF-1 is a peptide hormone produced by oligodendrocytes, Schwann cells, and muscle [60–62]. IGF-1 is a very potent trophic factor for motor neurons; it increases motor neuron survival both in vitro [63] and in an in vivo axotomy model [64]. IGF-1 also promotes motor neuron axonal sprouting, regeneration, and muscle innervation in vitro [65]. Targeting of IGF-1 to motor neurons slows the typical force decline seen in aging muscle [66]. Because IGF-1 is trophic for both motor neurons and muscle, there has been considerable interest in its potential protective capacity in various forms of MND. Most notably, viral delivery of IGF-1 dramatically slowed the progression of ALS in the SOD1 transgenic mouse model [67]. Additionally, the beneficial effects of IGF-1 in the Wobbler mouse model of MND are potentiated by glycosaminoglycans [68], and the neuroprotective effects of IGF-1 and GDNF act additively in the SOD1 mouse model of ALS [69]. IGF-1 can decrease the toxicity associated with polyQ-expanded AR in vitro by stimulating the Akt phosphoylation of the AR, thereby preventing ligand binding and receptor activation [70]. These trophic factors play an important role in protecting motor neurons from many of the cytotoxic insults that lead to motor neuron cell death.

Trophic effects of the AR

The trophic effects of androgens on reproductive organs are well established. AR signaling is essential for the normal development of male sexual features, including sexual organ development as well as the formation and maintenance of secondary sexual characteristics, including increased body hair and muscle mass [1]. Beyond sexual development, androgen signaling has been associated with neoplastic prostate growth [71,72] and male breast carcinoma [73], which demonstrates the strong trophism of androgens. Hormonal castration, the prevention of androgen signaling, and silencing prostate AR expression have all been demonstrated to retard cancerous growth of the prostate [74,75]. In this context, the trophic effects of androgens have been causally linked with the ability of the AR to stimulate VEGF expression, thereby increasing angiogenesis. However, androgens, as well as other sex hormones, have also demonstrated trophic actions in non-reproductive tissues. Immunohistochemical investigation has confirmed the presence of the AR in a wide variety of human fetal extra-genital tissues including the thymus, bronchial epithelium, cardiac valves and surrounding muscle, and in the spinal cord [76]. The presence of the AR in these early tissues suggests that androgen signaling might not simply affect sexual differentiation, but may be a broader signal for early growth and development of these tissues.

It is clear that AR expression in the spinal cord occurs as early as the first trimester and that high expression of AR within the spinal cord continues into adulthood. In a classic paper in 1977, Sar and Stumpf [77] demonstrated that androgen receptor expression is especially high in the ventral spinal cord. Therefore, it is reasonable to predict that AR signaling is important to the development and maintenance of this tissue, including especially spinal cord motor neurons. Studies of cell culture and animal models of spinal cord development have provided clues to the functions of androgens in such cell types. AR-expressing motor neuron-like cells in vitro exhibit changes in morphology in response to androgen treatment, including developing larger cell bodies and broader fields of neurite processes [78]. Further exploration of these effects indicates that this increased neurite outgrowth might be due to androgen-dependent up-regulation of neuritin, a protein previously demonstrated to be important for neurite elongation [79]. Another indication of the function of androgens in developing spinal cord motor neurons comes from careful investigation of the spinal nucleus of the bulbocavernosus (SNB), a sexually dimorphic nucleus of androgen-sensitive motor neurons in rodents that is analogous to Onuf's nucleus in humans. Androgen signaling has been demonstrated to influence soma size and dendrite length in SNB motor neurons [80]. These effects are linked to the expression of both BDNF and its receptor TrkB [81]. Furthermore, androgens and CNTF interact early in postnatal development to increase SNB motor neuron number [82]. These in vivo data confirm the in vitro observation that androgen signaling plays a crucial role in motor neuron development, especially with regard to the establishment of neurites (in vitro) and dendrites (in vivo). However, remaining questions are: to what degree does the AR maintain this trophic influence in adult motor neurons, and how might androgen signaling protect adult motor neurons from degeneration?

Trophism of adult neurons is frequently inferred from the ability of a trophic factor to protect neurons from a variety of insults. The AR has demonstrated a wide variety of neuroprotective effects. AR signaling protects many cells (including neuroblastoma cells [83], primary cerebellar granule cells [84] and striatal cells in vivo [85]) against oxidative stress-induced cell death. This protection may result from an AR-specific increase in catalase activity [83,84]. Another example of AR neuroprotection comes from an experiment in which the excitotoxin kainate was noted to kill more hippocampal neurons in gonadectomized male rats versus sham-operated controls; this cell death was then reversed by supplementation of the gonadectomized rats with DHT [86]. Androgens have even been shown to protect neurons from the toxic effects of the beta-amyloid peptide (Aβ1-42), believed to be a causative agent in Alzheimer's disease pathogenesis [87]. Both androgens and estrogen can protect neurons from Aβ toxicity by increasing the levels of the chaperone protein Hsp70, which is thought to prevent Aβ aggregate formation [88]. Additionally, androgens may protect against Aβ toxicity through a receptor-dependent activation of the MAPK/ERK signaling pathway in neurons, leading to downstream activation of Rsk and inactivation of Bad, a pro-apoptotic Bcl-2 family member [89].

Importantly, in the spinal cord, signaling through the AR can elicit specific motor neuron protection, both in vitro and in vivo. AR expressing motor neuron-like MN-1 cells not only exhibit larger somas and broader neurite arbors in response to androgens, but they are also protected from serum deprivation-induced cell death [26,78]. This seems to be a common function of AR signaling in neurons, as androgens promote the survival of human primary neurons in low serum conditions in a receptor-dependent fashion [90]. Evidence from in vivo motor neuron injury models indicates that AR signaling protects motor neurons from axotomy-induced death. Androgens interact with BDNF in the SNB to promote motor neuron survival and maintenance of the SNB dendritic arbor post-axotomy [80]. Furthermore, androgens are particularly trophic in a hamster facial motor neuron axotomy model, promoting survival of axotomized neurons and increasing the rate of functional recovery [91–93]. AR signaling is clearly involved in protecting adult neurons, including motor neurons, from toxicity, injury and death.

How might androgen signaling be promoting neuronal survival? Since the AR functions primarily as a transcription factor, it is logical to predict that this protective effect might be tied to the ability of the AR to induce the expression of genes that are involved in promoting motor neuron survival (Fig. 2). Indeed, AR mediated up-regulation of neuritin expression is directly responsible for neurite elongation in motor neuron-like cultures, as neuritin silencing by siRNA abolishes the trophic response to androgens [79]. Similarly, inhibition of neurotrophin and CNTF signaling prevents the sparing of SNB motor neurons normally observed after administration of androgens to neonatal rats [94]. Trophic factor signaling is thus an important aspect of AR trophism and might function downstream of androgen signaling.

Several trophic factors that are important for motor neuron biology have been associated with AR signaling. AR activation stimulates the production

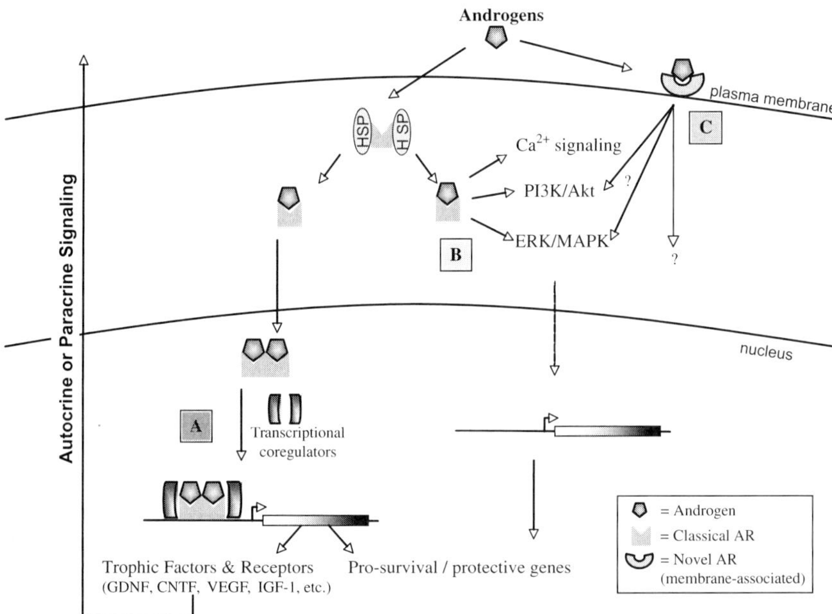

Fig. 2. Proposed mechanisms for androgen receptor (AR) protection of motor neurons. This figure summarizes three mechanisms by which AR may exert its trophic effects on motor neurons. (A) In the classical model of androgen receptor signaling, AR binds ligand, releasing it from its molecular chaperone and allowing it to undergo nuclear translocation to form homodimers. AR then associates with transcriptional co-regulators at androgen-responsive genes to promote their transcription. (B) In this non-genomic pathway of androgen receptor action, AR signaling does not involve direct interaction with genomic elements. Rather, ligand-bound AR interacts with second messenger signaling cascades, such as ERK/MAPK and PI3K/Akt, to influence the molecular status of the cell. This mechanism has not been validated yet in motor neurons. (C) Lastly, in the membrane-associated model for androgen receptor signaling, the authors postulate the interaction of androgens with putative novel membrane-associated ARs that would signal through second messenger signaling cascades.

of VEGF mRNA in prostate cancer cells [74]; and in vivo siRNA silencing of AR has been demonstrated to slow neoplastic prostate growth and repress VEGF expression [75]. AR stimulation of VEGF signaling increases BDNF levels and ultimately neurogenesis in the brains of adult songbirds [95], which demonstrates the possible multi-potency of AR-stimulated VEGF expression. Transgenic mice carrying a polyQ-expanded AR express less VEGF, and this reduction has been implicated in the pathology of SBMA [56]. In another mouse model of SBMA, polyQ-expanded AR is associated with decreased GDNF and IGF-1 expression [96]. Researchers have identified androgen response elements in the upstream promoter of the IGF-1 gene [97], and testosterone has been observed to stimulate IGF 1 transcription in prostate [98]. Interestingly, IGF-1 can facilitate AR signaling by de-repressing Foxo1 [99] or by stabilization of beta-catenin, an AR co-activator [100]. The authors' group, in collaboration with workers at the National Institutes of Health, has recently identified a mechanism through which IGF-1 prevents the deleterious effects of polyQ-expanded AR by stimulating Akt-mediated AR phosphorylation which blocks ligand binding and receptor activation [70]. These results indicate that while IGF-1 and AR signaling in motor neurons are intertwined, it is possible that AR stimulation of IGF-1 expression is a protective mechanism for motor neurons. CNTF is another important trophic factor that has been demonstrated to be androgen-responsive. Expression of the CNTF receptor alpha subunit is regulated by the AR in both spinal cord and muscle [101,102]. Furthermore, CNTF receptor knock-out mice do not exhibit the sexual dimorphism normally present in the SNB [103]; and SNB motor neuron death in androgen-insensitive rats can be prevented by CNTF administration [104]. These results, together with the previously noted observation that blocking CNTF signaling prevents the AR-mediated rescue of early SNB motor neurons, indicate that AR-mediated expression of the CNTF receptor is necessary for the sexually dimorphic sparing of SNB motor neurons in rodents. These data support a model in which AR-mediated expression of trophic factor signaling genes is a mechanism by which androgens convey their neuroprotection.

A complication of this interpretation comes from recent observations that AR signaling might not be restricted to direct genomic interaction and the subsequent regulation of transcription through binding of androgen response elements in the promoters of target genes (See Fig. 2). Indeed, it has been reported that the androgen antagonists flutamide and cyproterone acetate both exhibit agonist effects, including hippocampal neuroprotection, in an AR-dependent manner [105]. These antagonists have been shown to block AR DNA binding and disrupt AR co-regulator associations, respectively, ultimately preventing the transcriptional effects of the AR [106]. This suggests that either these compounds are not true anti-androgens or, more likely, that signaling through the AR is not limited to influencing transcription. Indeed, the AR, like many hormone receptors [107], can rapidly signal through ERK/MAPK and the PI3K/Akt pathways without direct genomic interaction [89,108–110]. These interactions could promote cell survival, however, rapid signaling of the AR through these second messenger pathways has not been directly observed in motor neurons. In addition, Gatson and colleagues [111] recently described the discovery of a novel membrane-associated androgen receptor action in a glial cell model. This membrane-associated receptor, triggered by a cell-impermeable BSA-conjugated DHT, was shown to have the opposite effect upon MAPK and Akt signaling pathways that had been elicited by non-BSA-conjugated DHT treatment. This group then further characterized their system in primary astrocyte cultures, and demonstrated that signaling through this potentially novel androgen pathway actually promotes astrocyte cell death [112]. These data indicate that despite years of research, there may be numerous aspects of AR signaling that are not fully understood.

Summary

Motor neurons are acutely dependent upon trophic factor support, as a variety of MND have responded very positively to trophic factor intervention. However, as most of these molecules are peptide hormones, there is the intrinsic problem of delivery across the blood-brain-barrier to the CNS. Many delivery paradigms have been employed with varying success – from systemic administration and use of motor neuron retrograde transport mechanisms, to viral and cellular delivery of specific trophic factors [113,114]. The cumulative data presented here suggest that these trophic signaling pathways might be prone to manipulation in other ways, including via signaling through the AR. Further supporting the involvement of AR in MND is evidence that AR signaling is perturbed not only in SBMA, but also in ALS. The incidence of ALS is strongly sexually dimorphic, with male predominance [115], and recently, Militello and colleagues [116] documented decreased serum levels of free testosterone in ALS patients. Completing the picture of how normal AR signaling promotes motor neuron health may be informative not only for SBMA, but also for other MND, including especially ALS.

The trophic effects of androgen signaling have been enumerated, but many questions still remain. One question is whether the beneficial effects of AR signaling in motor neurons occur by androgen acting directly upon the AR in the motor neurons themselves, or whether AR signaling in supporting cells, such as glia or muscle, might be promoting motor neuron health. As IGF-1 is produced by glial cells and muscle fibers, and IGF-1 expression is responsive to AR signaling, it is tempting to speculate that muscle production of IGF-1 drives AR-dependent trophic actions in a paracrine fashion to support motor neurons. There may also be a set of trophic autocrine signaling loops that are stimulated by AR activation. Future studies should test the ability of other steroid hormones to promote the protection of motor neurons. Finally, the relative contributions of the genomic and novel non-genomic signaling mechanisms of the AR on the neuroprotective functions of androgens on motor neurons needs to be resolved. Ultimately, there is a very compelling case that androgen signaling is protective in motor neurons. An understanding of AR biology in motor neurons will likely be required to fully appreciate the etiology of SBMA and other MND, and thereby devise effective treatments for these devastating disorders.

References

[1] Mooradian AD, Morley JE, Korenman SG. Biological actions of androgens. Endocr Rev 1987;8:1–28.

[2] Gelmann EP. Molecular biology of the androgen receptor. J Clin Oncol 2002;20:3001–15.

[3] Gottlieb B, Beitel LK, Wu JH, et al. The androgen receptor gene mutations database (ARDB): 2004 update. Hum Mutat 2004;23:527–33.

[4] Kennedy WR, Alter M, Sung JH. Progressive proximal spinal and bulbar muscular atrophy of late onset. A sex-linked recessive trait. Neurology 1968;18(7):671–80.

[5] Li M, Miwa S, Kobayashi Y, et al. Nuclear inclusions of the androgen receptor protein in spinal and bulbar muscular atrophy. Ann Neurol 1998;44:249–54.

[6] Kihira T, Yoshida S, Yoshimasu F, et al. Involvement of Onuf's nucleus in amyotrophic lateral sclerosis. J Neurol Sci 1997;147(1):81–8.

[7] Schroder HD, Reske-Nielsen E. Preservation of the nucleus X-pelvic floor motosystem in amyotrophic lateral sclerosis. Clin Neuropathol 1984;3(5):210–6.

[8] Olney RK, Aminoff MJ, So YT. Clinical and electrodiagnostic features of X-linked recessive bulbospinal neuronopathy. Neurology 1991;41:823–8.

[9] Barkhaus PE, Kennedy WR, Stern LZ, et al. Hereditary proximal spinal and bulbar motor neuron disease of late onset. A report of six cases. Arch Neurol 1982;39:112–6.

[10] Dejager S, Bry-Gauillard H, Bruckert E, et al. A comprehensive endocrine description of Kennedy's disease revealing androgen insensitivity linked to CAG repeat length. J Clin Endocrinol Metab 2002;87:3893–901.

[11] Arbizu T, Santamaría J, Gomez JM, et al. A family with adult spinal and bulbar muscular atrophy, X-linked inheritance and associated testicular failure. J Neurol Sci 1983;59:371–82.

[12] Fischbeck KH, Ionasescu V, Ritter AW, et al. Localization of the gene for X-linked spinal muscular atrophy. Neurology 1986;36:1595–8.

[13] La Spada AR, Wilson EM, Lubahn DB, et al. Androgen receptor gene mutations in X-linked spinal and bulbar muscular atrophy. Nature 1991;352:77–9.

[14] Zoghbi HY, Orr HT. Glutamine repeats and neurodegeneration. Annu Rev Neurosci 2000;23:217–47.

[15] Ordway JM, Tallaksen-Greene S, Gutekunst CA, et al. Ectopically expressed CAG repeats cause intranuclear inclusions and a progressive late onset neurological phenotype in the mouse. Cell 1997;91:753–63.

[16] Paulson HL, Bonini NM, Roth KA. Polyglutamine disease and neuronal cell death. Proc Natl Acad Sci USA 2000;97:12957–8.

[17] Schmidt BJ, Greenberg CR, Allingham-Hawkins DJ, et al. Expression of X-linked bulbospinal muscular atrophy (Kennedy disease) in two homozygous women. Neurology 2002;59:770–2.

[18] Thomas PS, Fraley GS, Damian V, et al. Loss of endogenous androgen receptor protein accelerates motor neuron degeneration and accentuates androgen insensitivity in a mouse model of X-linked spinal and bulbar muscular atrophy. Hum Mol Genet 2006;15:2225–38.

[19] Dragatsis I, Levine MS, Zeitlin S. Inactivation of Hdh in the brain and testis results in progressive neurodegeneration and sterility in mice. Nat Genet 2000;26:300–6.

[20] Leavitt BR, Guttman JA, Hodgson JG, et al. Wild-type huntingtin reduces the cellular toxicity of mutant huntingtin in vivo. Am J Hum Genet 2001;68:313–24.
[21] Rigamonti D, Bauer JH, De-Fraja C, et al. Wild-type huntingtin protects from apoptosis upstream of caspase-3. J Neurosci 2000;20:3705–13.
[22] Leavitt BR, van Raamsdonk JM, Shehadeh J, et al. Wild-type huntingtin protects neurons from excitotoxicity. J Neurochem 2006;96:1121–9.
[23] Gauthier LR, Charrin BC, Borrell-Pagès M, et al. Huntingtin controls neurotrophic support and survival of neurons by enhancing BDNF vesicular transport along microtubules. Cell 2004;118:127–38.
[24] Palhan VB, Chen S, Peng GH, et al. Polyglutamine-expanded ataxin-7 inhibits STAGA histone acetyltransferase activity to produce retinal degeneration. Proc Natl Acad Sci U S A 2005;102:8472–7.
[25] Donaldson KM, Li W, Ching KA, et al. Ubiquitin-mediated sequestration of normal cellular proteins into polyglutamine aggregates. Proc Natl Acad Sci USA 2003;100:8892–7.
[26] Lieberman AP, Harmison G, Strand AD, et al. Altered transcriptional regulation in cells expressing the expanded polyglutamine androgen receptor. Hum Mol Genet 2002;11:1967–76.
[27] Sendtner M, Holtmann B, Hughes RA. The response of motoneurons to neurotrophins. Neurochem Res 1996;21:831–41.
[28] Thoenen H, Hughes RA, Sendtner M. Trophic support of motoneurons: physiological, pathophysiological, and therapeutic implications. Exp Neurol 1993;124:47–55.
[29] Kilpatrick TJ, Soilu-Hänninen M. Molecular mechanisms regulating motor neuron development and degeneration. Mol Neurobiol 1999;19:205–28.
[30] Henderson CE, Phillips HS, Pollock RA, et al. GDNF: a potent survival factor for motoneurons present in peripheral nerve and muscle. Science 1994;266:1062–4.
[31] Zhao Z, Alam S, Oppenheim RW, et al. Overexpression of glial cell line-derived neurotrophic factor in the CNS rescues motoneurons from programmed cell death and promotes their long-term survival following axotomy. Exp Neurol 2004;190:356–72.
[32] Yan Q, Matheson C, Lopez OT. In vivo neurotrophic effects of GDNF on neonatal and adult facial motor neurons. Nature 1995;373:341–4.
[33] Yamamoto M, Mitsuma N, Inukai A, et al. Expression of GDNF and GDNFR-alpha mRNAs in muscles of patients with motor neuron diseases. Neurochem Res 1999;24(6):785–90.
[34] Henderson CE, Camu W, Mettling C, et al. Neurotrophins promote motor neuron survival and are present in embryonic limb bud. Nature 1993;363:266–70.
[35] DiStefano PS, Friedman B, Radziejewski C, et al. The neurotrophins BDNF, NT-3, and NGF display distinct patterns of retrograde axonal transport in peripheral and central neurons. Neuron 1992;8:983–93.
[36] Giménez y Ribotta M, Revah F, Pradier L, et al. Prevention of motoneuron death by adenovirus-mediated neurotrophic factors. J Neurosci Res 1997;48:281–5.
[37] Yan Q, Elliott J, Snider WD. Brain-derived neurotrophic factor rescues spinal motor neurons from axotomy-induced cell death. Nature 1992;360:753–5.
[38] Koliatsos VE, Clatterbuck RE, Winslow JW, et al. Evidence that brain-derived neurotrophic factor is a trophic factor for motor neurons in vivo. Neuron 1993;10:359–67.
[39] Estévez AG, Spear N, Manuel SM, et al. Nitric oxide and superoxide contribute to motor neuron apoptosis induced by trophic factor deprivation. J Neurosci 1998;18:923–31.
[40] Lindholm D, Dechant G, Heisenberg CP, et al. Brain-derived neurotrophic factor is a survival factor for cultured rat cerebellar granule neurons and protects them against glutamate-induced neurotoxicity. Eur J Neurosci 1993;5:1455–64.
[41] Shimohama S, Tamura Y, Akaike A, et al. Brain-derived neurotrophic factor pretreatment exerts a partially protective effect against glutamate-induced neurotoxicity in cultured rat cortical neurons. Neurosci Lett 1993;164:55–8.

[42] Ochs G, Penn RD, York M, et al. A phase I/II trial of recombinant methionyl human brain derived neurotrophic factor administered by intrathecal infusion to patients with amyotrophic lateral sclerosis. Amyotroph Lateral Scler Other Motor Neuron Disord 2000;1:201–6.
[43] Ikeda K, Klinkosz B, Greene T, et al. Effects of brain-derived neurotrophic factor on motor dysfunction in wobbler mouse motor neuron disease. Ann Neurol 1995;37:505–11.
[44] Negro A, Tolosano E, Skaper SD, et al. Cloning and expression of human ciliary neurotrophic factor. Eur J Biochem 1991;201:289–94.
[45] Sendtner M, Arakawa Y, Stöckli KA, et al. Effect of ciliary neurotrophic factor (CNTF) on motoneuron survival. J Cell Sci Suppl 1991;15:103–9.
[46] Clatterbuck RE, Price DL, Koliatsos VE. Further characterization of the effects of brain-derived neurotrophic factor and ciliary neurotrophic factor on axotomized neonatal and adult mammalian motor neurons. J Comp Neurol 1994;342:45–56.
[47] Tan SA, Déglon N, Zurn AD, et al. Rescue of motoneurons from axotomy-induced cell death by polymer encapsulated cells genetically engineered to release CNTF. Cell Transplant 1996;5:577–87.
[48] Gatzinsky KP, Holtmann B, Daraie B, et al. Early onset of degenerative changes at nodes of Ranvier in alpha-motor axons of Cntf null (-/-) mutant mice. Glia 2003;42:340–9.
[49] DeChiara TM, Vejsada R, Poueymirou WT, et al. Mice lacking the CNTF receptor, unlike mice lacking CNTF, exhibit profound motor neuron deficits at birth. Cell 1995;83:313–22.
[50] Azzouz M, Ralph GS, Storkebaum E, et al. VEGF delivery with retrogradely transported lentivector prolongs survival in a mouse ALS model. Nature 2004;429:413–7.
[51] Storkebaum E, Lambrechts D, Carmeliet P. VEGF: once regarded as a specific angiogenic factor, now implicated in neuroprotection. Bioessays 2004;26:943–54.
[52] Storkebaum E, Lambrechts D, Dewerchin M, et al. Treatment of motoneuron degeneration by intracerebroventricular delivery of VEGF in a rat model of ALS. Nat Neurosci 2005;8: 85–92.
[53] Van Den Bosch L, Storkebaum E, Vleminckx V, et al. Effects of vascular endothelial growth factor (VEGF) on motor neuron degeneration. Neurobiol Dis 2004;17:21–8.
[54] Hobson MI, Green CJ, Terenghi G. VEGF enhances intraneural angiogenesis and improves nerve regeneration after axotomy. J Anat 2000;197(Pt 4):591–605.
[55] Devos D, Moreau C, Lassalle P, et al. Low levels of the vascular endothelial growth factor in CSF from early ALS patients. Neurology 2004;62:2127–9.
[56] Sopher BL, Thomas PS, LaFevre-Bernt MA, et al. Androgen receptor YAC transgenic mice recapitulate SBMA motor neuronopathy and implicate VEGF164 in the motor neuron degeneration. Neuron 2004;41:687–99.
[57] Oosthuyse B, Moons L, Storkebaum E, et al. Deletion of the hypoxia-response element in the vascular endothelial growth factor promoter causes motor neuron degeneration. Nat Genet 2001;28:131–8.
[58] Terry PD, Kamel F, Umbach DM, et al. VEGF promoter haplotype and amyotrophic lateral sclerosis (ALS). J Neurogenet 2004;18(2):429–34.
[59] Zheng C, Nennesmo I, Fadeel B, et al. Vascular endothelial growth factor prolongs survival in a transgenic mouse model of ALS. Ann Neurol 2004;56(4):564–7.
[60] Wilkins A, Chandran S, Compston A. A role for oligodendrocyte-derived IGF-1 in trophic support of cortical neurons. Glia 2001;36:48–57.
[61] Hansson HA, Dahlin LB, Danielsen N, et al. Evidence indicating trophic importance of IGF-I in regenerating peripheral nerves. Acta Physiol Scand 1986;126:609–14.
[62] Dobrowolny G, Giacinti C, Pelosi L, et al. Muscle expression of a local Igf-1 isoform protects motor neurons in an ALS mouse model. J Cell Biol 2005;168:193–9.
[63] Ang LC, Bhaumick B, Munoz DG, et al. Effects of astrocytes, insulin and insulin-like growth factor I on the survival of motoneurons in vitro. J Neurol Sci 1992;109:168–72.
[64] Hughes RA, Sendtner M, Thoenen H. Members of several gene families influence survival of rat motoneurons in vitro and in vivo. J Neurosci Res 1993;36:663–71.

[65] Caroni P, Grandes P. Nerve sprouting in innervated adult skeletal muscle induced by exposure to elevated levels of insulin-like growth factors. J Cell Biol 1990;110:1307–17.
[66] Payne AM, Zheng Z, Messi ML, et al. Motor neurone targeting of IGF-1 prevents specific force decline in ageing mouse muscle. J Physiol 2006;570:283–94.
[67] Kaspar BK, Lladó J, Sherkat N, et al. Retrograde viral delivery of IGF-1 prolongs survival in a mouse ALS model. Science 2003;301:839–42.
[68] Gorio A, Lesma E, Madaschi L, et al. Co-administration of IGF-I and glycosaminoglycans greatly delays motor neurone disease and affects IGF-I expression in the wobbler mouse: a long-term study. J Neurochem 2002;81:194–202.
[69] Bilak MM, Corse AM, Kuncl RW. Additivity and potentiation of IGF-I and GDNF in the complete rescue of postnatal motor neurons. Amyotroph Lateral Scler Other Motor Neuron Disord 2001;2:83–91.
[70] Palazzolo I, Burnett BG, Young JE, et al. Akt blocks ligand binding and protects against expanded polyglutamine androgen receptor toxicity. Hum Mol Genet 2007;16:1593–603.
[71] Leav I, Lau KM, Adams JY, et al. Comparative studies of the estrogen receptors beta and alpha and the androgen receptor in normal human prostate glands, dysplasia, and in primary and metastatic carcinoma. Am J Pathol 2001;159(1):79–92.
[72] Waltregny D, Leav I, Signoretti S, et al. Androgen-driven prostate epithelial cell proliferation and differentiation in vivo involve the regulation of p27. Mol Endocrinol 2001; 15(5):765–82.
[73] Kidwai N, Gong Y, Sun X, et al. Expression of androgen receptor and prostate-specific antigen in male breast carcinoma. Breast Cancer Res 2004;6(1):R18–23.
[74] Sordello S, Bertrand N, Plouët J. Vascular endothelial growth factor is up-regulated in vitro and in vivo by androgens. Biochem Biophys Res Commun 1998;251:287–90.
[75] Compagno D, Merle C, Morin A, et al. SIRNA-directed in vivo silencing of androgen receptor inhibits the growth of castration-resistant prostate carcinomas. PLoS ONE 2007;2:e1006.
[76] Sajjad Y, Quenby S, Nickson P, et al. Androgen receptors are expressed in a variety of human fetal extragenital tissues: an immunohistochemical study. Asian J Androl 2007;9:751–9.
[77] Sar M, Stumpf WE. Androgen concentration in motor neurons of cranial nerves and spinal cord. Science 1977;197:77–9.
[78] Brooks BP, Merry DE, Paulson HL, et al. A cell culture model for androgen effects in motor neurons. J Neurochem 1998;70:1054–60.
[79] Marron TU, Guerini V, Rusmini P, et al. Androgen-induced neurite outgrowth is mediated by neuritin in motor neurones. J Neurochem 2005;92:10–20.
[80] Yang LY, Verhovshek T, Sengelaub DR. Brain-derived neurotrophic factor and androgen interact in the maintenance of dendritic morphology in a sexually dimorphic rat spinal nucleus. Endocrinology 2004;145:161–8.
[81] Ottem EN, Beck LA, Jordan CL, et al. Androgen-dependent regulation of brain-derived neurotrophic factor and tyrosine kinase B in the sexually dimorphic spinal nucleus of the bulbocavernosus. Endocrinology 2007;148(8):3655–65.
[82] Varela CR, Bengston L, Xu J, et al. Additive effects of ciliary neurotrophic factor and testosterone on motoneuron survival; differential effects on motoneuron size and muscle morphology. Exp Neurol 2000;165:384–93.
[83] Chisu V, Manca P, Lepore G, et al. Testosterone induces neuroprotection from oxidative stress. Effects on catalase activity and 3-nitro-L-tyrosine incorporation into alpha-tubulin in a mouse neuroblastoma cell line. Arch Ital Biol 2006;144:63–73.
[84] Ahlbom E, Prins GS, Ceccatelli S. Testosterone protects cerebellar granule cells from oxidative stress-induced cell death through a receptor mediated mechanism. Brain Res 2001;892:255–62.
[85] Tunez I, Feijoo M, Collado JA, et al. Effect of testosterone on oxidative stress and cell damage induced by 3-nitropropionic acid in striatum of ovariectomized rats. Life Sci 2007;80(13):1221–7.

[86] Ramsden M, Shin TM, Pike CJ. Androgens modulate neuronal vulnerability to kainate lesion. Neuroscience 2003;122:573–8.
[87] Magrané J, Smith RC, Walsh K, et al. Heat shock protein 70 participates in the neuroprotective response to intracellularly expressed beta-amyloid in neurons. J Neurosci 2004;24: 1700–6.
[88] Zhang Y, Champagne N, Beitel LK, et al. Estrogen and androgen protection of human neurons against intracellular amyloid beta1-42 toxicity through heat shock protein 70. J Neurosci 2004;24:5315–21.
[89] Nguyen TV, Yao M, Pike CJ. Androgens activate mitogen-activated protein kinase signaling: role in neuroprotection. J Neurochem 2005;94:1639–51.
[90] Hammond J, Le Q, Goodyer C, et al. Testosterone-mediated neuroprotection through the androgen receptor in human primary neurons. J Neurochem 2001;77:1319–26.
[91] Drengler SM, Handa RJ, Jones KJ. Effects of axotomy and testosterone on androgen receptor mRNA expression in hamster facial motoneurons. Exp Neurol 1997;146(2):374–9.
[92] Huppenbauer CB, Tanzer L, DonCarlos LL, et al. Gonadal steroid attenuation of developing hamster facial motoneuron loss by axotomy: equal efficacy of testosterone, dihydrotestosterone, and 17-beta estradiol. J Neurosci 2005;25(16):4004–13.
[93] Kujawa KA, Emeric E, Jones KJ. Testosterone differentially regulates the regenerative properties of injured hamster facial motoneurons. J Neurosci 1991;11(12):3898–906.
[94] Xu J, Gingras KM, Bengston L, et al. Blockade of endogenous neurotrophic factors prevents the androgenic rescue of rat spinal motoneurons. J Neurosci 2001;21:4366–72.
[95] Louissaint A, Rao S, Leventhal C, et al. Coordinated interaction of neurogenesis and angiogenesis in the adult songbird brain. Neuron 2002;34:945–60.
[96] Yu Z, Dadgar N, Albertelli M, et al. Androgen-dependent pathology demonstrates myopathic contribution to the Kennedy disease phenotype in a mouse knock-in model. J Clin Invest 2006;116:2663–72.
[97] Wu Y, Zhao W, Zhao J, et al. Identification of androgen response elements in the insulin-like growth factor I upstream promoter. Endocrinology 2007;148:2984–93.
[98] Pandini G, Mineo R, Frasca F, et al. Androgens up-regulate the insulin-like growth factor-I receptor in prostate cancer cells. Cancer Res 2005;65:1849–57.
[99] Fan W, Yanase T, Morinaga H, et al. Insulin-like growth factor 1/insulin signaling activates androgen signaling through direct interactions of Foxo1 with androgen receptor. J Biol Chem 2007;282:7329–38.
[100] Verras M, Sun Z. Beta-catenin is involved in insulin-like growth factor 1-mediated transactivation of the androgen receptor. Mol Endocrinol 2005;19:391–8.
[101] Xu J, Forger NG. Expression and androgen regulation of the ciliary neurotrophic factor receptor (CNTFRalpha) in muscles and spinal cord. J Neurobiol 1998;35:217–25.
[102] Forger NG, Wagner CK, Contois M, et al. Ciliary neurotrophic factor receptor alpha in spinal motoneurons is regulated by gonadal hormones. J Neurosci 1998;18:8720–9.
[103] Forger NG, Howell ML, Bengston L, et al. Sexual dimorphism in the spinal cord is absent in mice lacking the ciliary neurotrophic factor receptor. J Neurosci 1997;17:9605–12.
[104] Forger NG, Wong V, Breedlove SM. Ciliary neurotrophic factor arrests muscle and motoneuron degeneration in androgen-insensitive rats. J Neurobiol 1995;28:354–62.
[105] Nguyen TV, Yao M, Pike CJ. Flutamide and cyproterone acetate exert agonist effects: induction of androgen receptor-dependent neuroprotection. Endocrinology 2007;148: 2936–43.
[106] Berrevoets CA, Umar A, Brinkmann AO. Antiandrogens: selective androgen receptor modulators. Mol Cell Endocrinol 2002;198(1–2):97–103.
[107] Lösel R, Wehling M. Nongenomic actions of steroid hormones. Nat Rev Mol Cell Biol 2003;4:46–56.
[108] Kousteni S, Bellido T, Plotkin LI, et al. Nongenotropic, sex-nonspecific signaling through the estrogen or androgen receptors: dissociation from transcriptional activity. Cell 2001; 104:719–30.

[109] Michels G, Hoppe UC. Rapid actions of androgens. Front Neuroendocrinol 2007:10.1016/j.yfrne.2007.1008.1004. In press.

[110] Rahman F, Christian HC. Non-classical actions of testosterone: an update. Trends Endocrinol Metab 2007;18:371–8.

[111] Gatson JW, Kaur P, Singh M. Dihydrotestosterone differentially modulates the mitogen-activated protein kinase and the phosphoinositide 3-kinase/Akt pathways through the nuclear and novel membrane androgen receptor in C6 cells. Endocrinology 2006;147:2028–34.

[112] Gatson JW, Singh M. Activation of a membrane-associated androgen receptor promotes cell death in primary cortical astrocytes. Endocrinology 2007;148:2458–64.

[113] Federici T, Boulis NM. Gene-based treatment of motor neuron diseases. Muscle Nerve 2006;33(3):302–23.

[114] Nayak MS, Kim YS, Goldman M, et al. Cellular therapies in motor neuron diseases. Biochim Biophys Acta 2006;1762(11–12):1128–38.

[115] Beghi E, Logroscino G, Chiò A, et al. The epidemiology of ALS and the role of population-based registries. Biochim Biophys Acta 2006;1762:1150–7.

[116] Militello A, Vitello G, Lunetta C, et al. The serum level of free testosterone is reduced in amyotrophic lateral sclerosis. J Neurol Sci 2002;195:67–70.

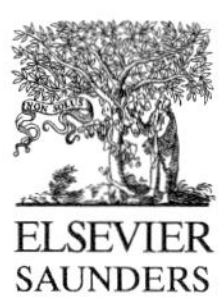

ELSEVIER
SAUNDERS

Phys Med Rehabil Clin N Am
19 (2008) 495–508

PHYSICAL MEDICINE AND REHABILITATION CLINICS OF NORTH AMERICA

Designing Clinical Trials in Amyotrophic Lateral Sclerosis

Jeremy M. Shefner, MD, PhD

Department of Neurology, State University of New York Upstate Medical University, 750 East Adams Street, Syracuse, NY 13210, USA

In recent years, much has been learned about pathogenic mechanisms of amyotrophic lateral sclerosis (ALS), leading to a proliferation of new targets for disease modification. Mitochondrial dysfunction, glutamate toxicity, protein misfolding, and microglial activation are just a few mechanisms that have been proposed. For each proposed mechanism, pharmacologic manipulation is possible. Targeted drug discovery programs can lead to new compounds, and re-evaluation of existing drugs may lead to recognition of properties not previously investigated. Recently, a collaborative effort jointly funded by the National Institute of Neurological Disorders and Stroke and the ALS Association tested more than 1,000 available compounds in 29 different assays to determine activity against a variety of different aspects of neurodegeneration [1]. Although the full results of this effort have not yet been published, individual laboratories have further investigated drugs identified by this screening program, with the first of these (ceftriaxone) entering clinical trials in 2006. At this writing, there are at least nine different compounds, either in human trials or about to be tested in human beings. All of these compounds target different aspects of the neurodegenerative process.

Given the plethora of potential therapeutic agents for a rare disease such as ALS, it is crucial that studies are performed in an efficient and effective manner. A well-designed trial can speed time to approval of a drug and identify efficacy, with the minimum number of patients exposed for the shortest possible time. In contrast, a poorly designed trial can fail to show an effect of an effective drug, can mistakenly suggest efficacy when there is no effect, can lead to patient distress and harm, or may simply delay time to approval. This article discusses a range of issues that relate to clinical trials. These include the choice of dose to be studied, the way in which disease progression is assessed, and the formal structure of the trial.

E-mail address: shefnerj@upstate.edu

1047-9651/08/$ - see front matter
doi:10.1016/j.pmr.2008.02.002 *pmr.theclinics.com*

Drug dose

Of all the issues surrounding the clinical investigation of an experimental therapeutic agent, dose would seem to be one of the least problematic. In fact, however, decisions about dose are not simple, and poor dose choices have lead to problems in many previously published ALS trials. Dose finding studies should start at the bench; in preclinical assays, drug activity should be assessed from a no-effect level to a point at which the drug causes clear toxicity. While drug concentrations achieved in vitro do not directly correlate to dose in either in vivo disease models or human trials, they do provide target tissue concentrations to which initial dosing studies should be aimed. Animal models should be used to establish maximum tolerated dose (MTD); disease related activity must be assessed in models that match the disease itself to the greatest extent possible. In ALS, the most commonly used model is the superoxide dismutase (SOD)1 transgenic mouse [2]. However, other models have been employed, including the progressive motor neuronopathy mouse [3], models of nerve injury such as facial axotomy [4,5], and viral diseases that result in motor neuron loss [6].

For many agents that have reached human trials, full dose exploration has not been performed on animal models. Full dose ranging was not performed using topiramate in the SOD1 mouse model [7], nor were celecoxib, creatine, or ceftriaxone studied at multiple doses [8–10]. In some cases, failure to find efficacy may have been the result of incorrect dose choice, while in other cases, efficacy was demonstrated but the most effective dose may not have been found. Failure to study a full range of doses at this level of investigation has lead to trials that may have reached erroneous conclusions.

Assuming MTD has been established in experimental models, as well as a range of doses that show activity against the target disease mechanism, dose ranges in the initial studies on human beings can be appropriately chosen. In ALS, this step has been problematic. For a number of compounds that have been previously studied in efficacy trials, the MTD has not been established. Thus, negative results have been reported for creatine and celecoxib [11–13], but the lack of a known MTD leads to the question of whether higher doses of either creatine or celecoxib could have demonstrated efficacy. In other studies, attempts were made to study compounds at doses close to MTD, but lower doses were not studied as well. This may have contributed to the fact that patients treated with topiramate at 800 mg per day progressed faster than placebo patients, and may also account for similar results in the recently reported minocycline trial [14–16].

Stages of drug development

The choice of trial design depends on the stage of development of a given drug. Phase I trials are performed to determine the appropriate dose range and dosing schedule, how the drug is metabolized or excreted, and to identify any acute or high frequency adverse events. Usually, phase I trials are performed on healthy volunteers. However, if there is reason to believe that specific aspects of a disease may have an impact on tolerability of a drug, phase I studies may also be performed on patients with disease. This is often the case in ALS; for example, a drug that causes moderate dizziness in normal subjects may result in frequent and serious falls in ALS patients. Usually, phase I studies are small and involve administration of the drug for only a short time period. Thus, low frequency events or effects of chronic administration are not measured. An important goal of phase I studies is to identify a dose above which adverse events preclude use, not to pick up events that will occur in a minority of patients.

Phase II trials are performed with the goal of gathering further safety information, especially related to long-term use of the drug. Pharmacokinetic evaluation of drug accumulation with long-term use is also commonly performed, and different schedules of drug dosing may be evaluated. Although not always the primary goal, some assessment of potential efficacy is often incorporated into phase II trials. In diseases associated with markers of activity (for example, CD4 counts or viral load in HIV), the effect of differing doses on these markers can be used to determine the dose choices for a phase III trial. In ALS, no such markers have been identified, so that attempts to gauge efficacy must be based on the outcomes typically employed in larger phase III trials. For this reason, the line between phase II and phase III trials is often blurred in ALS.

Decisions about dose are often made after phase II trials, so it is essential that multiple doses be evaluated. This has often not been done in phase II ALS trials, and when dose ranging is done, it is often inadequate. In a recently reported trial of pentoxyphylline in ALS, subjects were treated either with 1.2-g of pentoxyphylline or placebo. The trial showed increased mortality in the treated group. However, without any other tested doses, it is unknown whether a lower dose might have resulted in improved mortality. Similarly, topiramate was tested in a phase II study at a dose of 800 mg per day. Although there was no statistically significant effect on mortality, treated subjects lost an average of 10 lb more weight than placebo treated subjects and performed more poorly on functional and respiratory measurements [14]. From assessment of adverse events, it was clear that at this dose, topiramate was quite difficult to tolerate, and the results reported could easily have been a function of each subject's weight loss and other events. The lack of a lower dose group precludes any conclusion about the true efficacy of topiramate. The most recent example of the same difficulty is the recently reported trial of minocycline in ALS [15,16]. In both the phase I and II studies and the phase IIB study, more adverse events and poorer performance on outcome measures were noted in the treated group. Minocycline was intended to modulate a novel disease mechanism not previously tested in ALS; the fact that too high a dose may have been chosen means that it remains unclear whether this target is appropriate for further study.

Phase III trials are performed to determine the efficacy of a drug in treating the disease in question. Longer-term safety data are also gathered. In many diseases, phase III trials are expected to be positive, as they only are performed after clear evidence of efficacy is gathered from disease markers in phase II studies. This is obviously not the case in ALS research, as more than 10 years have elapsed and at least a dozen negative trials have been reported since efficacy of riluzole was reported in two phase III trials [17,18]. Depending on the preceding phase II studies, phase III trials may or may not involve multiple dose groups; however, negative studies that study only one dose level may not adequately test the hypothesis that the drug tested is effective in treating ALS.

Choice of outcome measures

As previously mentioned, no tissue based biomarkers currently exist to determine drug activity in ALS. Thus, clinical assessment of efficacy is based on measurement of a variety of aspects of disease. The gold standard outcome for ALS trials currently remains survival. Survival is obviously clinically meaningful and straightforward to measure. However, there are several reasons why other measures are being sought and why many current trials use outcomes other than survival. First, survival can be manipulated by many interventions that do not clearly alter the progression of underlying disease. Good nutrition and early use of percutaneous endoscopic gastrostomy clearly prolongs life [19–21]. Respiratory support with noninvasive positive pressure ventilation has been less well studied, but likely also prolongs life [22–25]. Beyond these clearly defined interventions, there is emerging evidence that patients cared for at multidisciplinary ALS clinics have prolonged survival as compared with community based controls [26–28]. As these interventions may not be applied uniformly across all sites in a clinical trial, conclusions based on survival may be confounded by these variables. Many trials stratify along certain treatment variables, but stratification can reduce the power of a trial to find a significant drug benefit.

In addition to the issues raised above, the use of survival as an endpoint mandates large trials that treat patients for long time periods. Unless patients are chosen late in the disease course, survival at 1 year ranges from 82% to 91% in recent studies [11,14]. Thus, very few patients will experience the event being measured. To show an 80% chance of seeing a 25% difference in mortality rate requires approximately 600 patients studied over 18 months (Schoenfeld, 2007, personal communication). This sample size is consistent with what was required to demonstrate efficacy of riluzole [18]. In the current environment, with many drugs to test in a limited population with a limited budget, other outcome measures that may demonstrate efficacy with smaller sample sizes are obviously desirable. Several of the measures currently in use are reviewed below. Table 1 summarizes the changes in these measures over time from several recently reported clinical trials.

Table 1
Rate of change of commonly used outcome measures in ALS

Measure	Mean change per month	Studies surveyed
ALS functional rating scale	0.77–1.07	[11,14,72,75]
%Forced vital capacity	1.04–2.46	[11,14,72,75]
Manual muscle testing	1.18	[75]
Maximum voluntary isometric contraction	0.075–0.99	[11,14]
Motor unit number estimation	2.20–2.35	[64,76]

Muscle strength

Muscle strength is a clinically relevant measure of disease progression in ALS. There are a variety of methods available to measure muscle strength. Both quantitative (maximum voluntary isometric contraction, or MVIC) and qualitative (Medical Research Council or MRC muscle grading) measures have been employed in past trials. Previous studies using MVIC employed an apparatus initially designed by Munsat and colleagues [29] that required many position changes on the part of the patient, was quite fatiguing, and took about 45 minutes to perform. More recently, hand held dynamometry (HHD) has been employed; with careful evaluator training, HHD can evaluate many muscles in a short period of time.

MVIC has proven useful as an outcome measure in natural history studies and clinical trials in ALS, and is a valid and reliable measure of disease progression [14,29–34]. Rather than evaluating individual muscle strength changes, strength for each muscle is normalized and averaged with other muscles of the same limb. This allows for the averaging of strength of small and large muscle groups, reduced variability, and greater linearity [29].

Intra- and inter-rater reliability of MVIC have been assessed in a number of clinical trials in ALS. With rigorous training of clinical evaluators, coefficient of variation between and within evaluators is less than 15% [29,35]. At least seven trials have used MVIC as the primary outcome measure. Rate of decline in MVIC was assessed slightly differently from trial to trial. However, the rate of change in MVIC was consistent in the placebo groups from these studies [14,32,33,36]. Data from the placebo treatment arms of two recent clinical trials with topiramate and creatine demonstrate that the rate of decline in MVIC is essentially linear, with only a small nonlinear component [14].

The above data were acquired using the original apparatus described by Munsat. More recent trials are employing HHD and studying a larger number of muscle groups. HHD has been directly validated against MVIC in ALS patients, and shown to change at a similar rate, with variability that is only slightly greater than MVIC [37]. For both upper and lower extremity muscles, correlations between MVIC and HHD measurements ranged between 0.84 and 0.92, with test retest variability that was extremely similar as well. The only strength level where correlation between HHD and

MVIC did not correlate well was when very strong muscles were assessed; while problematic in testing normal subjects, this is not likely to be a problem in an ALS clinical trial.

Manual muscle testing using the MRC grading scale has also been used in a number of ALS clinical trials. It involves measurement of muscle strength by a trained evaluator using standardized patient positioning. It was recently demonstrated that if enough muscles are tested, a decline in average grade can be determined early in the disease, and the variability of measurement approximates that of MVIC [38]. The advantages to manual muscle testing are speed, expense, and the lack of specialized equipment [39,40]. However, MRC grading is by nature nonlinear; the difference in isometric strength between grade 1 to grade 3 is a small fraction of the difference between grades 3 and 5. Grade 4 spans the bulk of the isometric range, so that large changes in strength are not reflected in changes in muscle grade. Thus, MRC strength grading has lower face validity than MVIC.

Pulmonary function

Respiratory failure is the primary cause of death in ALS, so its assessment has obvious clinical relevance. Vital capacity and maximal inspiratory and expiratory mouth pressures are the methods most commonly used. These measures are widely available, noninvasive, and portable. However, patients with significant bulbar involvement show great variability of measurement and require maximal respiratory muscle activation [41]. Bulbar or facial weakness can prevent the formation of a tight lip-seal around a mouthpiece so that a facemask or other seal must be used. Vocal cord spasms and excessive saliva and gagging can also interfere with study performance.

The forced vital capacity (FVC) measures volume of air forcefully expired in one breath. Usually, the FVC is reported as a percentage of a predicted vital capacity based on the subject's height, gender, and age. The FVC declines with time in patients with ALS and is a sensitive measure of disease progression. Both the baseline FVC and the rate of decline in FVC are predictive of survival [42–44].

Functional rating scales

Clinical rating scales that assess the activities of daily living are useful in both natural history studies of ALS and in clinical trials of experimental agents. Early examples are the Norris scale and the ALS severity scale, and the Appel ALS rating Scale. However, the scale that has achieved widest acceptance is the ALS functional rating scale (ALSFRS-R) [45]. The ALSFRS-R is now employed as a primary outcome measure in most ALS trials that do not employ survival as the primary endpoint.

The ALSFRS-R is a quickly administered ordinal rating scale used to determine a patient's assessment of their capability and independence in

12 functional activities. It assesses bulbar and respiratory functions, upper extremity functions (cutting food and dressing), lower extremity functions (walking and climbing), dressing hygiene, and ability to turn in bed. The instrument can be easily administered, and the patient's response is recorded to the closest approximation from a list of five choices. Each choice is scored from 0 to 4. The total score can range from 48 (normal function) to 0 (unable to attempt the task).

Initial validity was established by documenting that in ALS patients change in ALSFRS scores correlated with change in strength over time, as measured by MVIC, [36], and was closely associated with quality of life measures, and predicted survival [44–47]. With appropriate training, the ALSFRS can be administered with high inter-rater reliability and test-retest reliability. The test-retest reliability is greater than 0.88 for all test items.

The ALSFRS-R can be administered by phone, again with good inter-rater and test-retest reliability [48], thus obviating the need for some in-person visits for disease assessment. In addition, the ALSFRS-R can be administered to the patient directly when the patient is verbal, but as communication becomes more difficult, caregivers provide increasing assistance in providing responses. The equivalency of caregiver and patient responses has also not been established.

The ALSFRS was revised in 1999 to add assessments of respiratory dysfunction, including dyspnea, orthopnea, and the need for ventilatory support [46]. The revised ALSFRS (ALSFRS-R) was demonstrated to retain the properties of the original scale and show strong internal consistency and construct validity.

Motor unit number estimation

Although routine, nerve conduction studies and needle electromyography are essential for confirming lower motor neuron involvement in the initial diagnosis of motor neuron disease. However, they do not permit accurate measurement of motor neuron loss and compensatory reinnervation [49,50]. Motor unit number estimation (MUNE) quantifies the number of surviving motor units in the living human subject [51–56] and has emerged as an important potential marker in ALS [57–62] and other motor neuron disorders.

All techniques for counting motor units rely on the same basic premise. A maximum muscle response is generated to an electrical stimulus. Most often, the response measured is electrical, but force measurements have also been used. Then, the response amplitude of a single motor unit is estimated. Once a single motor unit amplitude estimate is made, this value is divided into the maximum response to yield a number reflecting the number of units that made up the response.

MUNE has been employed in two multicenter ALS trials as a secondary outcome measure [63,64]. Good intra-rater reliability was demonstrated and a reliable decline in MUNE was demonstrated. However, the method employed was laborious, and required the use of a particular EMG machine. A well quantified, easily performed method has been developed, and is now being employed in two ongoing trials. Coefficient of variation is less than 10%, significantly lower than the value seen in other MUNE methods.

Trial design

Phase I clinical trial design is fairly standard and will not be discussed here. Similarly, the goals of a phase III trial require a structure that is rigidly defined. The goal is to demonstrated efficacy of the therapeutic agent under study. Issues related to trial size and duration are related to the outcome measure chosen as the primary endpoint. For survival, as previously noted, approximately 600 subjects in two groups must be followed for 18 months to have an 80% chance of detecting a true difference in survival rate of 20%. As an example, if the placebo group has a 75% survival rate at 18 months, a 20% improvement would be a survival rate of 80%. In terms of actual events, a 25% death rate in 300 subjects would mean that 75 subjects died; an improvement in survival of 20% would result in 60 subjects in the treatment group dying. This example points out the problems inherent in survival studies; out of 600 subjects studied for 18 months, the entire treatment effect is determined by survival of 15 more subjects in the treatment group than the placebo group.

If multiple doses are to be studied, the required sample size would increase accordingly, requiring approximately 900 subjects to be studied in three groups, and so on. Clearly, studies requiring this sample size are expensive and limit the number of agents that can be concurrently studied. For these reasons, the alternate endpoints of muscle strength and ALSFRS-R have been employed. Sample size calculations depend on the rate and variability of decline for these measures; for both strength and ALSFRS-R, power analyses show that 150 to 200 subjects per group must be studied for 9 to 12 months to have an 80% chance of seeing a 25% difference in the rate of decline of either measure. While this is a clear improvement over the size and duration mandated by survival studies, further sample size reduction could be realized by the identification of an outcome measure that fell more rapidly or had lower variability. Preliminary data suggest that MUNE might offer these advantages. A biomarker based on fluid samples (blood, cerebrospinal fluid, urine) that showed changes over time with low variability would also allow for shorter trials; the search for such a biomarker is vigorous and ongoing [65–68].

Significantly more discussion has occurred regarding design options for phase II trials. In phase II, the goal is not necessarily to produce conclusive evidence of efficacy, and a suggestion of drug activity may be sufficient for a sponsor or investigator to decide that further studies are warranted. One possible approach is to apply what is called a "futility design" [69,70].

Rather than stating that the goal of the study is to show evidence of efficacy, the purpose of a futility study is to determine whether it is worthwhile going forward. There are certain possible outcomes of a small study that would make further investigation unwise; for example, if all treated subjects did worse on all measures than all placebo subjects, it is unlikely that the drug will show efficacy if more subjects were studied. In other words, futility has been demonstrated. Futility designs require that the traditional null hypothesis used in statistical comparisons be changed; the null hypothesis in a futility study is that it is not futile to go forward. If the null hypothesis is rejected, futility is proved. Demonstration of nonfutility requires far fewer subjects than demonstration of efficacy; however, depending on the measure used, nonfutility may be demonstrated even when two comparison groups are identical.

Another approach is to use what has been called an "adaptive design" to make decisions regarding what drug or dose level to test further in a phase III study. This design may or may not involve a placebo group, but compares several groups that may either be given different doses of the same drug or different drugs over a defined time period. At the end of the study, the best performing group is declared the "winner," and further studies are then performed using that drug or dose and comparing it to placebo in a phase III study. The potential advantages of such a design are that many doses or drugs can be tested concurrently; however, there are several drawbacks. First, there will always be a winner, so that even if chance dictates the best performing group, going forward with further testing is required. Second, especially if multiple drugs are compared together, it is possible that in fact more than one active compound is among the agents tested. In that situation, only one drug will be chosen for further testing even though two or more are active and potentially important. An adaptive trial design is currently being employed in a phase II clinical trial of coenzyme Q in ALS [71].

Lead-in or crossover designs have also been suggested for phase II studies. Crossover studies have not been deemed appropriate, as ALS is a progressive disease with properties that are likely to vary over time. Thus, a therapeutic agent that is neuroprotective is likely to have a more beneficial effect if given early in the disease than late, so that the effects of therapy after a crossover may not be the same as the effect noted before the crossover.

Lead-in studies involve enrolling patients into a trial, then following them with assessment of outcome measures for a period of time before starting active treatment. If the outcome measure chosen changes in a linear fashion, one can estimate the rate of change before active treatment, and use that rate of change as a covariate in the efficacy analysis, potentially reducing the sample size required to detect a given effect. However, most outcomes in ALS trials do not decline in a strictly linear fashion, so that behavior before institution of active treatment does not well predict the behavior of that outcome measure later in the study. Lead in designs also require that

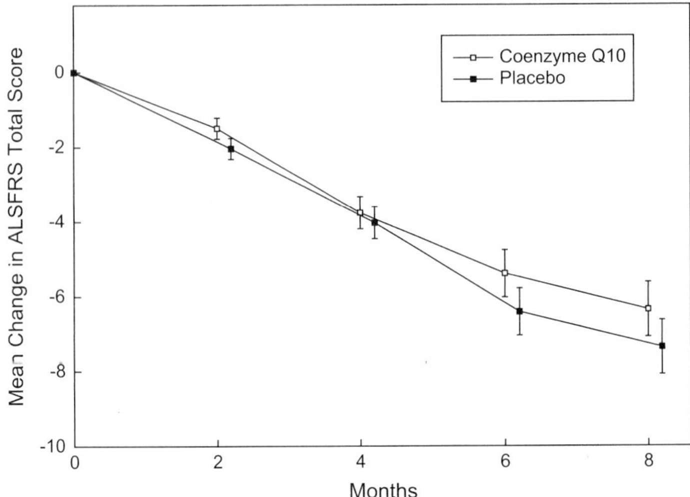

Fig. 1. Comparison of changes in ALSFRS-R of patients actively treated with coenzyme Q with historical controls taken from placebo group of a clinical trial of celecoxib in ALS. (*Data from* Cudkowicz ME, Shefner JM, Schoenfeld DA, et al. Trial of celecoxib in amyotrophic lateral sclerosis. Ann Neurol 2006;60:22; Ferrante KL, Shefner J, Zhang H, et al. Tolerance of high-dose (3,000 mg/day) coenzyme Q10 in ALS. Neurology 2005;65:1834.)

subjects receive treatment later than other designs, as all subjects have to be followed off treatment for a period of usually 3 to 6 months. Thus, if a drug is neuroprotective, administration later in the disease course may reduce the sensitivity of the study. A lead-in design was employed in a dose ranging study of TCH346; interestingly, all groups declined more rapidly during active treatment than during lead-in, even the placebo group [72].

Other options include the use of historical controls rather than a placebo group in phase II studies [73]. For this approach to be useful, the natural history of the rate of change of the outcome measure chosen must be well studied, and shown to not significantly change over time or from study to study. This requirement is clearly not met for survival studies, as the 1-year survival of ALS patients participating in studies from 1994 to 2007 has varied greatly [11,14,18]. However, both MVIC and ALSFRS-R have been quite stable over time. In particular, ALSFRS-R has been shown to decline between 0.9 and 1.0 points per month over a wide range of studies conducted over the past decade. In a phase II study of coenzyme Q, rates of decline in pulmonary function and ALSFRS-R closely matched that of a placebo group from a previous study (Fig. 1) [74].

Summary

Clinical trial design plays a crucial role in the development of new therapeutic agents. It is important to begin thinking about what an appropriate trial would look like far in advance of actual study initiation. Decisions regarding dose, outcomes to be measured, and duration of treatment all may have a critical impact on whether a new agent is found to be efficacious. Many of these decisions depend on adequate preclinical data; in their absence, trials may fail to show efficacy or even demonstrate harm to patients that could have been avoided.

References

[1] Heemskerk J. High throughput drug screening. Amyotroph Lateral Scler Other Motor Neuron Disord 2004;5(Suppl 1):19–21.
[2] Gurney ME, Pu H, Chiu AY, et al. Motor neuron degeneration in mice that express a human Cu,Zn superoxide dismutase mutation [see comments] [published erratum appears in Science 1995 Jul 14;269(5221):149]. Science 1994;264:1772–5.
[3] Pioro EP, Mitsumoto H. Animal models of ALS. Clin Neurosci 1995;3:375–85.
[4] Sendtner M, Gotz R, Holtmann B, et al. Endogenous ciliary neurotrophic factor is a lesion factor for axotomized motoneurons in adult mice. J Neurosci 1997;17:6999–7006.
[5] Sendtner M, Kreutzberg GW, Thoenen H. Ciliary neurotrophic factor prevents the degeneration of motor neurons after axotomy. Nature 1990;345:440–1.
[6] Deshpande DM, Kim YS, Martinez T, et al. Recovery from paralysis in adult rats using embryonic stem cells. Ann Neurol 2006;60:32–44.
[7] Maragakis NJ, Jackson M, Ganel R, et al. Topiramate protects against motor neuron degeneration in organotypic spinal cord cultures but not in G93A SOD1 transgenic mice. Neurosci Lett 2003;338:107–10.
[8] Drachman DB, Frank K, Dykes-Hoberg M, et al. Cyclooxygenase 2 inhibition protects motor neurons and prolongs survival in a transgenic mouse model of ALS. Ann Neurol 2002;52:771–8.
[9] Klivenyi P, Ferrante RJ, Matthews RT, et al. Neuroprotective effects of creatine in a transgenic animal model of amyotrophic lateral sclerosis. Nat Med 1999;5:347–50.
[10] Rothstein JD, Patel S, Regan MR, et al. Beta-lactam antibiotics offer neuroprotection by increasing glutamate transporter expression. Nature 2005;433:73–7.
[11] Cudkowicz ME, Shefner JM, Schoenfeld DA, et al. Trial of celecoxib in amyotrophic lateral sclerosis. Ann Neurol 2006;60:22–31.
[12] Groeneveld GJ, Veldink JH, van der Tweel I, et al. A randomized sequential trial of creatine in amyotrophic lateral sclerosis. Ann Neurol 2003;53:437–45.
[13] Shefner JM, Cudkowicz ME, Schoenfeld D, et al. A clinical trial of creatine in ALS. Neurology 2004;63:1656–61.
[14] Cudkowicz ME, Shefner JM, Schoenfeld DA, et al. A randomized, placebo-controlled trial of topiramate in amyotrophic lateral sclerosis. Neurology 2003;61:456–64.
[15] Gordon PH, Moore DH, Gelinas DF, et al. Placebo-controlled phase I/II studies of minocycline in amyotrophic lateral sclerosis. Neurology 2004;62:1845–7.
[16] Gordon PH, Moore DH, Miller RG, et al. Efficacy of minocycline in patients with amyotrophic lateral sclerosis: a phase III randomised trial. Lancet Neurol 2007;6:1045–53.
[17] Bensimon G, Lacomblez L, Meininger V, et al. A controlled trial of Riluzole in amyotrophic lateral sclerosis. N Engl J Med 1994;330:585–91.
[18] Lacomblez L, Bensimon G, Leigh P, et al. Dose-ranging study of riluzole in amyotrophic lateral sclerosis. Lancet 1996;347:1425–31.
[19] Mitsumoto H, Davidson M, Moore D, et al. Percutaneous endoscopic gastrostomy (PEG) in patients with ALS and bulbar dysfunction. Amyotroph Lateral Scler Other Motor Neuron Disord 2003;4:177–85.
[20] Thornton FJ, Fotheringham T, Alexander M, et al. Amyotrophic lateral sclerosis: enteral nutrition provision–endoscopic or radiologic gastrostomy? Radiology 2002;224:713–7.

[21] Kasarskis EJ, Scarlata D, Hill R, et al. A retrospective study of percutaneous endoscopic gastrostomy in ALS patients during the BDNF and CNTF trials. J Neurol Sci 1999;169:118–25.
[22] Gruis KL, Brown DL, Lisabeth LD, et al. Longitudinal assessment of noninvasive positive pressure ventilation adjustments in ALS patients. J Neurol Sci 2006;247:59–63.
[23] Heiman-Patterson TD, Miller RG. NIPPV: a treatment for ALS whose time has come. Neurology 2006;67:736.
[24] Lo Coco D, Marchese S, Pesco MC, et al. Noninvasive positive-pressure ventilation in ALS: predictors of tolerance and survival. Neurology 2006;67:761.
[25] Shoesmith CL, Findlater K, Rowe A, et al. Prognosis of amyotrophic lateral sclerosis with respiratory onset. J Neurol Neurosurg Psychiatry 2007;78:629.
[26] Kareus SA, Kagebein S, Rudnicki SA. The importance of a respiratory therapist in the ALS clinic. Amyotroph Lateral Scler 2007;8:1–4.
[27] Traynor BJ, Alexander M, Corr B, et al. Effect of a multidisciplinary amyotrophic lateral sclerosis (ALS) clinic on ALS survival: a population based study, 1996–2000. J Neurol Neurosurg Psychiatry 2003;74:1258–61.
[28] Zoccolella S, Beghi E, Palagano G, et al. ALS multidisciplinary clinic and survival. Results from a population-based study in Southern Italy. J Neurol 2007;254:1107–12.
[29] Andres P, Hedlund W, Finison L, et al. Quantitative motor assessment in amyotrophic lateral sclerosis. Neurol 1986;36:937–41.
[30] Andres PL, Finison L, Thibodeau LM, et al. Use of composite scores (megascores) to measure deficit in amyotrophic lateral sclerosis. Neurol 1988;38:405–8.
[31] Andres PL, Thibodeau LM, Finison LJ, et al. Quantitative assessment of neuromuscular deficit in ALS. Neurol Clin 1987;5:125–41.
[32] Miller R, Moore D, Young B, et al. Placebo-controlled trial of gabapentin in patients with amyotrophic lateral sclerosis. Neurology 1996;47:1383–8.
[33] Miller RG, Petajan JH, Bryan WW, et al. A placebo-controlled trial of recombinant human ciliary neurotrophic (rhCNTF) factor in amyotrophic lateral sclerosis. rhCNTF ALS Study Group. Ann Neurol 1996;39:256–60.
[34] Miller RG, Moore DH, Gelinas DF, et al. Phase III randomized trial of gabapentin in patients with amyotrophic lateral sclerosis. Neurology 2001;56:843–8.
[35] Hoagland R, Mendoza M, Armon C, et al. Reliability of maximal voluntary isometric contraction testing in a multicenter study of patients with amyotrophic lateral sclerosis. Muscle Nerve 1997;20:691–5.
[36] Group A-CTS. A double-blind placebo-controlled clinical trial of subcutaneous recombinant human ciliary neurotophic factor (rHCNTF) in amyotrophic lateral sclerosis. Neurology 1996;46:1244–9.
[37] Beck M, Giess R, Wurffel W, et al. Comparison of maximal voluntary isometric contraction and Drachman's hand-held dynamometry in evaluating patients with amyotrophic lateral sclerosis. Muscle Nerve 1999;22:1265–70.
[38] Group GLAS. A comparison of muscle strength testing techniques in amyotrophic lateral sclerosis. Neurology 2003;61:1503–6.
[39] Ziter FA, Allsop KG, Tyler FH. Assessment of muscle strength in Duchenne muscular dystrophy. Neurology 1977;27:981–4.
[40] Florence JM, Pandya S, King WM, et al. Clinical trials in Duchenne dystrophy. Standardization and reliability of evaluation procedures. Phys Ther 1984;64:41–5.
[41] Lyall RA, Donaldson N, Polkey MI, et al. Respiratory muscle strength and ventilatory failure in amyotrophic lateral sclerosis. Brain 2001;124:2000–13.
[42] Varrato J, Siderowf A, Damiano P, et al. Postural change of forced vital capacity predicts some respiratory symptoms in ALS. Neurology 2001;57:357–9.
[43] Stambler N, Charatan M, Cedarbaum JM. Prognostic indicators of survival in ALS. ALS CNTF Treatment Study Group. Neurology 1998;50:66–72.
[44] Magnus T, Beck M, Giess R, et al. Disease progression in amyotrophic lateral sclerosis: predictors of survival. Muscle Nerve 2002;25:709–14.

[45] Cedarbaum J. The amyotrophic lateral sclerosis functional rating scale (ALSFRS). Arch Neurol 1996;53:141–7.

[46] Cedarbaum JM, Stambler N, Malta E, et al. The ALSFRS-R: a revised ALS functional rating scale that incorporates assessments of respiratory function. BDNF ALS Study Group (Phase III). J Neurol Sci 1999;169:13–21.

[47] Clarke S, Hickey A, O'Boyle C, et al. Assessing individual quality of life in amyotrophic lateral sclerosis. Qual Life Res 2001;10:149–58.

[48] Kaufmann P, Levy G, Montes J, et al. Excellent inter-rater, intra-rater, and telephone-administered reliability of the ALSFRS-R in a multicenter clinical trial. Amyotroph Lateral Scler 2007;8:42–6.

[49] Shefner J, Brown RJ, Cole D, et al. Effect of neurophilin ligands on motor units in mice with SOD1 ALS mutations. Neurology 2001;57:1857–61.

[50] Shefner JM, Cudkowicz ME, Brown RH Jr. Comparison of incremental with multipoint MUNE methods in transgenic ALS mice. Muscle Nerve 2002;25:39–42.

[51] Bromberg MB, Forshew DA, Nau KL, et al. Motor unit number estimation, isometric strength, and electromyographic measures in amyotrophic lateral sclerosis. Muscle Nerve 1993;16:1213–9.

[52] Shefner JM, Cudkowicz ME, Zhang H, et al. The use of statistical MUNE in a multicenter clinical trial. Muscle Nerve 2004;30:463–9.

[53] Bromberg MB, Larson WL. Relationships between motor-unit number estimates and isometric strength in distal muscles in ALS/MND. J Neurol Sci 1996;139(Suppl):38–42.

[54] Bromberg MB, Abrams JL. Sources of error in the spike-triggered averaging method of motor unit number estimation (MUNE). Muscle Nerve 1995;18:1139–46.

[55] Doherty TJ, Brown WF. The estimated numbers and relative sizes of thenar motor units as selected by multiple point stimulation in young and older adults. Muscle Nerve 1993; 16:355–66.

[56] Lomen-Hoerth C, Olney RK. Comparison of multiple point and statistical motor unit number estimation. Muscle Nerve 2000;23:1525–33.

[57] Armon C, Brandstater ME. Motor unit number estimate-based rates of progression of ALS predict patient survival. Muscle Nerve 1999;22:1571–5.

[58] Felice KJ. A longitudinal study comparing thenar motor unit number estimates to other quantitative tests in patients with amyotrophic lateral sclerosis. Muscle Nerve 1997;20: 179–85.

[59] Yuen E, Olney R. Longitudinal study of fiber density and motor unit number estimate in patients with amyotrophic lateral sclerosis. Neurology 1997;49:573–8.

[60] Aggarwal A, Nicholson G. Detection of preclinical motor neurone loss in SOD1 mutation carriers using motor unit number estimation. J Neurol Neurosurg Psychiatry 2002;73:199–201.

[61] Daube JR. Estimating the number of motor units in a muscle. J Clin Neurophysiol 1995;12: 585–94.

[62] Olney RK, Lomen-Hoerth C. Motor unit number estimation (MUNE): how may it contribute to the diagnosis of ALS? Amyotroph Lateral Scler Other Motor Neuron Disord 2000; 1(Suppl 2):S41–4.

[63] Shefner J, Brown R, Cole D, et al. Neurophilin ligands enhance motor unit size in the FALS mouse. Neurology 2000;54(Suppl 3):A155.

[64] Shefner JM, Cudkowicz ME, Zhang H, et al. Revised statistical motor unit number estimation in the Celecoxib/ALS trial. Muscle Nerve 2007;35:228–34.

[65] Bowser R, Cudkowicz M, Kaddurah-Daouk R. Biomarkers for amyotrophic lateral sclerosis. Expert Rev Mol Diagn 2006;6:387–98.

[66] Kolarcik C, Bowser R. Plasma and cerebrospinal fluid-based protein biomarkers for motor neuron disease. Mol Diagn Ther 2006;10:281–92.

[67] Ranganathan S, Nicholl GC, Henry S, et al. Comparative proteomic profiling of cerebrospinal fluid between living and post mortem ALS and control subjects. Amyotroph Lateral Scler 2007;8:1–7.

[68] Ranganathan S, Williams E, Ganchev P, et al. Proteomic profiling of cerebrospinal fluid identifies biomarkers for amyotrophic lateral sclerosis. J Neurochem 2005;95:1461–71.
[69] Palesch YY, Tilley BC. An efficient multi-stage, single-arm Phase II futility design for ALS. Amyotroph Lateral Scler Other Motor Neuron Disord 2004;5(Suppl 1):55–6.
[70] Palesch YY, Tilley BC, Sackett DL, et al. Applying a phase II futility study design to therapeutic stroke trials. Stroke 2005;36:2410–4.
[71] Levy G, Kaufmann P, Buchsbaum R, et al. A two-stage design for a phase II clinical trial of coenzyme Q10 in ALS. Neurology 2006;66:660–3.
[72] Miller R, Bradley W, Cudkowicz M, et al. Phase II/III randomized trial of TCH346 in patients with ALS. Neurology 2007;69:776–84.
[73] Czaplinski A, Haverkamp LJ, Yen AA, et al. The value of database controls in pilot or futility studies in ALS. Neurology 2006;67:1827–32.
[74] Ferrante KL, Shefner J, Zhang H, et al. Tolerance of high-dose (3,000 mg/day) coenzyme Q10 in ALS. Neurology 2005;65:1834–6.
[75] Mitsumoto H, Ulug A, Pullman S, et al. Quantitative objective markers for upper and lower motor neuron dysfunction in ALS. Neurology 2007;68:1402–10.
[76] Mitsumoto H, Shungu DC, Ulug A, et al. Objective upper motor neuron and lower motor neuron markers of amyotrophic lateral sclerosis. Amyotroph Lateral Scler Other Motor Neuron Disord 2004;5(Suppl 2):34–5.

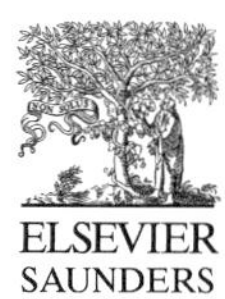
ELSEVIER
SAUNDERS

Phys Med Rehabil Clin N Am
19 (2008) 509–532

PHYSICAL MEDICINE
AND REHABILITATION
CLINICS OF
NORTH AMERICA

Motor Unit Number Estimation in the Assessment of Performance and Function in Motor Neuron Disease

Mark B. Bromberg, MD, PhD*,
Alexander A. Brownell, MS

Clinical Neuroscience Center, Department of Neurology, University of Utah Health Sciences Center, 175 North Medical Drive, Salt Lake City, UT 84132, USA

Motor unit number estimation (MUNE) is a unique electrophysiologic test used to estimate the number of surviving motor units in a muscle or group of muscles. It is used most frequently to monitor lower motor neuron loss in amyotrophic lateral sclerosis (ALS) and spinal muscle atrophy (SMA). Of particular interest is its use as an endpoint measure in clinical trials for these diseases.

The unique feature of MUNE is that it is not affected by collateral reinnervation. Other tests, including muscle strength (qualitative or quantitative) and compound muscle action potential (CMAP), are kept deceptively high by collateral reinnervation and do not fall in value until reinnervation cannot keep up with continuing denervation, which does not occur until 50% or more of motor units are lost. Needle electromyogram (EMG) is sensitive to denervation, as indicated by the presence of positive waves and fibrillation potentials, but the magnitude of abnormal spontaneous activity does not correlate with the degree of motor unit loss. Motor unit action potential morphology changes with collateral reinnervation, but the magnitude of motor unit action potential metric values (amplitude, duration, and complexity) does not correlate with the degree of denervation. Estimates of the degree of reduced motor unit recruitment during the needle examination are subjective and qualitative. Thus, MUNE is better suited than any other test to study the time course and degree of lower motor unit loss in motor neuron disease (MND).

* Corresponding author.
E-mail address: mbromberg@hsc.utah.edu (M.B. Bromberg).

1047-9651/08/$ - see front matter
doi:10.1016/j.pmr.2008.02.006

This article first describes the principles of MUNE and the factors that need to be considered. MUNE can be performed using several operational techniques that differ in approach, and this article reviews techniques that have been used in clinical trials and in monitoring progression. It then reviews experience with MUNE in clinical trials for ALS and SMA and discusses how MUNE correlates with measures of function.

Motor unit number estimation principles

MUNE is based on determining the size of an average surface-recorded motor unit potential (SMUP) and dividing that value into the maximal CMAP [1]:

$$\text{MUNE} = \frac{\text{Area}(\text{CMAP}_{\text{max}})}{\text{Area}\left(\text{SMUP}_{\text{average}}\right)} \text{ or MUNE} = \frac{\text{Amplitude}(\text{CMAP}_{\text{max}})}{\text{Amplitude}\left(\text{SMUP}_{\text{average}}\right)}$$

Although the principle underlying MUNE is simple in concept, many operational issues have been identified and extensively reviewed [1–5]. Several different MUNE techniques have been developed to manage these issues (Table 1). The techniques differ primarily in how the sample of SMUPs is obtained. Attention is directed to the proceedings of the First International Symposium on MUNE [5].

Muscle studied

MUNE is commonly applied to distal extremity muscles. In the lower extremities, the extensor digitorum brevis muscle can be assessed in isolation, but most MUNE determinations are estimates from a group of muscles

Table 1
Motor unit number estimation techniques

MUNE technique	Advantages	Disadvantages
Incremental stimulation	Applicable to any EMG machine Passive testing; patient cooperation not necessary	Alternation leading to an overestimate of the MUNE Applicable to distal muscles
Multiple point stimulation	Applicable to any EMG machine Avoids alternation Passive testing; patient cooperation not necessary	Applicable to distal muscles
Statistical	Samples range of nerve fibers Passive testing; patient cooperation not necessary	Assumes Poisson statistics Requires proprietary software Applicable to distal muscles
Spike-triggered averaging	Applicable to distal and proximal muscles Can provide quantitative intramuscular motor unit action potential data	Requires intramuscular needle EMG electrode Active testing; requires patient cooperation

Techniques differ in how SMUPs are obtained.

innervated by a nerve. In the assessment of the leg, study of the tibial-innervated abductor hallucis muscle also includes contributions from other intrinsic foot muscles. In the arm, study of the median-innervated thenar eminence and ulnar-innervated hypothenar eminence also includes contributions from multiple muscles. Proximal muscles, such as the biceps-brachii muscle group and trapezius muscle, can also be studied with certain MUNE techniques [4].

Recording electrode arrangements

The maximal CMAP is obtained using routine motor nerve conduction recording and stimulating techniques. The recording electrodes are left in place to record SMUPs. Positioning of the active recording electrode over the motor point to achieve maximal CMAP amplitude is important in serial MUNE studies to ensure reproducibility when the maximal CMAP is one of the metrics being followed [6]. However, if only MUNE values are being followed, variations from optimal recording electrode placement will be manifest equally in CMAP and SMUP waveforms, and MUNE values will not be affected [7].

Surface-recorded motor unit potential waveforms

SMUP waveforms vary in shape and size, and typically have an initial negative deflection followed by a terminal positive deflection (Fig. 1). Occasional SMUPs have almost entirely positive waveforms; these SMUPs are considered to represent volume-conducted motor units from adjacent muscles are usually not included in calculating the average SMUP value [5]. Total waveform duration is difficult to assess because onset and termination points cannot be determined easily. Peak-to-peak amplitude is readily measured. Negative peak amplitude and area are measured reliably by extending the prewaveform baseline across the negative portion of the waveform.

The size of SMUPs in normal muscle spans one order of magnitude, from approximately 20 to 200 μV peak-to-peak amplitude [7]. Low-amplitude SMUPs (negative peak amplitude $<$ 10 μV or negative peak area $<$ 25 μV*ms) are encountered but are considered to represent motor units from distant muscles, and are not included in calculating the average SMUP value [5]. SMUP amplitudes increase in denervated muscle because of collateral reinnervation, but the degree of enlargement (as measured in ALS) remains within the same order of magnitude as in normal subjects [7].

Phase cancellation

MUNE values can be calculated using CMAP and SMUP metrics based on peak-to-peak amplitude, negative peak amplitude, and negative peak area values. All metrics of the maximal CMAP incorporate the effects of phase cancellation between the constituent motor units; however, the effects

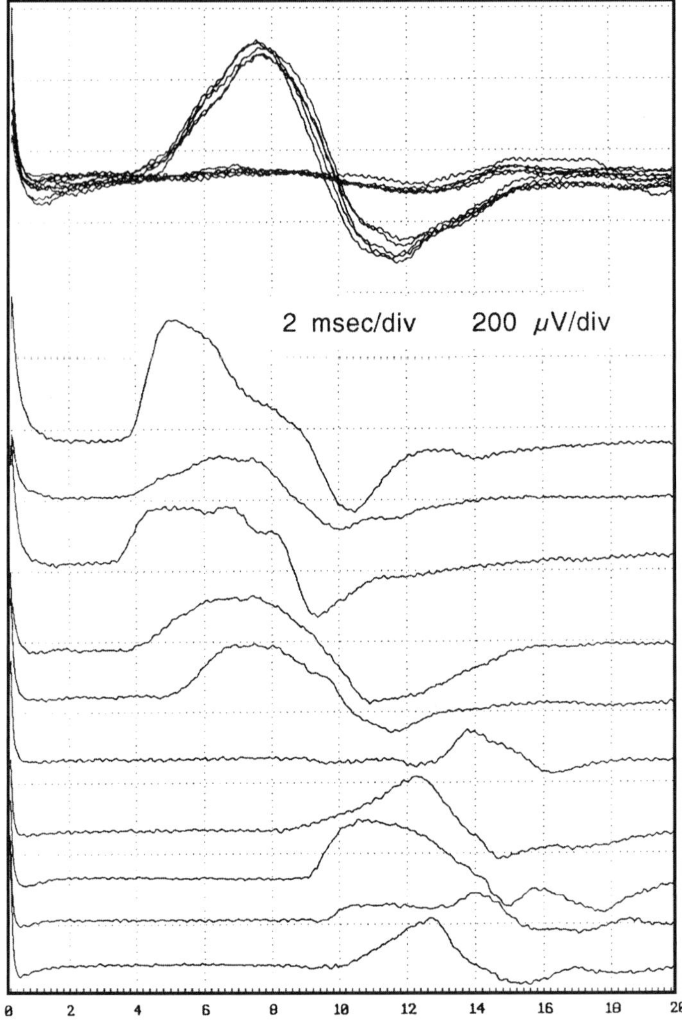

Fig. 1. Multiple point stimulation MUNE technique. (*Top*) All-or-none response. (*Bottom*) SMUP waveforms obtained at different stimulation sites.

of phase cancellation can affect the calculation of the average SMUP and, hence, the MUNE value. Factors that are included in phase cancellation include differences in conduction velocities of motor units from the site of stimulation to the recording electrode and differences in the shapes of SMUPs (relative position of peak negativity and positivity within the waveform). The metric of peak-to-peak amplitude will be most affected by phase cancellation; when the average SMUP is calculated by arithmetic addition of peak-to-peak amplitudes, phase cancellation will not be accounted for and the average SMUP value will be artificially high, leading to an artificially low MUNE value. Metrics of negative peak amplitude or negative peak area are less affected by phase cancellation [8].

It is preferable to determine the average SMUP by the technique of point-by-point averaging of individual SMUP waveforms. This technique includes the effects of phase cancellation but requires special computer software [5,8]. MUNE values from the same muscle calculated using different metrics (peak-to-peak amplitude, negative peak amplitude or area) result in a range of values differing by as much as 35% [8].

The effect of phase cancellation will be least problematic if all waveforms, including the CMAP and the sample of all SMUPs, are obtained from stimulation performed from one electrode site along the nerve, and will be most problematic if different stimulation sites along the nerve are used. When using one stimulation site is not possible, one method for neutralizing the effect of different conduction velocities is to obtain the maximal CMAP from a distal stimulation site along the nerve, to minimize the effect of phase cancellation due to temporal dispersion. Then, individual SMUP waveforms obtained by stimulation at different sites along the nerve can be aligned by the onset of the negative deflection before performing point-by-point averaging, to minimize the effect of temporal dispersion (see Fig. 1) [8].

Surface-recorded motor unit potential sample size and sample bias

Two important issues in MUNE are sample size and sample bias. Normal muscles are innervated by 120 to 400 (or more) motor units [4]. It is customary to sample less than 10% of the normal population (10 to 20 SMUPs) to determine the average SMUP, and the calculated MUNE values do not change substantially when more than 15 SMUPs are used to determine the SMUP value [9,10].

Most MUNE techniques rely on electric activation of the nerve, with graded currents in the range of threshold and just above. In vitro studies of single axons indicate that large-diameter axons have a lower threshold for electric stimulation, which was initially considered to impose a sampling bias in MUNE studies, particularly with techniques that are based on activating SMUPs with low current strengths. However, subsequent investigations comparing SMUP values obtained by various MUNE techniques indicate little bias [10,11]. The overall geometry of the nerve, including orientation of fascicles and overlying tissue, neutralizes the excitability relationship between axonal size and current intensity. Support for the lack of systematic bias comes from computer modeling studies of axon activation in whole nerves that incorporate axons of various diameters and excitability thresholds that show no systemic bias [12].

Test–retest reliability

Test–retest reliability has been assessed for most MUNE techniques in normal subjects and in those who have denervation (from ALS). When expressed as correlation coefficients (absolute value of the difference between the two test values divided by the average of the two values), test–retest reliability is 15% to 20%. Reliability is higher with reduced numbers of motor units [9,10].

Independent verification

No independent or anatomic method (gold standard) can count motor axons innervating a muscle, and MUNE values remain estimates [4,5]. Human autopsy studies counting axons require assumptions about the percentages of motor efferent and muscle afferent fibers within a motor nerve but show good correlations with MUNE values [13]. Animal studies have compared MUNE and anterior horn cell counts (identified by anatomic tracing techniques) and show high correlations [14].

Motor unit number estimation techniques

MUNE techniques differ in how SMUPs are obtained. Selection of an MUNE technique is guided by equipment availability, clinical experience, and study objectives. Direct comparisons among techniques show good concordance, with no technique listed in Table 1 markedly better than another [10,11,15].

Incremental stimulation motor unit number estimation technique

The incremental stimulation (IS) technique is the original MUNE technique [1] and is based on applying incremental increases in nerve stimulation intensity to generate an envelope of evoked responses. Each step in the envelope is considered to represent the activation of single motor axons that are serially added to the growing evoked response.

A maximal CMAP is recorded and the stimulating electrode remains fixed in the same position on the nerve, to record SMUPs. The display sensitivity is increased to 50 to 100 μV/div to help visualize the steps in the response envelope. The stimulus intensity is lowered to activate the first axon, indicated by an all-or-none response. By small increases in stimulation intensity, an envelope of responses is obtained with 8 to 10 discrete steps before the increments in the envelope become indistinguishable (Fig. 2). The number of steps is divided into the peak-to-peak amplitude of the envelope to determine the average amplitude of each step. This average value is considered to represent the average SMUP, and is used to calculate the MUNE value.

Advantages of IS include

- It can be used on any EMG machine.
- The stimulating electrode remains in the same position for the maximal CMAP and for determining the average SMUP, and the effects of phase cancellation are incorporated into CMAP and SMUP waveforms.

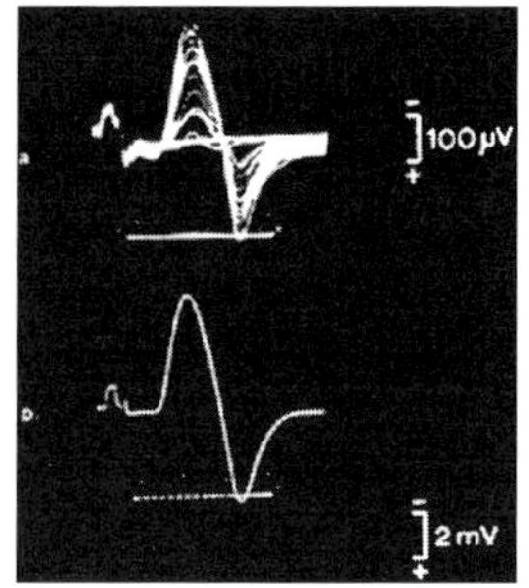

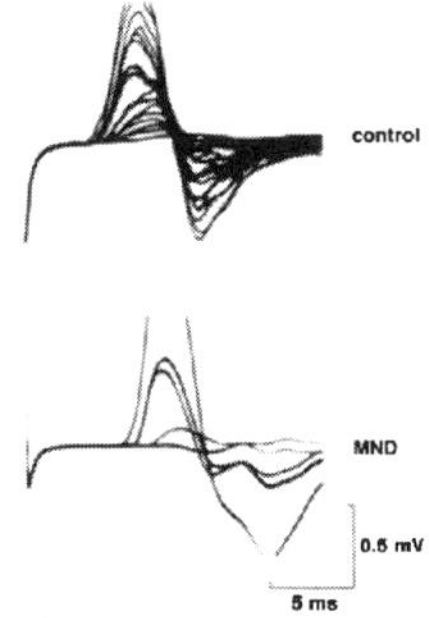

Fig. 2. Top half of figure modified from original description of IS technique. Upper waveforms show incremental response following electrical excitation of motor nerve from threshold to higher intensities. Lower waveform shows maximal compound muscle action potential. Numbers on the right show how average single motor unit potential is calculated and divided into the maximal potential to give the estimated motor unit count. Lower half of figure shows envelope of responses from a normal subject (*upper waveforms*) and those from a subject with ALS (*lower waveforms*). (*From* McComas A, Fawcett P, Campbell M, et al. Electrophysiological estimation of the number of motor units within a human muscle. J Neurol Neurosurg Psychiatry 1971;34:121–31; with permission).

Issues include

- Excitation of different combinations of axons (alternations) results in uncertainty in the number of steps that are truly represented in the envelope, which leads to a larger number of perceived steps and results in a smaller average SMUP and a larger MUNE value [1,2].

Multiple point stimulation motor unit number estimation technique

Multiple point stimulation (MPS) was developed to avoid the problem of alternation [16]. Alternation is avoided by activating only single axons, and other axons are activated by moving the stimulating electrode to different sites along the nerve [10,16].

Surface electrodes are placed and a maximal CMAP is recorded. The display sensitivity is raised to 50 to 100 µV/div to help visualize the low-amplitude SMUPs. The stimulus intensity is lowered to activate the first axon and verified by an all-or-none response to raising and lowering the stimulation current (see Fig. 1). The stimulating electrode is moved to a different site along the nerve and another all-or-none response is obtained. Ten to 15 responses are collected and averaged to obtain the average SMUP used to calculate the MUNE value.

Advantages of MPS include

- It avoids the problem of alternation.
- It can be used on any EMG machine.

Issues include:

- A suitable number of stimuli must be delivered to ensure that the response represents a single axon and does not fractionate into two smaller responses.
- The stimulating electrode is moved to different sites along the nerve to obtain single SMUPs, and if point-by-point averaging is used, the effects of phase cancellation from late-arriving waveforms will be problematic, unless the waveforms are aligned by their onset.

A modification of MPS combines IS and MPS, and is called the adapted MPS (AMPS) technique [17]. In traditional IS, the envelope includes as many SMUPs as can be discerned. With AMPS, an envelope of two or three SMUPs is elicited at one stimulation site and each waveform within the envelope is subtracted to determine if it represents a true single SMUP. The stimulating electrode is moved to multiple sites where the process is repeated until a suitable sample of SMUPs is obtained.

A similar modification does not rely on waveform subtraction but collects an envelope of three responses at each of three sites along the nerve. For each site, an average SMUP is calculated, and then the three averaged values are used to generate a grand average for the MUNE calculation [18].

Statistical motor unit number estimation technique

The statistical technique is a novel approach using Poisson statistics to determine the average response, based on the variability of the response [19,20]. When multiple stimuli are delivered at the same intensity, the evoked response varies from trial to trial (an envelope of responses), reflecting alternation as axons are added or lost, based on different probabilities of activation. The variance of the response amplitude or area can be determined by Poisson statistics; the variance is equal to the average unit of change, which can be used as a measure of the average SMUP amplitude or area.

Surface electrodes are placed and a maximal CMAP is recorded. The stimulating electrode is fixed and the nerve is "scanned" with a series of 30 stimuli delivered with increasing intensity from just subthreshold to just maximal, to generate the total envelope of evoked responses (Fig. 3).

This scan of the evoked response is used to identify the portions of the response envelope that will be sampled. Usually, three or four regions are sampled and the variance and SMUP amplitude value at each are determined. The variance of the response in each region is determined by applying sets of 30 stimuli. For each set of 30 stimuli, the variance is calculated and an average SMUP area is determined. Repeated sets of 30 stimuli are performed until the standard error of the different determinations is less than 10%. The average SMUP determined at each region is then used to calculate an MUNE value for that region. The other designated regions are similarly sampled. Regions selected for detailed study from the scan curve include regions with large steps, reflecting large-amplitude motor units, and one "average" region, considered to represent the unsampled region. An MUNE value is then calculated for the unsampled region using the smallest average SMUP value. Finally, all regional and unsampled MUNE values are combined for a total MUNE value.

Advantages of the statistical technique include

- The problem of alternation in the IS technique becomes the underlying basis of the statistical technique.
- A wide range of axon thresholds and their SMUPs are sampled.
- A degree of statistical robustness is included in the determination of the average SMUP for each region by repeatedly applying sets of 30 stimuli until the standard error of the response is less than 10% of the mean response.
- The stimulating electrode remains in the same position for the maximal CMAP and for determining the average SMUP, and the effects of phase cancellation are incorporated into the CMAP and SMUP waveforms.
- Negative peak area is the metric used for calculations.

Issues include

- It requires proprietary software.
- Assumption of Poisson distribution of response amplitudes (skewed to the left) is not always accurate [21].
- With denervation, enlarged SMUP may disproportionately reduce the MUNE value.
- SMUP values calculated from the variance represent putative SMUPs and not physiologic SMUPs.
- Many variables in how data are obtained influence the final MUNE calculation, and MUNE values from the same normal subject vary by more than 30% [21,22].
- Small variations in the response amplitude may be due to neuromuscular junction failures in patients who have ALS but may be misinterpreted by the algorithm as the addition or subtraction of axons, leading to some putative SMUPs of low amplitude that result in an erroneously high MUNE values in these subjects [23].

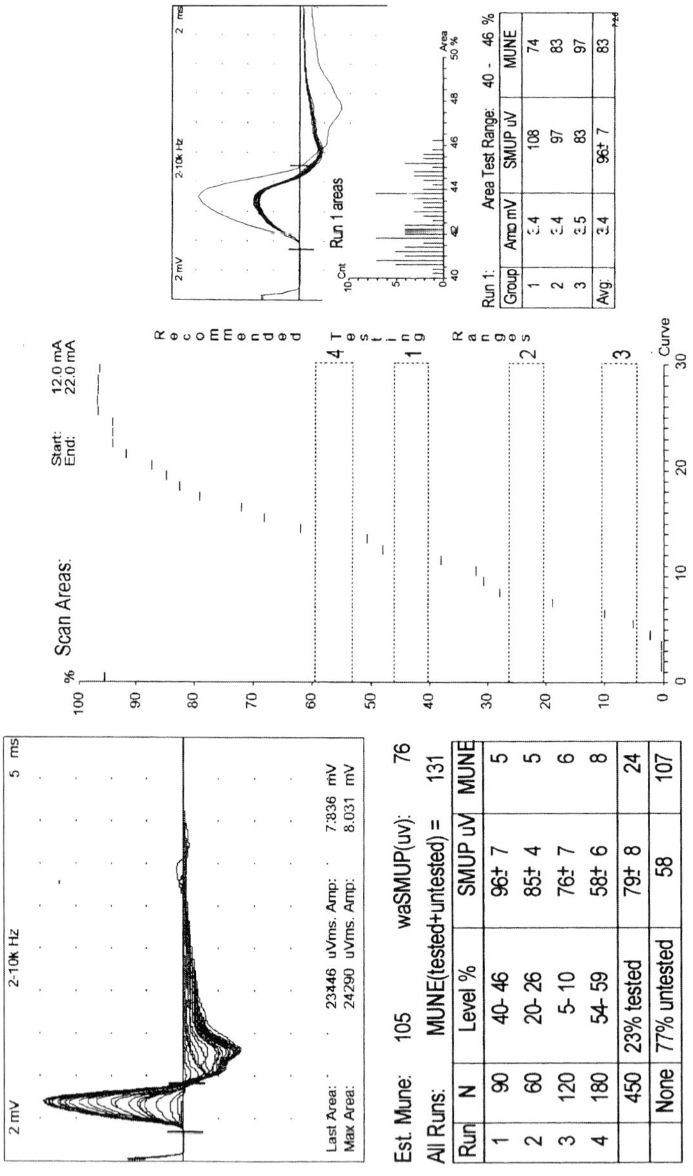
2 mV
2-10k Hz
5 ms
Last Area: 23446 uVms. Amp: 7.836 mV
Max Area: 24290 uVms. Amp: 8.031 mV
Est. Mune: 105
waSMUP(uv): 76
All Runs: MUNE(tested+untested) = 131
Run | N | Level % | SMUP uV | MUNE
1 | 90 | 40- 46 | 96± 7 | 5
2 | 60 | 20- 26 | 85± 4 | 5
3 | 120 | 5- 10 | 76± 7 | 6
4 | 180 | 54- 59 | 58± 6 | 8
| 450 | 23% tested | 79± 8 | 24
| None | 77% untested | 58 | 107
% Scan Areas:
Start: 12.0 mA
End: 22.0 mA
Recommended Testing Ranges
4
1
2
3
Curve
2 mV
2-10k Hz
2 ms
Cnt
Run 1 areas
Area
50 %
Run 1: Area Test Range: 40 - 46 %
Group | Amp mV | SMUP uV | MUNE
1 | 3.4 | 108 | 74
2 | 3.4 | 97 | 83
3 | 3.5 | 83 | 97
Avg: | 3.4 | 96± 7 | 83

The statistical technique has been modified in several ways:

- Different regions of the scan curve may be tested [21,24].
- Different approaches are proposed to detect outlying data [25].
- Different methods are used to calculate the average SMUP values that are used to determine the final MUNE [22].
- Different mathematic approaches are used to analyze the data [26–28].

Spike-triggered averaging motor unit number estimation technique

The IS, MPS, and statistical techniques rely on electric stimulation of the nerve to activate SMUPs. Spike-triggered averaging (STA) activates single motors by voluntary contraction of the muscle [29]. Individual motor units are identified from weak interference patterns and used to trigger a signal averager to extract the SMUP.

Two recording amplifiers and channels are used, one for surface recording and the other for intramuscular electrode recording. Surface electrodes are used to record the maximal CMAP and SMUPs. A weak interference pattern is generated and the intramuscular electrode is adjusted to isolate the discharge of one motor unit (Fig. 4). A voltage level trigger is set to detect the motor unit's discharge pattern, and the trigger signals from that motor unit are used for STA of the surface response of the motor unit. The intramuscular electrode is moved to another site in the muscle and another SMUP is obtained. Ten to 15 responses are collected and averaged to obtain the average SMUP used to calculate the MUNE value.

Advantages of STA include

- It can be used on any EMG machine with two amplifiers and signal averaging capabilities.

Fig. 3. Statistical MUNE technique. (*Upper left panel*) CMAP scan envelope from threshold to supramaximal response evoked by 30 graded stimuli. (*Middle panel*) Same scan, but CMAP amplitudes (*small horizontal marks*) displayed as percent of maximal response. Note the four regions selected by the algorithm for determining response variances. (*Right panel*) Top portion shows maximal CMAP and envelope of responses evoked by sets of 30 stimuli at a constant intensity to determine variance in zone 4. Middle plot shows response in histogram format to determine whether distribution of responses is appropriately skewed to the left. Lower chart shows calculated variance of the response to sets of 30 stimuli. The variance is equal to the mean change in response amplitude, which is considered to reflect the average SMUP amplitude for that region. A corresponding MUNE value is calculated. Three sets (groups) of 30 stimuli were required for the standard error to be less than 10% of the mean value (96±7). (*Lower left panel*) Results of testing all four regions (runs). An MUNE value is calculated for each region and summed, to give an overall MUNE value for the total percentage of the CMAP tested (23%). The untested percentage (77%) is assumed to be innervated by the smallest SMUPs, and an MUNE value is calculated accordingly. Tested and untested regions are summed, for a final MUNE value of 131. An alternative method is to weigh the tested regions to determine a weighted average SMUP value (waSMUP). This value is used to calculate an estimated MUNE value. See text for differences in final MUNE values from the different techniques.

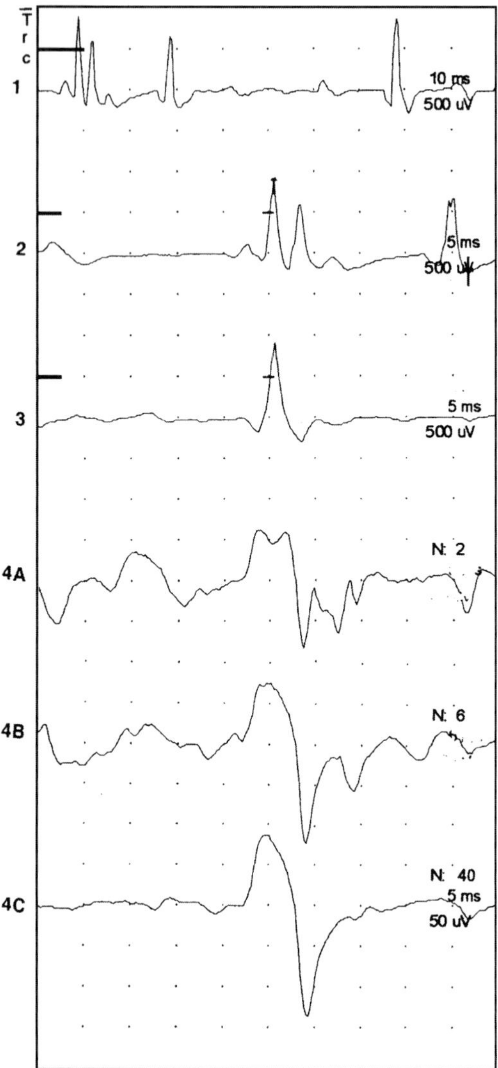

Fig. 4. STA MUNE technique. Determination of SMUPs by STA. (*Trace1*) Intramuscular needle EMG signal in free run mode. (*Trace 2*) Intramuscular needle EMG signal with isolation of single motor unit potential (middle of trace) by setting a voltage trigger (*horizontal line*). (*Trace 3*) Intramuscular needle EMG signal of isolated motor unit potential after averaging. Averaged motor unit potential can be assessed for quantitative EMG analysis. (*Trace 4A*) Surface EMG signal corresponding to intramuscular EMG signal isolated by spike triggering (averaged 2 times, N. 2). Note concurrent background surface EMG activity from other motor units. (*Trace 4B*) Surface signal averaged 6 times. (*Trace 4C*) Surface signal averaged 40 times. Note clear isolation of SMUP. Averaged SMUP can be assessed for negative peak amplitude and area.

- Quantitative motor unit action potential data from the intramuscular electrode are available.
- It can be applied to proximal muscles.

Issues include

- Care must be taken to avoid spurious trigger potentials [7].
- Potential sampling bias exists toward early recruited motor units [10,11].

A modification of STA has been developed, called decomposition-based quantitative EMG (DQEMG), which permits the collection of many SMUPs under controlled recruitment conditions. In conventional STA, single intramuscular potentials and their SMUP are isolated at each electrode site. Signal decomposition algorithms can identify four to eight single intramuscular potentials from the interference pattern, and each motor unit potential can be used for STA of the corresponding SMUPs (Fig. 5) [30–32]. DQEMG reduces the time necessary to obtain 10 to 15 SMUPs and increases the total number of SMUPs that can be obtained [33]. It is possible to use the surface EMG signal as a measure of the muscle contractile level and motor unit recruitment level, which are variables affecting the SMUP sample. Controlling for the level of contraction enhances MUNE reliability [33,34].

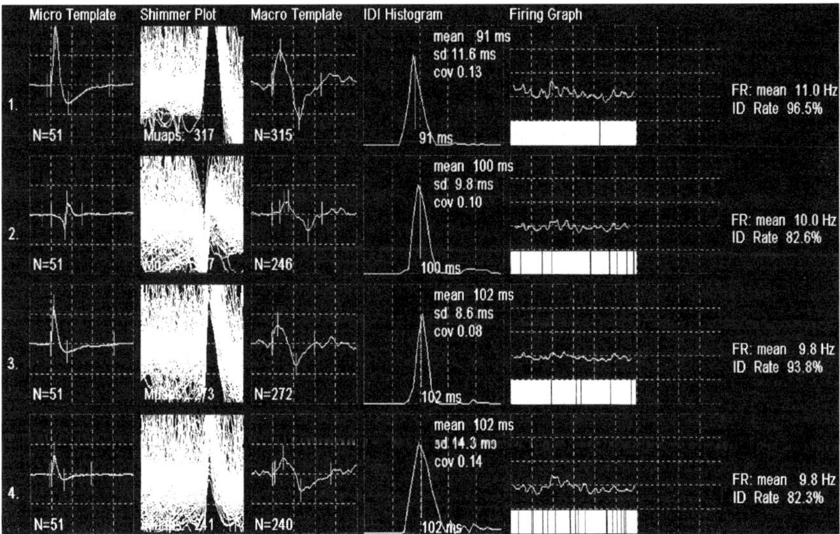

Fig. 5. Decomposition-enhanced STA MUNE technique. (*Micro Template panel*) Four intramuscular motor unit potentials isolated by the decomposition algorithm and averaged 51 times. (*Shimmer Plot panel*) Superimposition of all isolated motor unit potentials. (*Macro Template panel*) SMUPs associated with corresponding intramuscular potentials and averaged the indicated number of times. (*IDI Histogram panel*) Interdischarge interval (IDI) histogram of each motor unit discharge. (*Firing Graph panel*) Histogram display of same data. (*FR and ID rate panel*) Mean firing rate (FR) and identification (ID) rate for isolated motor units.

Motor unit number estimation in monitoring change in motor neuron disease

The ability of MUNE to assess lower motor neuron loss makes it attractive as a measure of change or progression in MND. Traditional efforts to measure the natural history of ALS and SMA have relied on muscle strength testing or functional measures. However, the effects of collateral reinnervation blunt the rate of change of strength or function and these measures do not provide true estimates of the underlying rates of lower motor neuron death. The effect of this blunting has been modeled in computer simulation studies [35]. When assumptions are made, based on physiologic data, about the magnitude of collateral reinnervation, the model shows that when a linear rate of loss of motor neurons is simulated, strength declines slowly until 50% of motor neurons are lost, after which a rapid loss of strength occurs (Fig. 6). When an exponential loss of lower motor neurons is simulated, with

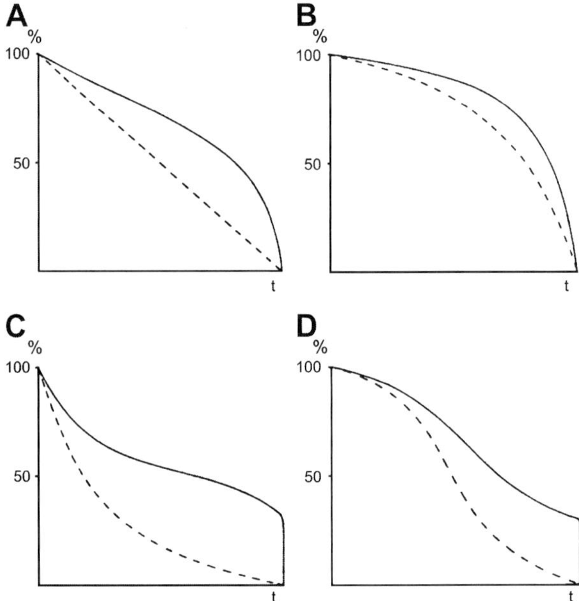

Fig. 6. Computer simulation model of rates of loss of muscle strength (*solid lines*) resulting from different rates of loss of motor neurons (*dashed lines*). Incorporated into the model are the effects of collateral reinnervation that include the extent and limitations on reinnervation. (*A*) Linear rate of loss of motor neurons results in an initial slow rate of loss of strength followed by a rapid loss when 50% of motor neurons are lost. (*B*) Curvilinear rate of motor neuron loss results in a curvilinear rate of strength loss. (*C*) Exponential rate of motor neuron loss, initial rapid and later slow, results in a uniform, sigmoidal rate of loss of strength. (*D*) Exponential rate of motor neuron loss, initial slow and later rapid, results in a uniform, sigmoidal rate of loss of strength. (*From* Kuether G, Lipinski HG. Computer simulation of neuron degeneration in motor neuron disease. In: Tsubaki T, Yase Y, editors. Amyotrophic lateral sclerosis: recent advances in research and treatment. Amsterdam: Elsevier Publishers; 1988; with permission).

an initial rapid loss and later slow loss, the rate of decline of strength is uniform until 80% of motor neurons are lost. Thus, mismatches are likely to exist between true rates of motor neuron death and metrics that include the effects of collateral reinnervation, and MUNE is the only measure that is not influenced by reinnervation.

Motor unit number estimation assessment of natural history in amyotrophic lateral sclerosis

The nature of ALS progression has been assessed by quantitative measurement of muscle strength or functional activities. Because weakness in ALS is focal at onset and progresses within a region and to other regions, strength measurements have been made from multiple muscle groups and combined into megascores. When megascores of strength in patients who have ALS are compared with normal control subjects and are standardized as z-scores, megascores show a linear decline, at least during the phase of the disease during which subjects are available for testing (Fig. 7) [36]. The ALS Functional Rating Scale-Revised (ALSFRS-R) assesses the ability to perform daily activities [37]. Assessments during the course of ALS show a linear decline [38]. Both of these metrics include the effects of collateral reinnervation. When MUNE determinations are made from single muscles in patients who have ALS, the rate of loss appears to be exponential, with an early and rapid depletion of a vulnerable motor neuron pool and a slow loss of a more robust pool (Fig. 8) [39]. The discrepancy between rates of progression as measured by strength and the ALSFRS-R, and the rate by MUNE, can be accounted for by the effects of collateral reinnervation in the computer modeling study discussed earlier.

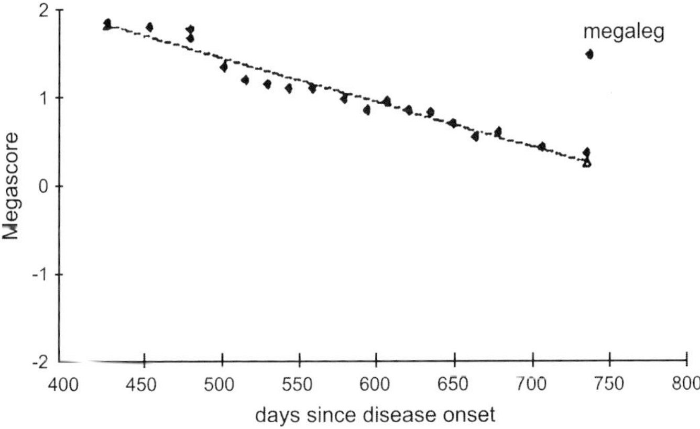

Fig. 7. Data from isometric strength measurements from leg muscles in subjects who have ALS summed as megascores, showing linear decline over time. (*From* Andres P, Finison L, Conlon T, et al. Use of composite scores (megascores) to measure deficit in amyotrophic lateral sclerosis. Neurology1988;38:405–8; with permission).

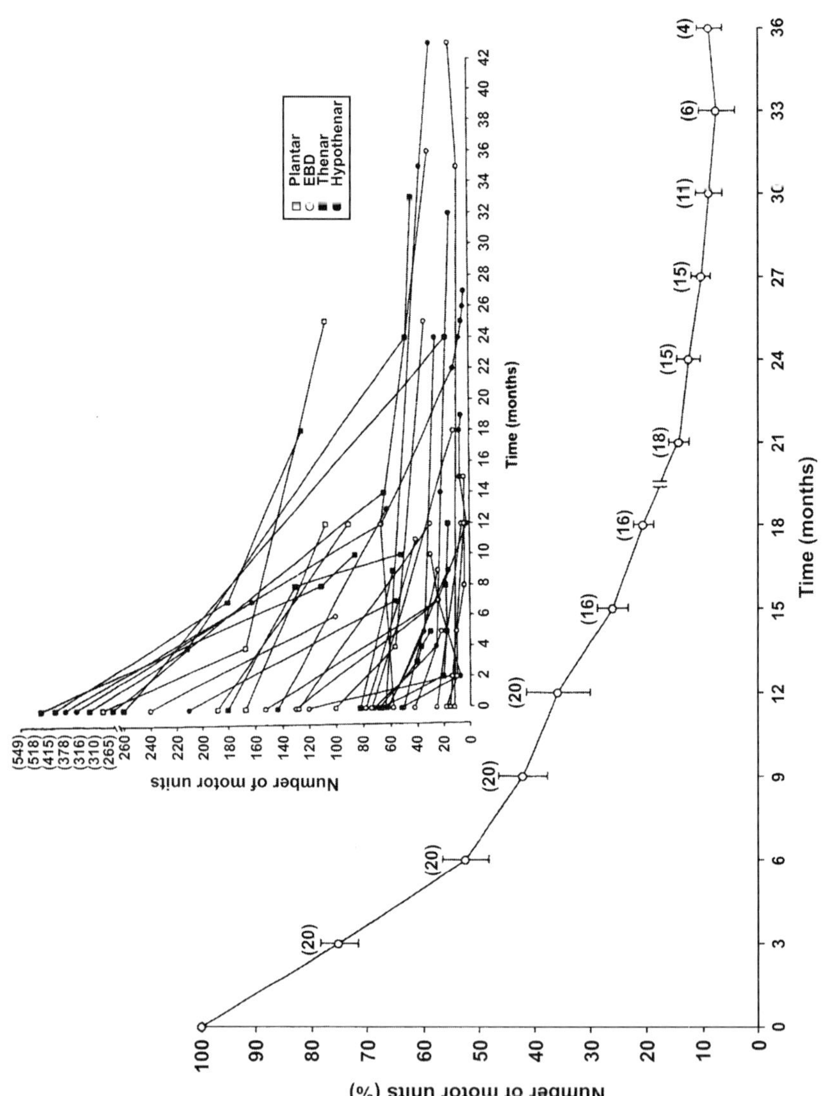
Number of motor units (%)
Time (months)
Number of motor units
Time (months)
Plantar
EBD
Thenar
Hypothenar

Motor unit number estimation assessment of natural history in spinal muscle atrophy

SMA is divided into clinical types, based on age of onset of weakness and early degree of weakness [40]. In type 1, strength at birth is usually normal but is lost rapidly (over weeks), followed by a period of stability; the degree of weakness precludes the ability to sit unaided. Types 2 and 3 have a longer period of normal strength followed by initial rapid loss of strength and, thereafter, a slow loss of strength. In type 2, strength is sufficient to allow sitting unaided but not standing, whereas in type 3, strength is sufficient to allow standing unaided. The IS MUNE technique has been used to study SMA, including in infants [41]. In a natural history study, MUNE determinations have been made in the different SMA types and over time (Fig. 9). MUNE determinations in presymptomatic infants who go on to a type 1 pattern have normal numbers of motor units. When they become symptomatic, motor unit numbers plummet to low values over a brief period of time (weeks) and remain largely unchanged. MUNE determinations made in symptomatic type 1 subjects are low and change little over time. MUNE determinations in symptomatic types 2 and 3 subjects show a marked degree of motor neuron loss (but greater MUNE values in type 3 than in type 2) and a slow decline over many months to years [42].

Another SMA natural history study by the Northeastern Clinical Trials Consortium in SMA is in progress and includes MUNE.

Motor unit number estimation correlations with other metrics

MUNE values show correlations with metrics related to general motor function, but the statistical robustness of the correlations varies markedly because of the effects of collateral reinnervation on each motor function. This variability was discussed earlier for megascores from quantitative strength testing and the ALSFRS-R scale. Correlations between rates of change of several metrics have been studied in ALS subjects. MUNE values fall at a more rapid rate than the ALSFRS-R, the Appel score [43], and forced vital capacity [44]. When MUNE values are compared with electrophysiologic metrics at a single point in time, correlations with single fiber measurement of fiber density are good, but those with macroEMG or motor unit action potential

Fig. 8. Time course of motor unit loss in ALS determined by the incremental MUNE technique. (*Inset*) MUNE values from different patients obtained at different time periods within the course of the disease and from different muscles (extensor digitorum brevis, hypothenar, thenar eminences). Note that patients who had high MUNE values at initial study had marked loss at subsequent studies, whereas patients who had low MUNE values at initial study had little further loss at subsequent studies. (*Bottom*) Averaged MUNE values over time, plotting patients whose initial values were above the lower limit of normal for that muscle. (*Modified from* Dantes M, McComas A. The extent and time course of motorneuron involvement in amyotrophic lateral sclerosis. Muscle Nerve 1991;14:416–21; with permission).

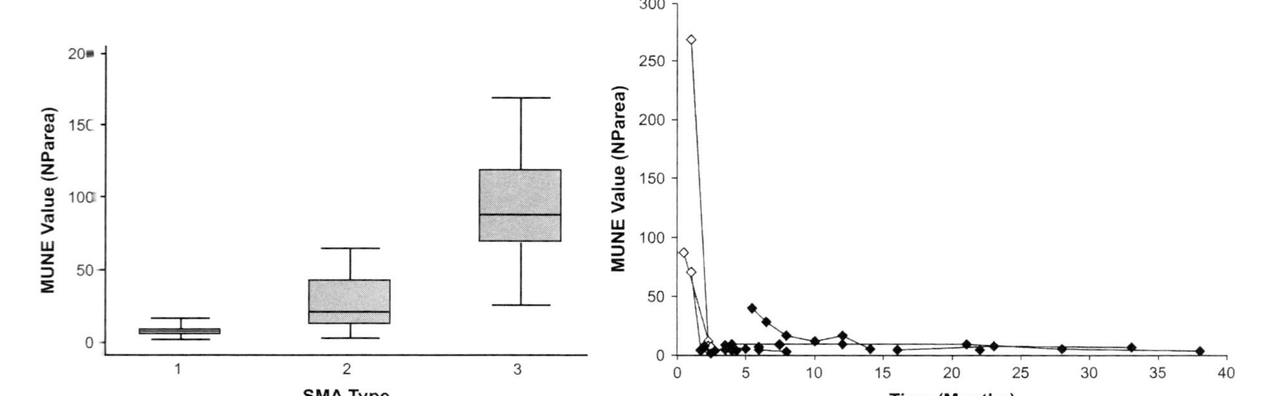

Fig. 9. MUNE values in SMA. (*Left*) Box-whisker plots showing mean (*dark line in box*), 75th percentile to 25th percentile (*box*), and range (*whiskers*) MUNE values for types 1, 2, and 3. (*Right*) Longitudinal MUNE values for type 1. Open diamonds represent genotyped but presymptomatic subjects. (*From* Swoboda K, Prior T, McNaught T, et al. Natural history of denervation in SMA: relation to age, SMN2 copy number, and function. Ann Neurol 2005;57:704–12; with permission).

amplitude are not [45]. Correlations between MUNE and the maximum CMAP will always be high because the CMAP is one of the mathematic determinants of MUNE. However, the average SMUP increases before the maximal CMAP falls, making the resultant MUNE value more sensitive to early change.

Motor unit number estimation in clinical drug trials in amyotrophic lateral sclerosis

MUNE is an attractive endpoint measure in ALS clinical drug trials because it directly assesses loss of lower motor neurons and has been shown to be more sensitive to progression than other measures of ALS (functional rating scales, strength, CMAP, forced vital capacity) [44]. However, the Food and Drug Administration feels at this time that MUNE is not suitable as a primary endpoint measure because it has not yet been sufficiently established as having clinical meaning, nor has it been shown to have the ability to predict clinical outcome [46]. MUNE has been used in several multicenter drug trials as a secondary endpoint measure. Because the trials were negative for drug efficacy, an opportunity has not arisen to compare MUNE to traditional primary endpoint measures for detecting differences due to drug effect. However, valuable experience has been gained from drug trials and this section reviews applications of MUNE in ALS.

Motor unit number estimation in familial amyotrophic lateral sclerosis

A unique opportunity to assess the sensitivity of MUNE for detecting the onset of motor unit loss in ALS is to study carriers of mutations of the superoxide dismutase 1 (SOD1) gene from presymptomatic to symptomatic stages. Statistical MUNE has been used to show, in the presymptomatic stage, that mutation carriers do not differ from control subjects and have consistent MUNE values during this time period [47]. In a longitudinal study with MUNE assessment at 6-month intervals, two carriers experienced 12% to 23% reductions in MUNE values in thenar or extensor digitorum brevis muscles in the setting of preserved strength. Evaluations several months later revealed further reductions in MUNE values, associated with clinical weakness [48]. Thus, MUNE was more sensitive in predicting the onset of the symptomatic stage than was strength.

Motor unit number estimation in clinical drug trials

MUNE has been used as a secondary endpoint measure in several multicenter drug trials. In a two-center, 6-month, placebo-controlled trial of amino acid therapy, STA MUNE was applied to the biceps brachii muscles at the beginning and end of the trial [49]. The trial showed no drug effect, and the combined data from both study arms (68 subjects) showed a fall in MUNE values during the course of the trial, but not to a significant degree. MUNE values showed considerable variability (32.6%), likely accounting for the lack of significance [45]. Weak correlations existed between MUNE values and electrodiagnostic measures of fiber density and macroEMG amplitude and with elbow flexion strength [45].

Statistical MUNE was applied to hypothenar and thenar muscle groups in a 14-center, 6-month trial of creatine versus placebo [50]. Formal training in MUNE resulted in good test–retest reliability in normal subjects (5%–20% variability). The trial showed no effect of creatine, and the combined data from both treatment groups (98 subjects) showed that MUNE values, measured monthly, fell by 23% during the course of the trial. However, several low-amplitude putative SMUPs were calculated in patients who had low CMAP amplitudes that resulted in larger MUNE values. This finding was felt to represent a statistical artifact caused by a small variability in single large motor unit responses with repeated activation, which reflected motor unit instability associated with reinnervation. Further study confirmed motor unit response variability in ALS subjects [23], which led to revisions in the statistical technique to reduce the chance of including small SMUPs. These revisions were incorporated into a multicenter trial of celecoxib [51] in which normal subjects showed good test–retest reliability (<20%). The trial showed no effect of celecoxib over placebo and combined data on 163 subjects studied during 12 months with seven MUNE determinations showed a 49% decline in MUNE values. However, with disease progression, SMUP values did not increase, whereas CMAP values fell, and the lower MUNE values were driven by the falling CMAP values. Again, the lack of increase in SMUP amplitude values was attributed to inclusion of putative small SMUPs reflecting motor unit instability despite the modifications. The conclusion from these experiences is that the statistical MUNE technique is inappropriate for use in clinical trials in which active reinnervation and motor unit instability are involved [51].

Motor unit number estimation in clinical trials in spinal muscle atrophy

The IS technique has been used by the American Spinal Muscular Atrophy Randomized Trials Consortium in an open-label phase II trial of riluzole in SMA types 1 and 2. The data have not been published.

The IS technique has also been used in an open-label phase I/II trial of valproic acid in symptomatic SMA subjects with types 1, 2, and 3 (K. Swoboda, 2007, personal communication). In type 1 subjects, MUNE values were low and did not fall during the 12 months, as would be expected from the natural history data, but CMAP and average SMUP values increased, reflecting some change. In types 2 and 3, although CMAP and average SMUP values increased, they did so disproportionately, and MUNE values fell. It is not known if valproic acid had a positive effect, but changes in CMAP and SMUP, at a minimum, likely reflect the natural history of the effects of collateral reinnervation.

Challenges for motor unit number estimation in clinical trials

The field of MUNE has shown major advances since its first description in 1971. Currently, one may choose from four major techniques, each with modifications. The choice depends largely on the intended application (see Table 1). Experience with MUNE in multicenter clinical drug trials is now considerable, and issues related to some MUNE techniques have emerged.

For MUNE to be used in multicenter trials, several practical requirements exist:

- Ease of operator understanding and use: It is desirable to have electrodiagnostic technologists perform MUNE studies in trials but, to date, physicians have preformed the studies. Techniques that are straightforward in concept and that require few operational judgments are important.
- Good test–retest reliability: Prestudy training and attainment of good test–retest reliability in normal and study subjects is essential. It is also important to have continuous review of data during the trial.
- Reasonable cost: The ability to perform studies on any EMG machine is desirable. If special software is required, it should function on any machine.
- Reasonable study time: The MUNE study should be able to be performed within 15 to 20 minutes.
- Subject tolerability: The study should entail minimal discomfort to ensure high completion rates in a trial.

Several challenges exist relating to MNDs that are independent of MUNE but will affect its usefulness and future as an endpoint measure:

- In ALS, motor neuron loss starts focally, resulting in various degrees of motor unit loss in the muscles studied by MUNE at entry into the trial. Thus, changes in MUNE with progression or with drug effect will vary among subjects. Whether MUNE measured from one muscle is sufficiently sensitive to show change remains to be seen.
- SMA, particularly type 1, involves profound motor unit loss and any slowing in the rate of loss will be challenging to document during a reasonable study duration. MUNE may be a good measure in genotyped, but presymptomatic, subjects.

Finally, and most important, it will take a positive drug trial to determine the sensitivity of MUNE as an endpoint measure. It is likely that until then, MUNE will be a secondary endpoint measure and comparisons will have to be made to other endpoint measures to determine sensitivity.

References

[1] McComas A, Fawcett P, Campbell M, et al. Electrophysiological estimation of the number of motor units within a human muscle. J Neurol Neurosurg Psychiatry 1971;34:121–31.

[2] Brown W, Milner-Brown H. Some electrical properties of motor units and their effects on the methods of estimating motor unit numbers. J Neurol Neurosurg Psychiatry 1976;39: 249–57.
[3] Slawnych M, Laszlo C, Hershler C. A review of techniques employed to estimate the number of motor units in a muscle. Muscle Nerve 1990;13:1050–64.
[4] McComas A. Invited review: motor unit estimation: methods, results, and present status. Muscle Nerve 1991;14:585–97.
[5] Bromberg M, editor. Motor unit number estimation (MUNE). Amsterdam: Elsevier; 2003. Supplements to Clinical Neurophysiology; No. 55.
[6] Bromberg M, Spiegelberg T. The influence of active electrode placement on CMAP amplitude. Electroencephalogr clin Neurophysiol 1997;105:385–9.
[7] Bromberg M, Abrams J. Sources of error in the spike-triggered averaging method of motor unit number estimation (MUNE). Muscle Nerve 1995;18:1139–46.
[8] Doherty T, Stashuk D, Brown W. Determinants of mean motor unit size: impact on estimates of motor unit number. Muscle Nerve 1993;16:1326–31.
[9] Bromberg M. Motor unit estimation: reproducibility of the spike-triggered averaging technique in normal and ALS subjects. Muscle Nerve 1993;16:466–71.
[10] Doherty T, Brown W. The estimated numbers and relative sizes of thenar units as selected by multiple point stimulation in young and older adults. Muscle Nerve 1993;16:355–66.
[11] Stein R, Yang J. Methods for estimating the number of motor units in human muscles. Ann Neurol 1990;28:487–95.
[12] Major L, Jones K. Simulations of motor unit number estimation techniques. J Neural Eng 2005;2:17–34.
[13] Feinstein B, Lindegård B, Nyman E, et al. Morphologic studies of motor units in normal human muscle. Acta Anat (Basel) 1955;23:127–43.
[14] Arasaki K, Tamaki M, Hosoya Y, et al. Validity of electromyograms and tension as a means of motor unit number estimation. Muscle Nerve 1997;20:552–60.
[15] Lomen-Hoerth C, Olney R. Comparison of multiple-point and statistical motor unit number estimation. Muscle Nerve 2000;23:1525–33.
[16] Kadrie H, Yates S, Milner-Brown H, et al. Multiple point electrical stimulation of ulnar and median nerves. J Neurol Neurosurg Psychiatry 1976;39:973–85.
[17] Wang F, Delwaide P. Number and relative size of thenar motor units estimated by an adapted multiple point stimulation method. Muscle Nerve 1995;18:969–79.
[18] Simionescu L, Mosquera R, Shefner JM. Reliability of a standardized form of modified multipoint MUNE. Amyotroph Lateral Scler Other Motor Neuron Disord 2007;8 (Suppl 1):41.
[19] Daube J. Estimating the number of motor units in a muscle. J Clin Neurophysiol 1995;12: 585–94.
[20] Lomen-Hoerth C, Slawnych M. Statistical motor unit number estimation: from theory to practice. Muscle Nerve 2003;28:263–72.
[21] Lomen-Hoerth C, Olney R. Effect of recording window and stimulation variables on the statistical technique of motor unit number estimation. Muscle Nerve 2001;24:1659–64.
[22] Shefner J, Jillapalli D, Bradshaw D. Reducing intersubject variability in motor unit number estimation. Muscle Nerve 1999;22:1457–60.
[23] Jillapalli D, Shefner J. Single motor unit variability with threshold stimulation in patients with amyotrophic lateral sclerosis and normal subjects. Muscle Nerve 2004;30:578–84.
[24] Olney R, Yuen E, Engstrom J. Statistical motor unit number estimation: reproducibility and sources of error in patients with amyotrophic lateral sclerosis. Muscle Nerve 2000;23:193–7.
[25] Miller T, Kogelnik A, Olney R. Proposed modification to data analysis for statistical motor unit number estimate. Muscle Nerve 2004;29:700–6.
[26] Blok J, Visser G, de Graaf S, et al. Statistical motor unit number estimation assuming a binomial distribution. Muscle Nerve 2005;31:182–91.

[27] Ridall PG, Pettitt AN, Henderson RD, et al. Motor unit number estimation–a Bayesian approach. Biometrics 2006;62(4):1235–50.
[28] Henderson RD, Ridall GR, Pettitt AN, et al. The stimulus-response curve and motor unit variability in normal subjects and subjects with amyotrophic lateral sclerosis. Muscle Nerve 2006;34(1):34–43.
[29] Brown W, Strong M, Snow R. Methods for estimating numbers of motor units in biceps-brachialis muscles and losses of motor units with aging. Muscle Nerve 1988;11: 423–31.
[30] Stashuk D. Decomposition and quantitative analysis of clinical electromyographic signals. Med Eng Phys 1999;21:389–404.
[31] Doherty T, Stashuk D. Decomposition-based quantitative electromyography: methods and initial normative data in five muscles. Muscle Nerve 2003;28:204–11.
[32] Lawson V, Bromberg M, Stashuk D. Comparison of conventional and decomposition-enhanced spike triggered averaging techniques. Clin Neurophysiol 2004;115:564–8.
[33] Boe S, Stashuk D, Brown W, et al. Decomposition-based quantitative electromyography: effect of force on motor unit potentials and motor unit number estimates. Muscle Nerve 2005;31:365–73.
[34] Boe S, Stashuk D, Doherty T. Motor unit number estimation by decomposition-enhanced spike-triggered averaging: control data, test-retest reliability, and contractile level effects. Muscle Nerve 2004;29:693–9.
[35] Kuether G, Lipinski H-G. Computer simulation of neuron degeneration in motor neuron disease. Amsterdam: Elsevier; 1988.
[36] Andres P, Finison L, Conlon T, et al. Use of composite scores (megascores) to measure deficit in amyotrophic lateral sclerosis. Neurology 1988;38:405–8.
[37] Cedarbaum J, Stambler N, et al. The ALSFRS-R: a revised ALS functional rating scale that incorporates assessments of respiratory function. J Neurol Sci 1999;169:13–21.
[38] Traynor BJ, Zhang H, Shefner JM, et al. Functional outcome measures as clinical trial endpoints in ALS. Neurology 2004;63(10):1933–5.
[39] Dantes M, McComas A. The extent and time course of motorneuron involvement in amyotrophic lateral sclerosis. Muscle Nerve 1991;14:416–21.
[40] Munsat T, Davies K. Spinal muscular atrophy. 2nd edition. London: Royal Society of Medicine Press; 1997.
[41] Bromberg M, Swoboda K. Motor unit number estimation in infants and children with spinal muscular atrophy. Muscle Nerve 2002;25:445–7.
[42] Swoboda K, Prior T, McNaught T, et al. Natural history of denervation in SMA: relation to age, SMN2 copy number, and function. Ann Neurol 2005;57:704–12.
[43] Appel V, Stewart S, Smith G, et al. A rating scale for amyotrophic lateral sclerosis: description and preliminary experience. Ann Neurol 1987;22:328–33.
[44] Felice K. A longitudinal study comparing thenar motor unit number estimates to other quantitative tests in patients with amyotrophic lateral sclerosis. Muscle Nerve 1997;20: 179–85.
[45] Bromberg M, Forshew D, Nau K, et al. Motor unit number estimation, isometric strength, and electromyographic measures in amyotrophic lateral sclerosis. Muscle Nerve 1993;16: 1213–9.
[46] Bryan W. MUNE as an endpoint in clinical trials. In: Bromberg M, editor. Motor unit number estimation (MUNE), vol. 55Amsterdam: Elsevier; 2003. p. 324–8.
[47] Aggarwal A, Nicholson G. Normal complement of motor units in asymptomatic familial (SOD1 mutation) amyotrophic lateral sclerosis carriers. J Neurol Neurosurg Psychiatry 2001;71(4):478–81.
[48] Aggarwal A, Nicholson G. Detection of preclinical motor neurone loss in SOD1 mutation carriers using motor unit number estimation. J Neurol Neurosurg Psychiatry 2002;73(2): 199–201.

[49] Bromberg M, Fries T, Forshew D, et al. Electrophysiologic endpoint measures in a multicenter ALS drug trial. J Neurol Sci 2001;184:51–5.
[50] Shefner J, Cudkowicz M, Zhang M, et al, Northeast ALS Consortium. The use of statistical MUNE in a multicenter clinical trial. Muscle Nerve 2004;30:463–9.
[51] Shefner JM, Cudkowicz ME, Zhang H, et al. Revised statistical motor unit number estimation in the Celecoxib/ALS trial. Muscle Nerve 2007;35(2):228–34.

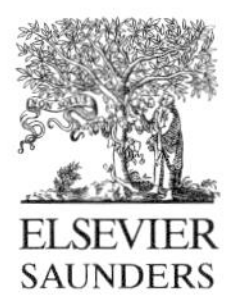

ELSEVIER
SAUNDERS

Phys Med Rehabil Clin N Am
19 (2008) 533–543

PHYSICAL MEDICINE
AND REHABILITATION
CLINICS OF
NORTH AMERICA

Fatigue in Amyotrophic Lateral Sclerosis

Jau-Shin Lou, MD, PhD

ALS Center of Oregon, Oregon Health & Science University, 3181 SW Sam Jackson Park Road, CR120, Portland, OR 97239, USA

The hallmark of amyotrophic lateral sclerosis (ALS) is progressive muscular weakness that leads to immobility, loss of ability to speak and swallow, and eventual respiratory failure [1]. Because there are no effective treatments for the disease and the only approved pharmacologic treatment (Riluzole) extends survival by only 2 months, the focus of ALS care is supportive care to palliate symptoms and improve quality of life. There are two primary examples of supportive care interventions in ALS. Percutaneous endoscopic gastrostomy (PEG) is used for administering tube feedings to prevent the negative effects of dehydration and starvation in people with ALS who are losing the ability to swallow [2]. Noninvasive positive pressure ventilation (NIPPV), delivered via a mask strapped over the mouth and nose, is used to maintain oxygenation when respiratory muscle function is impaired. This intervention extends survival and improves quality of life through beneficial effects on sleep and emotional status [3].

Fatigue is an understudied clinical problem in ALS and is often overlooked by clinicians who care for people with ALS. About 20% of ALS patients indicate that they have severe suffering [4]. Because it is a rapidly progressive and fatal disease without a cure [5], some patients with the option of physician-assisted suicide will choose to do so. In Oregon, where physician-assisted suicide is legal, ALS patients are 25 times more likely than those dying of other terminal illnesses to die by lethal ingestion [6]. In the Netherlands, 20% of all people with ALS die by euthanasia or physician-assisted suicide [7]. In addition, many ALS patients decline treatments that both sustain life and improve quality of life (QoL), such as noninvasive ventilation and PEG [8]. It is possible that more people with ALS would accept life-sustaining treatments and be less interested in physician-assisted dying if symptoms, such as fatigue, were better addressed to improve quality

E-mail address: louja@ohsu.edu

1047-9651/08/$ - see front matter
doi:10.1016/j.pmr.2008.02.001

of life. Thus, it is imperative for health care providers to understand the mechanisms of fatigue and treat fatigue effectively to improve quality of life in patients with ALS.

Approaching fatigue in ALS

One can evaluate fatigue systematically following the chart in Fig. 1 [9]. The first step in assessing fatigue in ALS is to use a questionnaire to evaluate subjective fatigue. Questionnaires commonly used for fatigue include the Multidimensional Fatigue Inventory (MFI), the Fatigue Severity Scale (FSS), the Piper Fatigue Scale, and the Visual Analog Scale of fatigue. The author prefers to use the MFI because it is a multidimensional instrument that evaluates physical fatigue and mental fatigue independently. After one establishes that subjective physical fatigue is present, one can use a continuous supramaximal force exercise paradigm or an intermittent submaximal force exercise paradigm to quantify physical fatigue objectively in a laboratory setting. While questionnaires assess the severity of subjective fatigue over days to weeks, exercise protocols assess the severity of physical fatigue over seconds to minutes. Therefore, the severity of subjective fatigue

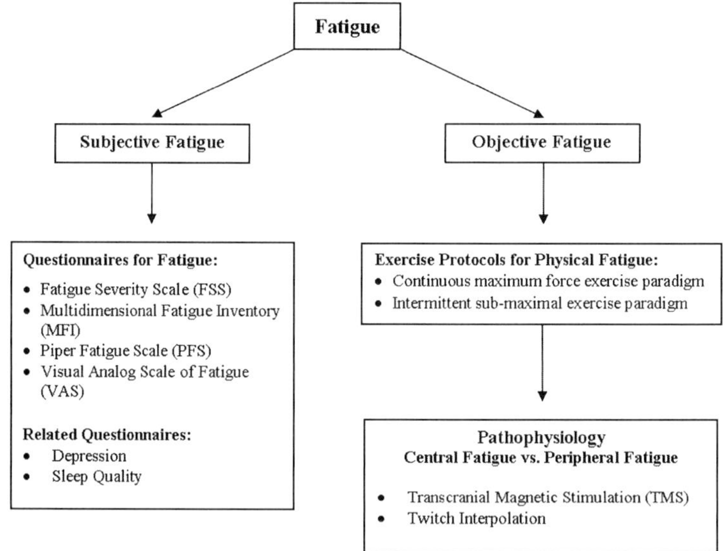

Fig. 1. Approaching fatigue in ALS. Fatigue has many different components. Fatigue studies can address subjective (how the patients feels) or objective (measured in a laboratory setting) fatigue. Subjective fatigue is studied using questionnaires. Objective fatigue is measured using force exercise paradigms. Further study of fatigue pathophysiology can elucidate if fatigue is central (upper and lower motor neurons) or peripheral (neuromuscular junction or muscle). Transcranial magnetic stimulation and twitch interpolation can also be used to study pathophysiology of fatigue.

as measured by questionnaires may not correlate with the severity of physical fatigue measured by exercise protocols.

To further understand the pathophysiology of physical fatigue, one can use additional techniques, such as twitch interpolation and transcranial magnetic stimulation, to identify whether the fatigue is peripheral (in the neuromuscular junction or the muscles) or central (in upper motor neurons and lower motor neurons).

Though research into fatigue in ALS has been limited, a number of studies have scratched the surface by employing each of these techniques. However, it is not clear if fatigue in ALS: (a) remains an independent symptom that is treatable after treating other symptoms, such as depression, pain, or dyspnea; (b) simply reflects the effects of other pathophysiologic constructs, such as sleep problems, dyspnea, or depression; or (c) is associated with other symptoms because they share a common cause [10].

ALS subjects report more subjective fatigue than normal controls

The author has used the MFI to compare the fatigue in ALS subjects with normal controls and examined the influence of fatigue on QoL, as measured by the McGill Quality of Life (MQoL) questionnaire [11]. The MFI is a 20-item self-report instrument designed to measure fatigue [12]. The 20 items cover five dimensions of fatigue: general fatigue, physical fatigue, mental fatigue, reduced motivation, and reduced activity. This study demonstrated that subjects with ALS reported more fatigue than normal controls, and fatigue severity correlated inversely with QoL. Compared with normal controls, ALS subjects reported more general fatigue, physical fatigue, and reduced activity, but not mental fatigue or reduced motivation (Fig. 2). Most importantly, the author found that the severity of fatigue and depression did not correlate with disease severity, as measured by the ALS functional rating scale (ALSFRS), muscle strength, or disease duration. Severity of general fatigue contributed significantly to more severe physical symptoms, as measured by a subscale in the MQoL. Higher depression scores were correlated with increased mental fatigue but not physical fatigue. This cross-sectional pilot study demonstrated that fatigue and depression in ALS subjects are important predictors of QoL and that fatigue and depression are independent of physical function. Although the author and colleagues still do not have an effective treatment for ALS, treating fatigue and depression aggressively in ALS patients may improve their QoL.

In addition to muscle weakness, depression, poor pulmonary function, and poor quality of sleep might contribute to fatigue in ALS patients. Depression is common in ALS patients: more than 40% of ALS subjects in two studies had depressive symptoms [13,14]. Approximately 10% of ALS subjects met criteria for major depressive disorder [4,15]. The author and colleagues need further study to examine if treating depression aggressively will reduce fatigue in ALS patients.

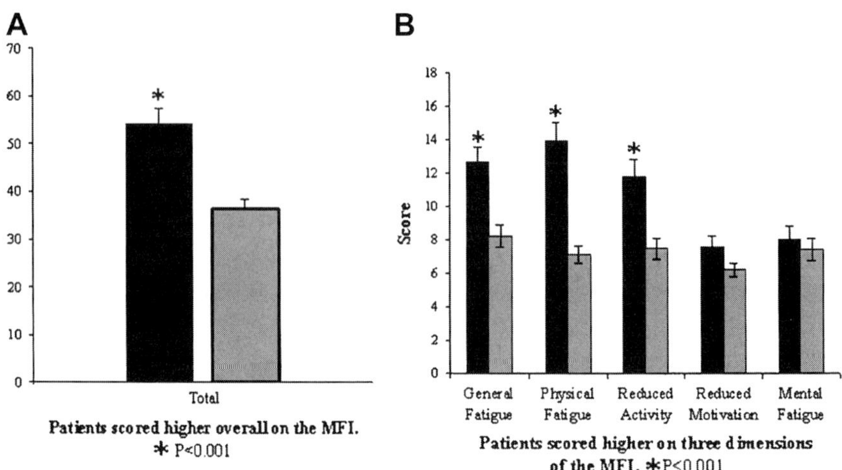

Fig. 2. Comparisons of total scores and subscores between patients ($n = 25$) and control groups ($n = 32$). Black bars = patients, gray bars = controls. (*A*) MFI total scores (mean ± standard error). (*B*) Subscores for the five dimensions of the MFI (mean ± standard error). (*Reprinted from* Lou JS, Reeves A, Benice T, et al. Fatigue and depression are associated with poor quality of life in ALS. Neurology 2003;60(1):122–3, with permission.)

Poor pulmonary function might cause fatigue through mechanisms such as insomnia, hypersomnia, and exercise intolerance. Standard pulmonary function testing has been used to assess the progression of respiratory muscle weakness in ALS. Forced vital capacity (FVC) is indicative of both inspiratory and expiratory muscle strength. Peak inspiratory pressures are more specific indicators of diaphragmatic function, which correlates with a subject's ability to ventilate, and are inversely correlated with the frequency and degree of sleep-disordered breathing. Lower peak inspiratory pressures are associated with lower QoL in ALS patients [16].

Poor quality of sleep and excessive daytime somnolence might also contribute to fatigue in ALS. ALS patients have reduced total sleep time, reduced sleep efficiency, and increased apneas and hypopneas [17]. Whether specific aspects of sleep affect fatigue in ALS patients remains unknown.

ALS subjects have more objective fatigue than normal controls

Physical fatigue in ALS cannot be totally attributed to muscle weakness. Sanjak and colleagues [18] examined the relationship between weakness and fatigue in 54 ALS subjects compared with normal controls. Subjects performed 30 seconds of sustained maximal voluntary isometric contraction of elbow flexors, knee extensors, and ankle dorsiflexors, using a computerized force measurement system and standardized testing procedures. They used a continuous maximum force exercise paradigm to calculate the Fatigue Index (Fig. 3B). Fatigue was greater in ALS subjects than in normal

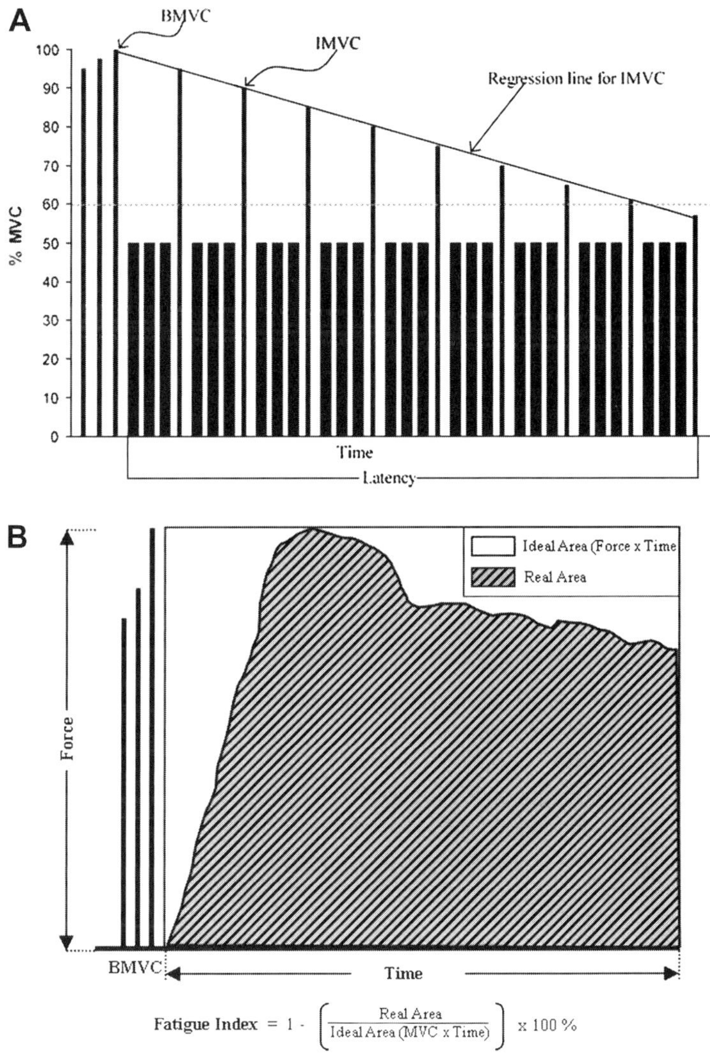

Fig. 3. The intermittent submaximal force exercise paradigm versus the continuous maximum force exercise paradigm. At the beginning of the trial, the subject is encouraged to generate as much force as possible. The largest force of three attempts is the maximal voluntary contraction (MVC) or baseline MVC (BMVC). (*A*) In the intermittent paradigm, each subject then performs cycles of exercise lasting for 10 seconds to 7 seconds of muscle contraction at 50% of BMVC and 3 seconds of rest. An interval maximal voluntary contraction (IMVC) is performed after every three cycles. This continues until the subject develops fatigue, defined as the inability to generate an IMVC greater than 60% of BMVC. (*B*) In the continuous maximum force paradigm, subjects try to maintain the muscle contraction at the maximal force for a period of time (for example, 30 seconds). The actual force generated (the curved line) will decline because of development of fatigue. The fatigue index is calculated as 1 minus the real area divided by the ideal area (time × MVC) times 100%. A higher Fatigue Index indicates more fatigue. (*Reprinted from* Lou JS, Kearns G, Benice T, et al. Levodopa improves physical fatigue in Parkinson's disease—a double blind, placebo-controlled crossover study. Mov Disord 2003;18(10):1108–14; with permission.)

controls (mean = 23% versus 15%, $p<.001$) in all muscles, including muscles that were not clearly weak. They found that muscle weakness and fatigue were poorly correlated in ALS subjects.

Both peripheral fatigue and central fatigue contribute to physical fatigue in ALS. Voluntary force generation in the maximal or submaximal exercise paradigm results from a sequence of events, and each of these is a potential site for developing fatigue [19]. These events (Fig. 4) include all central nervous system processes influencing excitation and activation of the upper motor neurons, including motivational factors and integration of sensory information, the conduction along the pyramidal tract, activation of lower motor neurons in the anterior horn of the spinal cord, the signal transfer along the lower motor neuron, and across the neuromuscular junction. In

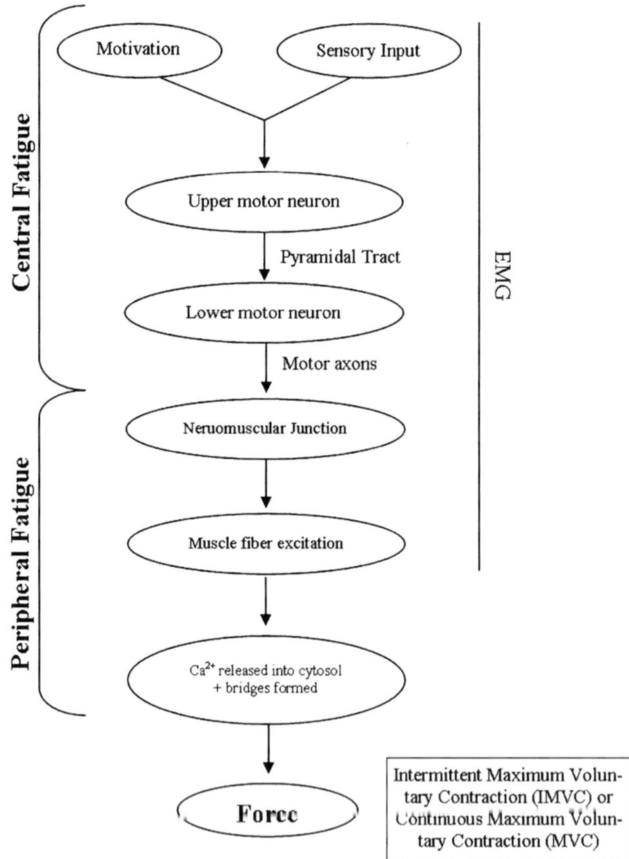

Fig. 4. Central and peripheral aspects of fatigue. Central fatigue is defined as fatigue originating at or proximal to the anterior horn cells. Peripheral fatigue occurs at or distal to the neuromuscular junction. EMG, twitch interpolation, and transcranial magnetic stimulation can be used to determine if fatigue (measured by IMVC or MVC) is central or peripheral.

addition, events occurring in the muscle during exercise can cause fatigue. Central fatigue refers to reduced force generation caused by events proximal to the neuromuscular junction. Peripheral fatigue refers to the failure at or beyond the neuromuscular junction.

Peripheral fatigue

Using an intermittent submaximal isometric contraction protocol (see Fig. 3A), Sharma and colleagues [20,21] showed that physical fatigue in ALS subjects is caused by peripheral fatigue. Both maximum voluntary force and tetanic force induced by electrical stimulation declined more in ALS subjects than in normal controls, suggesting that ALS patients have more objective physical fatigue. The similar decline in voluntary force and tetanic force indicated that most physical fatigue was peripheral in origin, located at a site distal to lower motor neurons. Furthermore, they demonstrated that evoked compound muscle action potential (CMAP) amplitude did not decline, indicating ALS patients have no neuromuscular transmission failure. In spite of greater fatigability, changes during exercise in energy metabolites and proton signal intensity tended to be less in ALS subjects compared with controls, suggesting impaired muscular activation. They concluded that the greater muscle fatigue in ALS patients results from impaired muscle activation, caused in part to alterations distal to the muscle membrane [20].

Sharma and Miller [21] subsequently demonstrated that increased muscle fatigability in ALS patients is partly because of dissociation between electrical and mechanical muscle properties. They compared motor unit potentials, muscle force, and muscle fatigability in subjects with ALS and controls, using low to moderate intensity voluntary contraction. The enlarged motor units in subjects negatively correlated to the muscle force and positively correlated to muscle fatigability. Furthermore, after an average 9-month follow-up, the decline in force was greater than the decline in the amplitude of the CMAP, suggesting a relative dissociation between electrical and mechanical properties. They concluded that increased fatigue in ALS patients is associated with enlarged motor units that are mechanically less efficient and fatigue faster than normal muscles.

Using a continuous maximal exercise protocol and power spectrum analysis of surface EMG, Sanjak and colleagues [22] showed that the dissociation between mechanical and myoelectrical signals contributed to peripheral fatigue in ALS. During the MVC, the power spectrum analysis of the surface EMG showed changes in two variables: amplitude and frequency. The decline in the amplitude of the power spectrum indicates central fatigue, and a shift of power spectrum toward a lower frequency fatigue indicates peripheral fatigue [23]. Sanjak and colleagues [22] showed that in ALS subjects, the reduction in IMVC during 30-second contractions is much higher than that in normal controls. However, the shift in the frequency of the power spectrum in ALS patients was much less than that of the normal controls. Sanjak and colleagues suggested that the dissociation between the reduction in IMVC and the shift in power spectrum indicated that excessive fatigue in the ALS patients is caused by peripheral fatigue because of a reduction in muscle fiber conduction velocity. They further suggested that group atrophy observed in both type I and II muscle fibers and muscle fiber grouping into large motor units may lead to a reduction in IMVC, but less shift in the power spectrum frequency.

Changes in axonal excitability after MVC also cause peripheral fatigue in ALS. Vucic and colleagues [24] recently studied nerve excitability changes before and after MVC in ALS and normal subjects. There was a greater increase in threshold after MVC in ALS subjects, accompanied by a reduction in the amplitude of the CMAP generated by a submaximal stimulus. In addition, activity-dependent hyperpolarization is more prominent in ALS subjects than in normal controls.

Central fatigue

Central fatigue also plays a role in increased objective physical fatigue in ALS patients. Kent-Braun and Miller [25] used the technique of twitch interpolation and compared voluntary and electrically stimulated force, central and peripheral indices of muscle activation, and intramuscular energy metabolism before and during intermittent submaximal isometric ankle dorsiflexion in seven ALS subjects and six normal controls. In the technique of twitch interpolation, an electrical stimulus is delivered to the muscle or nerve to evoke a maximal evocable force (MEF). The MEF is the force generated by a muscle when additional electrical stimulation does not increase force. Based on this technique, central fatigue can be defined as any exercise-induced reduction in maximal voluntary contraction force that is not accompanied by the same reduction in MEF. In peripheral fatigue, there is a parallel decrease in MVC and MEF. Using this technique, Kent-Braun and Miller demonstrated that at the end of fatiguing exercise, only the ALS group had an increase in the added force in response to a stimulus train imposed during MVC, indicating significant central fatigue in ALS.

In summary, the severity of physical fatigue in ALS does not correlate with muscle weakness. Physical fatigue in ALS has both central and peripheral components.

Treatment of fatigue in ALS

No double-blind, placebo-controlled trials have been performed for the treatment of fatigue in ALS. Carter and colleagues [26], studied the effect of modafinil in ALS in an open-label study. Fifteen ALS subjects took 200-mg or 400-mg modafinil in an open label fashion for 2 weeks. Following treatment, mean scores on the FSS decreased from 51.3 plus or minus 9.2 to 42.8 plus or minus 10.2. On the Epworth Sleepiness Scale (ESS), mean scores decreased from 8.2 plus or minus 2.0 to 4.5 plus or minus 2.4. Reductions in both the FSS and the ESS were significant ($p<.001$). Mean scores on the self-report version of the Functional Independence Measure increased from 115.2 plus or minus 5.6 to 118.1 plus or minus 5.4, with $p<.01$. No patients dropped out because of side effects. Reported side effects included diarrhea, headache, nervousness, and insomnia. This pilot study suggests that modafinil is well tolerated and may reduce symptoms of fatigue in ALS. Further blinded, controlled studies of modafinil in larger numbers of ALS patients are therefore warranted.

Other studies have used fatigue as a secondary outcome measure. NIPPV reduced fatigue in ALS subjects [27]. The study assessed the impact of NIPPV on pulmonary function studies, QoL, and survival in patients with ALS. The severity of fatigue was assessed by a subscore of the Chronic Respiratory Index Questionnaire. This index evaluates quality of life along four dimensions: dyspnea, fatigue, emotional, and sense of control over the disease (mastery). It was administered before and after initiation of NIPPV. Of 47 subjects started on NIPPV, 23 were tolerant and 24 were intolerant. Tolerance of NIPPV was strictly defined as the ability to sleep with the device for at least four consecutive hours nightly. NIPPV did not change the rate of decline of the FVC. Fatigue and mastery scores were improved by NIPPV. Median survivals in subjects intolerant and tolerant of NIPPV were 5 and 20 months, respectively ($p = .002$). Although NIPPV has no impact on the rate of decline of lung function, it may improve fatigue.

High-frequency chest wall oscillation (HFCWO) decreased fatigue measured by the FSS and showed a trend toward slowing the decline of forced vital capacity in patients with impaired breathing [28]. HFCWO was well tolerated, considered helpful by a majority of patients, and decreased symptoms of breathlessness. In HFCWO, a high-frequency oscillation applied to the chest wall transmits reversing oscillatory pressures rapidly through the chest wall and into the airways. This technique dramatically increases mucous clearance and enhanced gas exchange in the lung [29,30]. Forty-six subjects participated in this 12-week randomized, controlled trial of HFCWO and 35 completed the trial. HFCWO users ($n = 19$) had less breathlessness and coughed more at night at 12 weeks compared with baseline. There were no significant differences in FVC change. When patients with FVC between 40% and 70% predicted were analyzed, HFCWO subjects showed less decrease in FVC and less increased fatigue and breathlessness than subjects not receiving HFCWO.

Resistance exercise did not reduce fatigue measured by FSS but improved function, as measured by total ALSFRS, upper and lower extremity subscale scores, and quality of life in a 6-month long trial [31]. Of 33 subjects screened for the study, 27 were randomly assigned (resistance = 13; usual care = 14) to study groups. Eight resistance exercise subjects and 10 usual care subjects completed the trial. At 6 months, the resistance exercise group had significantly higher ALSFRS and SF-36 physical function subscale scores. No adverse events related to the intervention occurred. More than 30% of the subjects dropped out of the study, mostly because of the progression of the disease.

Summary

Research of fatigue in ALS is still at an early stage. It is imperative for clinicians to better understand fatigue in ALS and develop effective treatment for fatigue. Doing so may improve quality of life in ALS patients. There is no effective treatment for fatigue in ALS; however, a small open label study showed modafinil may be helpful. Interventions, such as noninvasive ventilation or high-frequency chest wall oscillation, may also reduce fatigue. Further study is needed to evaluate if treating depression or improving nutrition with PEG will reduce fatigue. Additional exploration of fatigue in ALS should focus on whether it remains an independent symptom that is treatable after treating other symptoms, whether it simply reflects the effects of other pathophysiologic constructs, or whether it is associated with other symptoms because they share a common cause [10].

Acknowledgments

The author thanks Grace Arnold for her skillful editing.

References

[1] Rowland LP, Shneider NA. Amyotrophic lateral sclerosis. N Engl J Med 2001;344(22): 1688–700.

[2] Mitsumoto H, Davidson M, Moore D, et al. Percutaneous endoscopic gastrostomy (PEG) in patients with ALS and bulbar dysfunction. Amyotroph Lateral Scler Other Motor Neuron Disord 2003;4(3):177–85.

[3] Bourke SC, Bullock RE, Williams TL, et al. Noninvasive ventilation in ALS: indications and effect on quality of life. Neurology 2003;61(2):171–7.

[4] Ganzini L, Johnston WS, Hoffman WF. Correlation of suffering in amyotrophic lateral sclerosis. Neurology 1999;52(7):1434–40.

[5] Mitsumoto H, Del Bene M. Improving the quality of life for people with ALS: the challenge ahead. Amyotroph Lateral Scler Other Motor Neuron Disord 2000;1(5):329–36.

[6] Sixth annual report on Oregon's Death with Dignity Act. Oregon Department of Human Services; 2004.

[7] Veldink JH, Wokke JH, van der Wal G, et al. Euthanasia and physician-assisted suicide among patients with amyotrophic lateral sclerosis in the Netherlands. N Engl J Med 2002; 346(21):1638–44.

[8] Bradley WG, Anderson F, Bromberg M, et al. Current management of ALS-comparison of the ALS CARE database and the AAN practice parameter. Neurology 2001;57(3):500–4.

[9] Lou JS. Approaching fatigue in neuromuscular diseases. Phys Med Rehabil Clin N Am 2005; 16(4):1063–79.

[10] Barsevick AM, Dudley W, Beck S, et al. A randomized clinical trial of energy conservation for patients with cancer-related fatigue. Cancer 2004;100(6):1302–10.

[11] Lou JS, Kearns G, Benice T, et al. Levodopa improves physical fatigue in Parkinson's disease—a double blind, placebo-controlled crossover study. Mov Disord 2003;18(10): 1108–14.
[12] Smets EM, Garssen B, Bonke B, et al. The multidimensional fatigue inventory (MFI) psychometric quantities of an instrument to assess fatigue. J Psychosom Res 1995;39(3):315–25.
[13] Lou JS, Reeves A, Benice T, et al. Fatigue and depression are associated with poor quality of life in ALS. Neurology 2003;60(1):122–3.
[14] Boynton De Sepulveda L. Identification of psychological well-being and depression in an ALS population and factors influencing its presentation. The ALS CARE Program Physician Notes. 2002;26(4):193–203.
[15] Rabkin JG, Wagner GJ, Del Bene M. Resilience and distress among amyotrophic lateral sclerosis patients and caregivers. Psychosom Med 2000;62(2):271–9.
[16] Bourke SC, Shaw PJ, Gibson GJ. Respiratory function vs. sleep-disordered breathing as predictors of QOL in ALS. Neurology 2001;57(11):2040–4.
[17] Ferguson KA, Strong MJ, Ahmad D, et al. Sleep-disordered breathing in amyotrophic lateral sclerosis. Chest 1996;110(3):664–9.
[18] Sanjak M, Brinkmann J, Belden DS, et al. Quantitative assessment of motor fatigue in amyotrophic lateral sclerosis. J Neurol Sci 2001;191(1–2):55–9.
[19] Vollestad NK. Measurement of human muscle fatigue. J Neurosci Methods 1997;74(2): 219–27.
[20] Sharma KR, Kent-Braun JA, Majumdar S, et al. Physiology of fatigue in amyotrophic lateral sclerosis. Neurology 1995;45(4):733–40.
[21] Sharma KR, Miller RG. Electrical and mechanical properties of skeletal muscle underlying increased fatigue in patients with amyotrophic lateral sclerosis. Muscle Nerve 1996;20(4):469–78.
[22] Sanjak M, Konopacki R, Capasso R, et al. Dissociation between mechanical and myoelectrical manifestation of muscle fatigue in amyotrophic lateral sclerosis. Amyotroph Lateral Scler Other Motor Neuron Disord 2004;5(1):26–32.
[23] Dimitrova NA, Dimitrov GV. Interpretation of EMG changes with fatigue: facts, pitfalls, and fallacies. J Electromyogr Kinesiol 2003;13(1):13–36.
[24] Vucic S, Krishnan AV, Kiernan MC. Fatigue and activity dependent changes in axonal excitability in amyotrophic lateral sclerosis. J Neurol Neurosurg Psychiatry 2007;78(11): 1202–8.
[25] Kent-Braun J, Miller RG. Central fatigue during isometric exercise in amyotrophic lateral sclerosis. Muscle Nerve 2000;23(6):909–14.
[26] Carter GT, Weiss MD, Lou JS, et al. Modafinil to treat fatigue in amyotrophic lateral sclerosis: an open label pilot study. Am J Hosp Palliat Care 2005;22(1):55–9.
[27] Aboussouan LS, Khan SU, Banerjee M, et al. Objective measures of the efficacy of noninvasive positive-pressure ventilation in amyotrophic lateral sclerosis. Muscle Nerve 2001;24(3):403–9.
[28] Lange DJ, Lechtzin N, Davey C, et al. High-frequency chest wall oscillation in ALS: an exploratory randomized, controlled trial. Neurology 2006;67(6):991–7.
[29] Rubin EM, Scantlen GE, Chapman GA, et al. Effect of chest wall oscillation on mucus clearance: comparison of two vibrators. Pediatr Pulmonol 1989;6(2):122–6.
[30] Harf A, Zidulka A, Chang HK. Nitrogen washout during tidal breathing with superimposed high-frequency chest wall oscillation. Am Rev Respir Dis 1985;132(2):350–3.
[31] Bello-Haas VD, Florence JM, Kloos AD, et al. A randomized controlled trial of resistance exercise in individuals with ALS. Neurology 2007;68(23):2003–7.

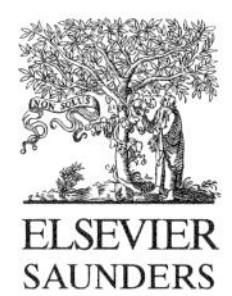
ELSEVIER
SAUNDERS

Phys Med Rehabil Clin N Am
19 (2008) 545–557

PHYSICAL MEDICINE
AND REHABILITATION
CLINICS OF
NORTH AMERICA

The Role of Exercise in Amyotrophic Lateral Sclerosis

Amy Chen, MD, PhD[a,*],
Jacqueline Montes, PT, MA, NCS[b],
Hiroshi Mitsumoto, MD, DSc[c,d]

[a]*Department of Neurology, Columbia University, 710 West 168th Street, 9th Floor, New York, NY 10032, USA*
[b]*SMA Clinical Research Center, Department of Neurology, Columbia University, 180 Ft. Washington Avenue, 5th Floor, New York, NY 10032, USA*
[c]*College of Physicians and Surgeons, Columbia University, 710 West 168th Street, New York, NY 10032, USA*
[d]*Neuromuscular Diseases Division, Eleanor & Lou Gehrig MDA/ALS Center, Columbia University, 710 West 168th Street, New York, NY 10032, USA*

Amyotrophic lateral sclerosis (ALS) is a neurodegenerative disease affecting the motor nervous system, involving the cortex, brainstem, and spinal cord. It causes progressive and cumulative physical disabilities in patients, and leads to eventual death due to respiratory muscle failure. The incidence of ALS is 1 to 2 cases per 100,000 population per year, and the prevalence is 4 to 7 cases per 100,000 population because of the short mean survival time [1]. It is estimated that 10,000 to 25,000 people are affected by ALS in the United States at any time. The disease is diverse in its presentation, course, and progression. We do not yet fully understand the cause or causes of the disease, nor the mechanisms for its progression; thus, we lack effective means for treating it. Currently, we rely on a multidisciplinary approach to manage and care for patients who have ALS symptomatically [2]. Rehabilitation plays an essential role in the care of patients who have ALS, along with pharmacologic interventions, respiratory support, nutritional supplements, communication devices, and social and psychologic support [3]. In

This work was supported in part by MDA Wings Over Wall Street; the MDA Center Block Fund; the Judith & Jean Page Adams Charitable Foundation; Spina Family Golf for Life, Ride for Life; the Bowen Gold Outing; and other philanthropic donations.

* Corresponding author.
E-mail address: achen@neuro.columbia.edu (A. Chen).

1047-9651/08/$ - see front matter. Published by Elsevier Inc.
doi:10.1016/j.pmr.2008.02.003

the authors' experience, one of the most frequently asked questions by patients who have ALS is whether exercise is beneficial.

In this article, the authors review the literature on the role of exercise in patients who have ALS, and briefly compare what is known about exercise in other neuromuscular diseases. Specifically, they ask

1. What types of exercise (stretching, resistance/strengthening, and aerobic/endurance training) have been examined in patients who have ALS?
2. What kinds of exercise regimens (intensity, duration, and frequency) are beneficial for patients who have ALS?
3. What are the demonstrated benefits and how are they measured?

The authors also reviewed animal studies for comparison. They hope to determine whether clinicians may safely recommend a structured exercise regimen as a treatment intervention for patients who have ALS.

Importance of exercise for the general public

Exercise is widely promoted to the general population because of its great benefit to health and wellbeing. In 1996, the American Surgeon General published a health report [4] recommending (1) regular physical activity, consisting of moderate-intensity exercise for at least 30 minutes on most days of the week, for the general population of all ages; (2) more vigorous intensity of physical activity and of longer duration for greater health benefit; and (3) strength-developing exercises at least twice a week for most adults, to supplement the benefits of cardiorespiratory endurance exercise.

The health benefits of physical activity include enhancement of the cardiovascular, respiratory, musculoskeletal, and endocrine function, and psychologic wellbeing [5]. Moreover, exercise lowers the risks of developing chronic diseases that are associated with inflammation, such as coronary heart disease [6], hypertension [7], colon cancer [8], and diabetes mellitus [9]. The authors briefly discuss the potential mechanisms by which exercise improves health and reduces inflammation, based on data that are mostly derived from healthy people and animal studies.

Mechanisms by which exercise benefits health

Myofiber remodeling

During exercise, myofibers are activated, either by mechanochemical or mechanoelectric signals, which lead to an increased intracellular calcium concentration and subsequent signaling cascades. An intricate network of coordinated gene expressions, which are not yet fully understood, is then responsible for myofiber remodeling. Type I slow-twitch oxidative myofibers are induced after exercise training, as evidenced by the induction of myoglobin, troponin I slow, and myosin heavy chain type I molecules [10]. The transition of myofibers from type II to type I may allow for enhanced muscle adaptability and a greater insulin-induced glucose uptake, thus presenting a lower risk for developing diabetes mellitus [11].

With exercise also comes an enhanced beta-oxidation of fatty acids, which is caused by the induction of the peroxisome proliferator activated receptor and its coactivator 1 (PGC-1α) [12]. This results in an enhanced metabolism of fat and a reduction of adipose tissues, and, conceivably, contributing to the consequent reduction of inflammation associated with sedentary lifestyle. Resistance training also causes muscle hypertrophy, which is mediated by insulin-like growth factor (IGF-1) and the target of rapamycin (TOR) signaling pathway [13,14].

Antioxidative and anti-inflammatory adaptation

Besides modifying the muscle fiber types and mass, exercise also causes an initial increase in free radical production and oxidative stress, which is counteracted by the subsequent activation of the endogenous antioxidative defense mechanism [15,16]. A new homeostasis is achieved; thus, regular exercise of moderate intensity appears to result in a lower basal state of oxidative stress level [17–19]. Depending on the duration and intensity of the exercise and the age of the person, the myokine interleukin-6 is produced following exercise. It contributes to health by activating downstream anti-inflammatory pathways and enhancing the metabolic and immunologic response [20–22], which ultimately benefits the cardiovascular system in healthy and disease states [23].

Central nervous system stimulation and plasticity

Exercise has an effect on the central nervous system; reorganization and an increase in motor neuron excitability have been demonstrated in the motor cortex and the spinal cord following resistance training [24,25]. The central nervous system thus has a role in contributing to increased strength following exercise training.

Neuroendocrine effect

Exercise also activates the hypothalamic-pituitary-adrenal (HPA) axis, increases the production of cortisol and catecholamines, and enhances cellular metabolism [26]. However, the interplay of exercise on the neuroendocrine system, including the HPA axis, the thyroid function, and the reproductive hormones, is complex. The response of the neuroendocrine system depends on the intensity, type, and duration of exercise, as well as the age, gender, and fitness level of the person. Although exercise in general benefits health, in some cases such as chronic intense training, it may affect the neuroendocrine system negatively [27]. This possibility should be borne in mind whenever exercise regimens are being recommended.

Exercise and neuromuscular diseases

In a recent meta-analysis by the Cochrane review group of 35 exercise trials in muscle diseases from 1966 to 2002, only two studies met rigorously defined criteria for inclusion [28]. To be included, studies have to be randomized, use a nonintervention group as a comparison, and have a standardized training protocol of at least 10 weeks' duration. One study involved patients who had fascioescapulohumeral muscular dystrophy and the other, myotonic dystrophy. The investigators concluded that in patients who had either of these two diseases, moderate intensity strength training showed no significant benefit or harm.

A more inclusive review of exercise studies in patients who had neuromuscular diseases found 58 studies to be of sufficient methodological quality for analysis [29]. The investigators examined the effects of strengthening exercise, aerobic exercise, or a combination of the two, in diseases of the anterior horn cells, nerves, and muscles. Nearly all the studies included an individualized, progressive strengthening protocol as defined by established guidelines for healthy adults [30] and the protocols were of moderate intensity. Despite variations in the types of exercises and muscle used, the interventions in nearly all disease groups caused no adverse effects. The investigators concluded that the combination of strengthening and aerobic exercises is likely to be effective (level II evidence) in patients who have muscle diseases, and that aerobic exercises may be effective (level III evidence) for patients who have muscle diseases. In addition, breathing exercises may be effective (level III evidence) for patients who have myasthenia gravis and neuromuscular diseases. Evidence was insufficient of a beneficial effect of strengthening alone in all neuromuscular diseases included in the review.

Rehabilitation for patients who have stroke and multiple sclerosis deserves some mentioning here, because these patients often exhibit spasticity, which is also commonly seen in patients who have ALS. A systematic review of progressive resistance strength training in poststroke patients showed that such training can increase muscle strength without increasing spasticity or reducing range of movement [31]. A review of the literature on physical training and multiple sclerosis also showed that exercise is beneficial for these patients, without adverse effects [32,33]. These findings are encouraging and suggest that exercise may be safely applied to ALS patients who have spasticity.

Exercise and amyotrophic lateral sclerosis (human studies)

Below, the authors review studies of exercise, grouped by the types of exercise regimen, in patients who have ALS.

Stretching exercise

Stretching, or exercises that improve flexibility, can maintain muscle and soft tissue extensibility and joint mobility, and can prevent contractures [34].

Muscle weakness in ALS can cause an imbalance between agonist and antagonist muscle groups, predisposing patients who have ALS to muscle shortening, joint contractures, and poor posture. Claw hand deformity is a good example of this disparity and occurs in ALS patients. Stretching weakened and unaffected muscle groups prevents contractures, maintains good postural alignment, reduces pain from hypomobility, and helps lessen the potential complexities of functional mobility and performing activities of daily living. Because stretching does not impact muscle strength, it is often used as a placebo or a control in studies examining the benefits of other types of exercise in ALS (Table 1). It, itself, has not been randomized against nonstretching in the study of exercise in ALS.

Resistance/strengthening exercise

Strengthening exercise, or exercises that are used to maintain or improve a muscle's ability to generate force, helps maintain function, avoid injury, and prevent disability [34]. Skeletal muscle weakness is the cardinal sign and symptom of motor neuron degeneration in ALS. Strengthening exercises can be tailored for weak and strong muscle groups and can be performed with or without resistance [34].

One of the first published reports of the beneficial effects of strengthening in ALS was a case study using upper extremity resistive exercise for 75 days [35]. Isometric strength, assessed with a strain gauge, demonstrated improvements in 14 upper extremity muscle groups and diminished strength in 4 muscle groups, resulting in a subjective report of functional improvement.

The first prospective, randomized study examining the effect of strengthening exercise in patients who have ALS was done in 2001 [36]. The investigators randomized 25 patients to either an exercise or a nonexercise group. A moderate-intensity exercise program was developed for the individual and performed by patients at home for 15 minutes twice a day. At 3 months, differences in functional improvements were noted between the exercise and control groups, as measured by the ALS Functional Rating Scale (ALSFRS) and the Ashworth Spasticity Scale, but not in manual muscle testing scores or reports of fatigue and quality of life. At 6 months, no significant difference was noted between the groups on any measures. Unfortunately, the investigators did not define the training regimen or the length of the training regimen more specifically, making it difficult to duplicate or use for comparison.

A multicenter, prospective, randomized study published in 2007 using 27 subjects who had ALS was the first to use a scientifically defined training protocol recognized by the American College of Sports Medicine [37]. Subjects were assigned to one of two groups: a treatment group consisting of an individually tailored, home resistance exercise program three times weekly along with a daily stretching program, or a control group consisting of a daily stretching program only, for 6 months. The exercise group had

Table 1
Exercise studies in amyotrophic lateral sclerosis

Types of exercise	Studies	Outcomes
Stretching	No RCT	
Enhances connective tissue		
Strengthening	Bohannon et al, [35] case study	Improved isometric strength in 14 U/E muscles
Myofiber remodeling		Decreased isometric strength in 4 muscles
Reduces inflammation		Subjective improvement of functions
Enhances metabolism	Drory et al, [36] randomized	Improved function (ALSFRS) at 3 months
CNS adaptation		Improved spasticity (ASS) at 3 months
		No changes in MMT, fatigue, and QOL
	Bello-Haas et al, [37] randomized	Improved function (total and subtotal ALSFRS-R) at 6 months
		Improved QOL (SF36) at 6 months
Aerobic	Sanjak et al, [40] case control	Examined biophysical and metabolic responses:
Myofiber remodeling		Increased oxygen cost of work
Reduces inflammation		Decreased lipid metabolism
Enhances metabolism	Pinto et al, [42] case control	Improved the rate of functional decline (Spinal Norris)
CNS adaptation		Improved QOL on FIM scale, but not Bartels
	Siciliano et al, [43,44] case control	Increased lactate and lipid peroxides
		Precocious anaerobic threshold achieved

Abbreviations: ALSFRS, ALS Functional Rating Scale; ALSFRS-R, ALS Functional Rating Scale-Revised; ASS, Ashworth Spasticity Scale; CNS, central nervous system; FIM, Functional Independence Measure; MMT, manual muscle testing; QOL, quality of life; RCT, randomized controlled trial; U/E, upper extremity.

significantly higher functions (as measured by the total ALSFRS and combined upper and lower extremity subtotal ALSFRS scores) and an improved qualify of life, (as measured by the 36-Item Short Form Health Survey Physical Function Subscale) at 6 months. This exercise study in ALS is the best to date, providing class II evidence of the positive effect of exercise for these patients, as defined by the American Academy of Neurology [38]. The number of subjects who were recruited and who completed the study was small; this problem is commonly encountered in ALS research, and it should be addressed in future studies.

Aerobic/endurance exercise

Aerobic exercise has been shown to maintain cardiorespiratory fitness and to benefit mood, appetite, and sleep in healthy people [39]. Few studies have been done that address whether aerobic exercise affects the functional outcomes in patients who have ALS. Instead, most of these studies were performed to examine the immediate physiologic and metabolic responses of ALS patients to exercise. The first such study was done in 1987, when investigators studied 35 ALS patients and compared their physiologic response to bicycle ergometer aerobic exercise with healthy controls [40]. They found that the autonomic response (heart rate and ventilatory response) to exercise was similar in patients and controls. However, the use of oxygen and metabolism of lipid in response to exercise is altered in patients who have ALS. It is therefore logical to ensure adequate oxygenation, aeration, and carbohydrate loads when recommending exercise for patients who have ALS. The last is especially important because studies have shown that carbohydrate supplementation in healthy subjects reduces oxidative stress load [41].

In 1999, one study was published whereby ALS patients were asked to perform a ramp treadmill exercise up to an anaerobic threshold, either with the assistance of a noninvasive ventilation (bilevel positive airway pressure) or without [42]. The investigators then measured the respiratory function, Barthel score, Functional Independence Measure Scale, and Spinal and Bulbar Norris scores. The purpose of this study was to determine if the compensation of alveolar hypoventilation with noninvasive ventilation support in ALS patients during exercise can achieve a greater conditioning effect. Their results demonstrated significant differences between the exercise group and a nonexercise control group in the rate of decline and absolute values on the Spinal Norris scale, a functional rating scale not widely used. Quality of life was different as measured by Functional Independence Measure, but not by Barthel scores. Their results suggest that exercise may be beneficial in ALS and may be performed even when respiratory insufficiency is present, with the support of noninvasive ventilation.

In subsequent years, two other studies were done to examine the oxidative stress responses in ALS patients versus controls after an incremental bicycling test, by measuring the lactate and lipoperoxide levels [43,44]. Both studies were small, with 11 and 10 patients, respectively. The investigators found that baseline lactate and lipoperoxide levels were higher in ALS patients than in controls, and that the anaerobic threshold was precociously activated in ALS patients, suggesting that mitochondrial dysfunction occurs in the exercising skeletal muscle of ALS patients.

Based on the authors' analysis, only two class II studies of exercise as a therapeutic intervention in ALS have been done [36,37]. Although both studies were small, and only single blinded, they allowed the authors to conclude that individualized strengthening exercise during the early stage of the disease is probably effective in improving the function of patients who have ALS, and such a recommendation should be considered. Although cardiovascular exercise appears safe in the early and late stages of ALS, the data are insufficient at this time to make further recommendations regarding endurance training for ALS patients (see Table 1).

Exercise and amyotrophic lateral sclerosis (animal studies)

Because only a few studies in humans on exercise and ALS have been published, one must turn to animal studies to further our understanding of the effects of exercise on ALS. Transgenic mice overexpressing the human superoxide dismutase gene, G93A-SOD1, are used as an animal model of ALS, because these mice exhibit hindlimb weakness, spasticity, and atrophy at 3 months of age, and progress to paralysis within 4 to 5 months of age [45]. All four animal studies used treadmill running (aerobic/endurance training) as the mode of exercise, in contrast to the human studies, in which resistance training was used.

Veldink's group [46] randomized 65 low-copy SOD1 transgenic mice and 16 wild-type controls to either treadmill exercise or a sedentary group. The animals were trained from 8 weeks of age, when they were presymptomatic, to a median age of 26 weeks throughout the disease course, running on a treadmill at 16 m/min, for 45 minutes daily, 5 days per week. The outcome measurements were onset of disease (measured by hindpaw extension reflex), progression of disease (measured by beam balance test and the loaded grid test), and survival. In this study, it was found that moderate exercise starting at a presymptomatic stage delayed the disease onset in the low-copy SOD1 female mice by 48 days. When the investigators repeated the study using 20 high-copy SOD1 female mice, they found that the survival was prolonged by 4 days compared with the sedentary female mice. The outcome measurements for the male SOD1 mice showed no statistically significant differences.

Another study performed by Kirkinezos' group [47] showed that 10 weeks of treadmill training (from age 7 weeks to 17 weeks) in SOD1 mice, with 13 m/min of treadmill running for 30 minutes, 5 days per week, expanded the average lifespan for the male mice from 129 days to 139 days, and for the female mice from 139 days to 144 days. In this study, the beneficial effect in expanding life expectancy was statistically significant for the male mice but not for the female mice. The investigators proposed that this finding may be caused by the effect of testosterone on muscle build-up. However, it is unclear as to why the effect of sex on exercise and survival outcome is different for these two animal studies. Parenthetically, no data in humans suggest that men and women with ALS respond differently to exercise regimens.

In another study, performed by Mahoney and colleagues [48], SOD1 mice were trained from 6 weeks of age onward with a high-intensity endurance treadmill exercise, running to a peak of 22 m/min, 45 minutes per day, 5 times per week, until the mice were symptomatic and unable to maintain running at 9 m/min for 45 minutes. The investigators found that such high-intensity endurance training does not affect the age or probability of disease onset in either male or female SOD1 mice but it hastened death by 11 days in SOD1 male mice.

Finally, Liebetanz and colleagues [49] studied lifetime vigorous exercise, consisting of 400 minutes of daily treadmill running (40 $\times$ 10 minutes running at 3.4 m/min interspersed with 5-minute rest intervals) in SOD1 mice, starting at 5 weeks of age. The investigators did not find a deleterious effect on the onset or progression of motor degeneration. Instead, a nonsignificant positive survival trend was found for the exercise group.

The authors conclude from these animal studies that (1) SOD1 mice may have an inverse response of survival to the exercise intensity, with a lower treadmill running speed (3.4 to 16 m/min) prolonging survival [46,47,49] and an intense treadmill running speed (22 m/min) decreasing survival [48] and (2) prolonged exercise is not necessarily harmful to the survival of SOD1 mice, as long as the exercise periods are regularly interspersed with rest periods, allowing for proper physiologic adaptations [49].

Whether one may extrapolate the above findings to humans remains to be demonstrated, because the SOD1 gene mutation explains only 2% of all human ALS cases. The treadmill running protocols were also initiated early in mice, equivalent to the teenage years in humans. The positive effect of "prehabilitation" with moderate endurance training in prolonging survival will be practically impossible to replicate in humans, except for a few identified familial ALS cases.

The debate surrounding strenuous physical activity and amyotrophic lateral sclerosis

The issue of whether highly intense and strenuous physical activity leads to an increased risk for ALS is still debated. Case reports and retrospective studies have shown a link between intense physical activity and ALS, as in professional soccer players and war veterans [50,51]. However, it is difficult to ascertain the relative risk ratio from retrospective analyses [52–54]. People have proposed that other common factors, such as a genetic predisposition, may exist between high levels of athleticism and the pathogenesis of ALS, rather than the act of intense physical exertion itself as a causative factor for the development of ALS. Although investigators have shown that the resting energy expenditures in ALS patients are higher than in controls [55,56], it is not clear if the hypermetabolic state is a causative or correlated feature of the disease. Further studies are needed to clarify the questions raised here.

Summary

Based on the authors' review of the few human and animal studies of exercise and motor neuron degeneration, they conclude that exercise is likely to be more beneficial than deleterious for patients who have ALS. In particular, they recommend individualized and carefully monitored, progressive resistance exercise in patients who have early ALS, for functional improvement. This recommendation is based on the positive results of two class II studies [36,37].

Studies are needed to examine stretching and endurance training, and a combination of endurance and strengthening exercises as therapeutic means for patients who have ALS. Lessons learned from SOD1 mice suggest that it is important for future studies of endurance training in humans to define the training protocol clearly, including the intensity, duration, and frequency of training, and the pretraining functional status of the patients. It is to be hoped that such measures will help standardize the investigative effort and further our understanding about how each type of exercise may affect patients who have ALS. Finally, it remains unknown whether oral and breathing exercises would help the bulbar and respiratory function in patients who have ALS. Studies are clearly needed in this respect. The authors hope this article stimulates further discussions and investigations among neurologists, physiatrists, physical therapists, researchers, and scientists in addressing the important question as to whether and how exercise may be used to alter the course of the disease and to improve the strength, function, and quality of life for people who have ALS.

References

[1] Mitsumoto H, Chad DA, Pioro EP. Amyotrophic lateral sclerosis, vol. 49. Philadelphia: F.A. Davis Company; 1998.

[2] Mitsumoto H, Del Bene M. Improving the quality of life for people with ALS: the challenge ahead. Amyotroph Lateral Scler Other Motor Neuron Disord 2000;1(5):329–36.

[3] Van den Berg JP, Kalmijn S, Lindeman E, et al. Multidisciplinary ALS care improves quality of life in patients with ALS. Neurology 2005;65(8):1264–7.

[4] Physical activity and health: a report of the surgeon general. Atlanta (GA): US Department of Health and Human Services, Public Health Service, CDC, National Center for Chronic Disease Prevention and Health Promotion; 1996.

[5] Bauman AE. Updating the evidence that physical activity is good for health: an epidemiological review 2000–2003. J Sci Med Sport 2004;7(1 Suppl):6–19.
[6] Linke A, Erbs S, Hambrecht R. Exercise and the coronary circulation-alterations and adaptations in coronary artery disease. Prog Cardiovasc Dis 2006;48(4):270–84.
[7] Pescatello LS. Exercise and hypertension: recent advances in exercise prescription. Curr Hypertens Rep 2005;7(4):281–6.
[8] Hardman AE. Physical activity and cancer risk. Proc Nutr Soc 2001;60(1):107–13.
[9] Sato Y. Diabetes and life-styles: role of physical exercise for primary prevention. Br J Nutr 2000;84(Suppl 2):S187–90.
[10] Bassel-Duby R, Olson EN. Signaling pathways in skeletal muscle remodeling. Annu Rev Biochem 2006;75:19–37.
[11] Ryder JW, Bassel-Duby R, Olson EN, et al. Skeletal muscle reprogramming by activation of calcineurin improves insulin action on metabolic pathways. J Biol Chem 2003;278(45): 44298–304.
[12] Muoio DM, Koves TR. Skeletal muscle adaptation to fatty acid depends on coordinated actions of the PPARs and PGC1 alpha: implications for metabolic disease. Appl Physiol Nutr Metab 2007;32(5):874–83.
[13] Rennie MJ, Wackerhage H, Spangenburg EE, et al. Control of the size of the human muscle mass. Annu Rev Physiol 2004;66:799–828.
[14] Goldspink G. Changes in muscle mass and phenotype and the expression of autocrine and systemic growth factors by muscle in response to stretch and overload. J Anat 1999;194(Pt 3):323–34.
[15] Vollaard NB, Shearman JP, Cooper CE. Exercise-induced oxidative stress: myths, realities and physiological relevance. Sports Med 2005;35(12):1045–62.
[16] Ji LL. Exercise-induced modulation of antioxidant defense. Ann N Y Acad Sci 2002;959: 82–92.
[17] Balakrishnan SD, Anuradha CV. Exercise, depletion of antioxidants and antioxidant manipulation. Cell Biochem Funct 1998;16(4):269–75.
[18] Brites FD, Evelson PA, Christiansen MG, et al. Soccer players under regular training show oxidative stress but an improved plasma antioxidant status. Clin Sci (Lond) 1999;96(4): 381–5.
[19] Wang JS, Huang YH. Effects of exercise intensity on lymphocyte apoptosis induced by oxidative stress in men. Eur J Appl Physiol 2005;95(4):290–7.
[20] Pedersen BK. The anti-inflammatory effect of exercise: its role in diabetes and cardiovascular disease control. Essays Biochem 2006;42:105–17.
[21] Fischer CP. Interleukin-6 in acute exercise and training: what is the biological relevance? Exerc Immunol Rev 2006;12:6–33.
[22] Pedersen BK, Fischer CP. Physiological roles of muscle-derived interleukin-6 in response to exercise. Curr Opin Clin Nutr Metab Care 2007;10(3):265–71.
[23] Stewart KJ. Exercise training and the cardiovascular consequences of type 2 diabetes and hypertension: plausible mechanisms for improving cardiovascular health. JAMA 2002;288(13): 1622–31.
[24] Adkins DL, Boychuk J, Remple MS, et al. Motor training induces experience specific patterns of plasticity across motor cortex and spinal cord. J Appl Physiol 2006;101(6):1776–82.
[25] Aagaard P, Simonsen EB, Andersen JL, et al. Neural adaptation to resistance training: changes in evoked V-wave and H-reflex responses. J Appl Physiol 2002;92(6):2309–18.
[26] Leal-Cerro A, Gippini A, Amaya MJ, et al. Mechanisms underlying the neuroendocrine response to physical exercise. J Endocrinol Invest 2003;26(9):879–85.
[27] Mastorakos G, Pavlatou M. Exercise as a stress model and the interplay between the hypothalamus-pituitary-adrenal and the hypothalamus-pituitary-thyroid axes. Horm Metab Res 2005;37(9):577–84.
[28] van der Kooi EL, Lindeman E, Riphagen I. Strength training and aerobic exercise training for muscle disease. Cochrane Database Syst Rev 2005;(1):CD003907.

[29] Cup EH, Pieterse AJ, Ten Broek-Pastoor JM, et al. Exercise therapy and other types of physical therapy for patients with neuromuscular diseases: a systematic review. Arch Phys Med Rehabil 2007;88(11):1452–64.

[30] American College of Sports Medicine position stand. The recommended quantity and quality of exercise for developing and maintaining cardiorespiratory and muscular fitness, and flexibility in healthy adults. Med Sci Sports Exerc 1998;30(6):975–91.

[31] Morris SL, Dodd KJ, Morris ME. Outcomes of progressive resistance strength training following stroke: a systematic review. Clin Rehabil 2004;18(1):27–39.

[32] Gallien P, Nicolas B, Robineau S, et al. Physical training and multiple sclerosis. Ann Readapt Med Phys 2007;50(6):373–6.

[33] White LJ, Dressendorfer RH. Exercise and multiple sclerosis. Sports Med 2004;34(15): 1077–100.

[34] Kisner C, Colby LA. Therapeutic exercise: foundations and techniques. 5th edition. Philadelphia: F.A. Davis; 2007.

[35] Bohannon RW. Results of resistance exercise on a patient with amyotrophic lateral sclerosis. A case report. Phys Ther 1983;63(6):965–8.

[36] Drory VE, Goltsman E, Reznik JG, et al. The value of muscle exercise in patients with amyotrophic lateral sclerosis. J Neurol Sci 2001;191(1–2):133–7.

[37] Bello-Haas VD, Florence JM, Kloos AD, et al. A randomized controlled trial of resistance exercise in individuals with ALS. Neurology 2007;68(23):2003–7.

[38] Edlund W, Gronseth G, So Y, et al. Clinical practice guideline process manual. Available at: www.aan.com/globals/axon/assets/2535.pdf.

[39] Karani R, McLaughlin MA, Cassel CK. Exercise in the healthy older adult. Am J Geriatr Cardiol 2001;10(5):269–73.

[40] Sanjak M, Paulson D, Sufit R, et al. Physiologic and metabolic response to progressive and prolonged exercise in amyotrophic lateral sclerosis. Neurology 1987;37(7):1217–20.

[41] Gleeson M. Can nutrition limit exercise-induced immunodepression? Nutr Rev 2006;64(3): 119–31.

[42] Pinto AC, Evangelista T, de Carvalho M, et al. Respiratory disorders in ALS: sleep and exercise studies. J Neurol Sci 1999;169(1–2):61–8.

[43] Siciliano G, D'Avino C, Del Corona A, et al. Impaired oxidative metabolism and lipid peroxidation in exercising muscle from ALS patients. Amyotroph Lateral Scler Other Motor Neuron Disord 2002;3(2):57–62.

[44] Siciliano G, Pastorini E, Pasquali L, et al. Impaired oxidative metabolism in exercising muscle from ALS patients. J Neurol Sci 2001;191(1–2):61–5.

[45] Chiu AY, Zhai P, Dal Canto MC, et al. Age-dependent penetrance of disease in a transgenic mouse model of familial amyotrophic lateral sclerosis. Mol Cell Neurosci 1995;6(4): 349–62.

[46] Veldink JH, Bar PR, Joosten EA, et al. Sexual differences in onset of disease and response to exercise in a transgenic model of ALS. Neuromuscul Disord 2003;13(9):737–43.

[47] Kirkinezos IG, Hernandez D, Bradley WG, et al. Regular exercise is beneficial to a mouse model of amyotrophic lateral sclerosis. Ann Neurol 2003;53(6):804–7.

[48] Mahoney DJ, Rodriguez C, Devries M, et al. Effects of high-intensity endurance exercise training in the G93A mouse model of amyotrophic lateral sclerosis. Muscle Nerve 2004; 29(5):656–62.

[49] Liebetanz D, Hagemann K, von Lewinski F, et al. Extensive exercise is not harmful in amyotrophic lateral sclerosis. Eur J Neurosci 2004;20(11):3115–20.

[50] Longstreth WT, McGuire V, Koepsell TD, et al. Risk of amyotrophic lateral sclerosis and history of physical activity: a population-based case-control study. Arch Neurol 1998; 55(2):201–6.

[51] Scarmeas N, Shih T, Stern Y, et al. Premorbid weight, body mass, and varsity athletics in ALS. Neurology 2002;59(5):773–5.

[52] Armon C. An evidence-based medicine approach to the evaluation of the role of exogenous risk factors in sporadic amyotrophic lateral sclerosis. Neuroepidemiology 2003;22(4): 217–28.

[53] Armon C. Sports and trauma in amyotrophic lateral sclerosis revisited. J Neurol Sci 2007; 262(1–2):45–53.

[54] Brooks BR. Risk factors in the early diagnosis of ALS: North American epidemiological studies. ALS CARE Study Group. Amyotroph Lateral Scler Other Motor Neuron Disord 2000;1(Suppl 1):S19–26.

[55] Desport JC, Preux PM, Magy L, et al. Factors correlated with hypermetabolism in patients with amyotrophic lateral sclerosis. Am J Clin Nutr 2001;74(3):328–34.

[56] Gonzalez A, Morales R, Pageot N, et al. ALS patients have a significant hyperactivity at all ages: results of a prospective study. Toronto: International Symposium on ALS/MND; 2007.

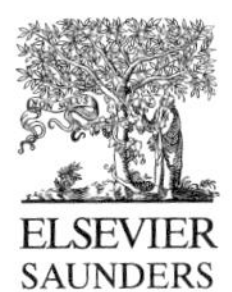
ELSEVIER
SAUNDERS

Phys Med Rehabil Clin N Am
19 (2008) 559–572

PHYSICAL MEDICINE
AND REHABILITATION
CLINICS OF
NORTH AMERICA

Respiratory Treatment of Amyotrophic Lateral Sclerosis

Joshua O. Benditt, MD[a],*, Louis Boitano, MS, RRT[b]

[a]*University of Washington Medical Center, Pulmonary and Critical Care Medicine, 1959 NE Pacific Street, Box 356522, Seattle, WA 98195-6522*

[b]*Respiratory Care Department, University of Washington Medical Center, Seattle, WA, USA*

Amyotrophic lateral sclerosis pathogenesis and respiratory system effects

Amyotrophic lateral sclerosis (ALS), or Lou Gehrig disease, is a progressive neurodegenerative disease of unknown cause. Approximately 1.4 individuals per 100,000 develop ALS annually and the peak incidence occurs between the ages of 55 and 75 [1]. The disease affects all races, but men are affected 1.5 times as often as women. Although the cause of ALS is unknown, many potential causes have been proposed, including exposure to neurotoxic agents, genetic or autoimmune disease, deficiencies of nerve growth factors, and viral infection, to name a few [2–6]. Regardless of the initiating event, ALS has a characteristic pattern of damage to the nervous system, with involvement of the motor neurons of the brainstem, the anterior horn area of the spinal cord, and the large pyramidal neurons of the motor cortex.

The usual clinical presentation is that of an individual with gradually progressive asymmetric weakness associated with hyperreflexia and muscle fasciculations. The disease presents with equal frequency in the upper and lower limbs (~40%) and less frequently with bulbar muscle involvement (~20%) [1]. Difficulty with walking, balance, picking up objects, and, ultimately, any limb muscle movement can occur. Patients who have bulbar muscle involvement suffer difficulty with swallowing, cough, and protection of the airway. The diagnosis is made on the basis of history, physical examination revealing upper and lower motor neuron signs, and electromyography demonstrating signs of denervation and true fasciculations. Other disease processes, such as myasthenia gravis, myelopathies, heavy metal intoxication, and vitamin deficiencies, must be aggressively excluded.

* Corresponding author.
E-mail address: benditt@u.washington.edu (J.O. Benditt).

1047-9651/08/$ - see front matter
doi:10.1016/j.pmr.2008.02.007

pmr.theclinics.com

Respiratory system involvement in amyotrophic lateral sclerosis

ALS has no direct effect on the lung, but the mechanical respiratory system is significantly involved. ALS affects all the major muscle groups of the mechanical respiratory system: (1) upper airway muscles (abnormal swallowing and cough); (2) expiratory muscles (inadequate cough); and (3) inspiratory muscles (inadequate maintenance of ventilation). Therefore, all patients who have ALS are at significant risk for respiratory complications; the leading cause of death in this population is respiratory failure.

Upper airway muscle dysfunction

Patients who have ALS frequently develop bulbar muscle dysfunction because of motor neuron involvement in the brainstem. Dysfunction of the lips, tongue, and pharyngeal and laryngeal muscles can result in an increased risk for aspiration and difficulty with generating adequate glottic closure for effective cough function. Swallowing may be impaired, and ingesting adequate nutrition can be trying for the patient and family alike. Choking episodes are common and may even be triggered by saliva. Secretion management is a particularly difficult issue because secretions may become viscous because of inadequate hydration [7]. Sialorrhea (drooling) is due to inadequate handling of secretions, rather than the amount of secretions; in fact, salivary secretions in ALS appear to be less than in normal subjects [8]. Malnutrition due to inadequate protein-calorie intake can occur and rapid weight loss should signal the clinician to assess the swallowing mechanism carefully [9]. Speech and swallowing are often affected and patients may require assistive technology to communicate effectively. Choice boards and computer-assisted speech devices are available for patients who have neuromuscular speech difficulties. The authors have found referral to a speech and swallowing clinic to be helpful in diagnosing swallowing and airway protection problems and for instructing patients and their families in steps they can take to reduce the risk for aspiration.

Expiratory muscle dysfunction

Cough is an essential airway protection reflex. Particles are expelled from the airway through a complex set of nerve and muscle responses to cough stimulation, through receptors located predominantly in the upper airway [10]. Cough receptor stimulation results in inhalation to approximately 60% of maximum vital capacity (inspiratory phase). The glottis then closes and the abdominal muscles contract, resulting in markedly elevated intrathoracic pressures without airflow (compressive phase). The glottis opens shortly thereafter and gas is propelled through the airways at high velocities, resulting in airway clearance (expiratory phase). The individual who has ALS may experience cough impairment in any one, or all three, of the stages of cough, including reduction in the inspired volume due to diaphragm weakness, inability to close the glottis completely during the compressive phase due to bulbar muscle dysfunction, and inability to compress and expel intrathoracic gas because of expiratory muscle weakness. Polkey and colleagues [11] performed a careful investigation of cough function in patients who had ALS. They studied 26 patients who had ALS, 16 of whom had respiratory symptoms and 9 of whom did not. They found that the ability to generate cough was related to expiratory muscle strength, as gauged by a balloon placed in the stomach measuring gastric pressure. This finding appeared to be a threshold phenomenon. Cough was not lost until substantial levels of expiratory muscle strength were lost. Maximal expiratory pressure, a commonly used clinical measure of expiratory muscle strength, did not correlate well with the presence or absence of cough generation. Inspiratory muscle strength also did not correlate well with cough generation. Endoscopic evaluation of the patients who had respiratory symptoms revealed only 2 patients with obvious glottic dysfunction, indicating that the presence of glottic function alone did not ensure effective cough. Some have suggested that the measurement of peak cough flow (PCF) is an effective, noninvasive assessment of cough function [12–14]. In the experience of these investigators, a measured PCF of less than 160 L per minute during illness and less than 270 L per minute while well was associated with poor cough and a high risk for respiratory infection.

Inspiratory muscle dysfunction

ALS often affects the inspiratory muscles, including the diaphragm and external intercostal muscles, which leads to a reduction in respiratory muscle strength, restrictive lung disease, and, ultimately, carbon dioxide retention and frank respiratory failure. In some cases, respiratory muscle dysfunction leading to respiratory failure may be the presenting clinical picture for the patient who has ALS [15–18]. Usually, the symptoms of respiratory muscle insufficiency, such as dyspnea, occur gradually over time and may defy diagnosis. Pulmonary function testing is invaluable in assessing the level of respiratory impairment, in following disease progression, and in assessing prognosis in ALS. Fallat and colleagues [19] evaluated comprehensive pulmonary function testing over time in 218 patients who had ALS. All their patients showed evidence of restrictive lung disease, with reductions in total lung capacity, forced vital capacity (FVC), forced expiratory volume in 1 second, and maximum voluntary ventilation. The FVC averaged 80% of predicted at presentation to their clinic. They were able to follow pulmonary function tests over time in 103 patients, which showed significant decrements in all values over time. Black and Hyatt [20] studied respiratory muscle function in ALS with dyspnea and near-normal vital capacity. Maximal inspiratory and maximal expiratory pressures were markedly reduced (34% and 47%, respectively). Reduction in maximal muscle strength correlated well with sensation of dyspnea in their patients. These respiratory muscle strength measures correlated with dyspnea in their patients despite near-normal vital capacity. In patients in whom oral bulbar weakness may limit the ability to accurately measure maximum inspiratory pressure by mouth, sniff nasal inspiratory pressure has been found to be a reliable alternative [21]. Maximal inspiratory pressure and sniff nasal inspiratory pressure may be inaccurate measures of inspiratory muscle strength when significant bulbar weakness affects the test maneuver because of an inadequate oral seal or upper airway collapse.

Nocturnal hypoventilation and sleep-disordered breathing is a common problem for patients who have ALS [22–26] and can occur even when respiratory muscle function is only mildly affected and daytime gas exchange remains normal. Neural output to the respiratory muscles decreases during sleep. Even mild muscle weakness, coupled with the normal decreases in ventilatory drive, can result in nocturnal hypoventilation and disturbed sleep architecture [27]. Symptoms and signs of nocturnal hypoventilation can manifest at night and during the day. Nighttime symptoms include air hunger, observed apneas, orthopnea, cyanosis, restlessness, and insomnia. Daytime findings include excessive sleepiness, morning headaches or drowsiness, polycythemia, and pulmonary hypertension. The health care provider should be vigilant for these symptoms. Sleep studies can be helpful in elucidating sleep-disturbed breathing in these patients if doubt remains.

Hypercarbia and atelectasis can lead to lower than expected arterial oxygen levels, but primary oxygenation problems are not common in ALS, except in the final stages, when pneumonia intervenes. Oxygen as a primary therapy for respiratory insufficiency is not recommended. However, oxygen therapy in an attempt to relieve dyspnea in the hospice setting may be appropriate.

Monitoring and treatment of respiratory complications in amyotrophic lateral sclerosis

Patients who have ALS present a challenging set of issues for the clinician and the health care system. A neurologist usually accomplishes diagnosis of ALS, although diagnosis is often delayed because of the insidious onset of the disease. Unfortunately, neither cure nor truly effective treatment is yet available for ALS. Riluzole, an antagonist of glutamergic neurotransmission, has been shown to increase the time to death or mechanical ventilation by approximately 3 months only [28]. Therefore, health care for these individuals focuses on maintenance of quality of life and adaptation to advancing disability due to muscle weakness. A rehabilitation medicine specialist can provide invaluable input into the care of the patient who has ALS. The management of devices needed for locomotion, medications for muscle spasm, and prevention of contractures and skin breakdown, and assistive communication technologies, are all areas that require careful oversight. The respiratory specialist is integral to the care of the patient who has

ALS because of the multiple effects of this disease on the respiratory system. Frequent monitoring of pulmonary function gives valuable information on prognosis and gives input into the timing of interventions and discussions of long-term mechanical ventilation. At their institution, the authors have found that the most efficient way of delivering health care to these individuals is through a multidisciplinary clinic that involves care providers from rehabilitation medicine, neurology, and respiratory medicine, and therapists for speech and swallowing. The following discussion focuses on the monitoring and management of respiratory issues related to ALS.

Aspiration/pneumonia risk

The risk for aspiration and development of pneumonia in patients who have ALS is due primarily to problems with upper airway function and cough. Pharyngeal and laryngeal muscle dysfunction can lead directly to aspiration of oral contents into the lungs. Other than surgical diversion of the airway, no treatment directly aimed at the laryngeal and glottic function is available. However, reduction of the amount of salivary secretions is possible through the use of several medications and modalities (Box 1) [29–31]. Teaching proper swallowing technique to avoid aspiration is also helpful and involves keeping the head downward and using straws; drinking thicker, rather than thin, liquids; concentrating on eating during mealtime (no television, reading, and so forth); and maintaining hydration with at least two quarts of water per day. In addition, when patients who have ALS develop significant dysphagia and aspiration with solids or liquids, many experts recommend placement of a percutaneous endoscopic gastrostomy tube [32,33], which may prevent large-volume aspiration and is associated

Box 1. Therapeutic options for sialorrhea

Pharmacologic options
Amitriptyline (Elavil)
Glycopyrrolate (Robinul)
Benztropine (Cogentin)
Scopolamine (Transdermal Hyoscine)
Trihexyphenidyl hydrochloride (Artane)
Atropine
B-blocker (thick secretions)
Guaifensin (thick secretions)

Nonpharmacologic options
Salivary gland resection
Parotid gland irradiation
Airway diversion

with improvement in hydration and nutritional status. Although the American Academy of Neurology practice parameter recommends placing the tube before decrease of the FVC below 50%, the authors have been able to place percutaneous endoscopic gastrostomy tubes in patients with an FVC as low as 13% [34].

Cough function, which depends in large part on expiratory muscles, can be mechanically assisted when adequate bulbar function exists. Bach [14] postulates that cough function is adequate when the patient can generate at least 3 L per second of PCF [14]. PCF can be measured with a simple device in the clinic (Fig. 1) and the authors routinely perform this procedure during clinic visits. When PCF drops below 270 L per minute, they carefully evaluate potential interventions to improve cough function. These interventions may include teaching the caregivers manually assisted cough and the Heimlich maneuver. Inspiratory-related cough weakness can be supported with manual insufflation. A one-way valve mouthpiece circuit combined with a self-inflating resuscitator bag (Fig. 2) can be used to insufflate the lungs by applying a series of breath-stacking maneuvers. Manual insufflation alone has been shown to improve cough function, and when combined with abdominal thrust, can further improve cough strength [35]. When bulbar function is good but the patient has significant expiratory muscle weakness, mechanical in-exsufflation (Cough Assist Respironics Inc., Murrysville, Pennsylvania) can be used to augment cough function (Fig. 3). This device mimics the normal cough and has been shown to be helpful in patients who have ALS and other neuromuscular diseases [36]. Mechanical pressure-targeted insufflation and manual hyperinflation may also be beneficial to neuromuscular patients in maintaining lung compliance, decreasing the work of breathing, and managing atelectasis. Lechtzin and colleagues [37] measured lung compliance by esophageal balloon monitoring in a cohort of patients who had ALS, before and after brief periods of pressure-targeted hyperinflation [37]. They were able to show that patients who had

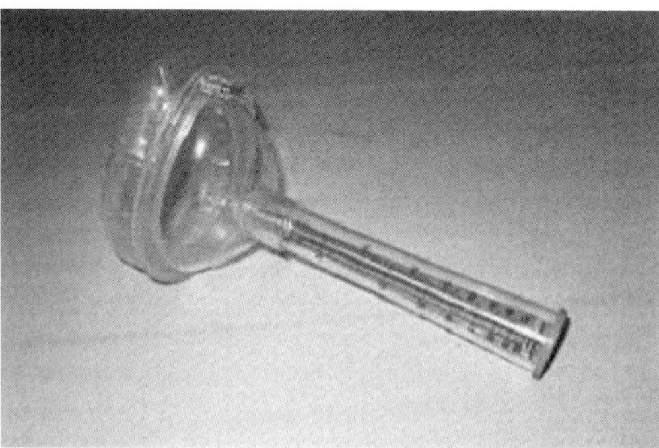

Fig. 1. A device to measure peak expiratory cough flow, combining an air cushion face mask with a Monaghan peak flow meter. (*Courtesy of* Monaghan Medical Corp., Plattsburgh, NY; with permission).

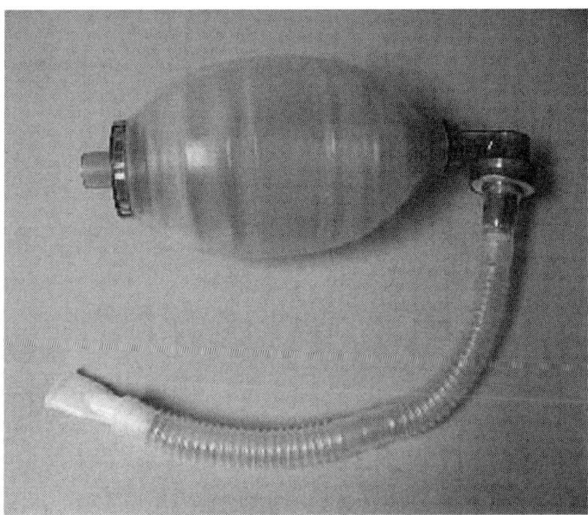

Fig. 2. Manual insufflation device, combining a one-way valve mouthpiece circuit with a self-inflating resuscitator bag.

diaphragmatic weakness had decreased lung compliance and that intermittent pressure-targeted insufflation could improve compliance. Hyperinflation maneuvers can be administered by either manual hyperinflation or mechanical insufflation using the cough-assist device. The effectiveness of this therapy is limited by the degree of bulbar impairment. As bulbar and cough function deteriorate, the risk for pneumonia may increase to the point where tracheostomy will be necessary.

Ventilatory failure

Progressive inspiratory muscle weakness in ALS inevitably leads to carbon dioxide retention and hypercarbic respiratory failure. In fact, the major

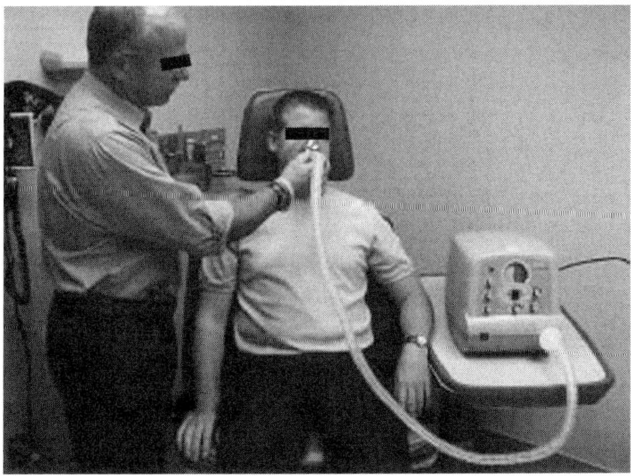

Fig. 3. The application of mechanical in-exsufflation using the Cough Assist Device with an air cushion facemask circuit. (*Courtesy of* Respironics Corp., Murrysville, PA; with permission).

cause of death in ALS is respiratory failure. Predicting when respiratory failure will occur in the patient who has ALS is important for planning appropriate clinical interventions and for helping patients and their families address crucial questions concerning long-term mechanical ventilation and end-of-life issues. Unfortunately, accurately predicting impending respiratory failure is a difficult task. Assessing symptoms of respiratory insufficiency, such as dyspnea and orthopnea, on each visit is important. Nocturnal hypoventilation often occurs before the onset of daytime problems and therefore, symptoms of sleep-disordered breathing, such as frequent awakening, vivid nightmares, night sweats, morning headaches, and daytime hypersomnolence, should be sought. Objective measurements of pulmonary function can be helpful but are not entirely predictive of either impending respiratory failure or death [19]. Upright and supine vital capacity, FVC, maximal inspiratory pressure [19], and even transdiaphragmatic pressure measurements [11] have been used to predict respiratory failure. Stambler and colleagues [38] looked at several clinical variables to predict death in ALS. They found that serum chloride was a sensitive predictor of time to death in these patients. Serum chloride levels decreased rapidly in the months before death, which the investigators postulate represents compensation for developing respiratory acidosis. The authors rarely obtain arterial blood gases because $Paco_2$ can be maintained until immediately prior to respiratory failure. Most investigators agree that, although it is impossible to predict accurately the lifespan of any given individual who has ALS, severe restrictive disease with an FVC of less than 50% should prompt careful discussions with the patient concerning medical interventions in the event of respiratory failure [8]. The frequency at which FVC measurements should be taken has not been established, but every 3 months appears to be a reasonable timeframe. This measurement can easily be performed in clinic with portable spirometry equipment. Patients who have oral muscle weakness may need to perform the spirometry maneuver through an air cushion facemask to obtain reliable measurements. Bulbar-related upper airway obstruction that results in an uneven forced expiratory flow-volume pattern can portend a poor prognosis related to airway protection, cough effectiveness, and tolerance for, and benefit from, noninvasive respiratory therapies.

Mechanical ventilator support with noninvasive positive pressure ventilation (NPPV) and has been shown to be effective in improving quality and duration of life [39–44]. Improvements in cognitive function have been shown in patients who have ALS who are receiving nocturnal NPPV [45]. Recently, a randomized controlled trial of noninvasive ventilation was done in a cohort of patients who had ALS, which measured survival and quality of life [44]. Ninety-two patients were assessed every 2 months and randomly assigned to noninvasive ventilation (22) or standard care (19) when either orthopnea developed with a maximum inspiratory pressure of less than 60% of predicted or when symptomatic hypercarbia occurred. NPPV improved quality of life and survival in all patients who did not have bulbar symptoms and in a subset of patients who had mild bulbar symptoms. In patients who had more severe bulbar symptoms, NPPV produced some improvement in quality of life but did not improve survival.

The practice parameters of the American Academy of Neurology suggest that all patients who have ALS and respiratory symptoms or an FVC of less than 50% predicted should be offered the use of NPPV [8]. NPPV is usually initiated at night because of the high frequency of sleep-disordered breathing. Sleep studies may be helpful if symptoms are unclear and FVC is greater than 50%, although they are not necessary to initiate treatment. However, patients will often begin using NPPV during the day as their disease progresses and the authors have had several patients who have used this modality for 24 hours per day. The authors have adapted wheelchairs to carry these machines so that patients can leave the house with NPPV. Portable daytime NPPV can be provided most easily by using a bi-level pressure ventilator in conjunction with a less obtrusive interface, either a nasal cannula or nasal pillow interface. A small subset of patients who have slow-progressing limb onset disease and no bulbar symptoms may benefit from portable daytime mouthpiece ventilation (MPV) (Figs. 4 and 5). Portable MPV can be supported using a bi-level pressure ventilator but is administered most effectively using a pressure-triggered volume-cycled home ventilator. The benefits of MPV include progressive ventilatory support and sigh and cough augmentation through the use of breath-stacking maneuvers. A survey that assessed the use of NPPV during the years 1996 to 1999 (before the issuance

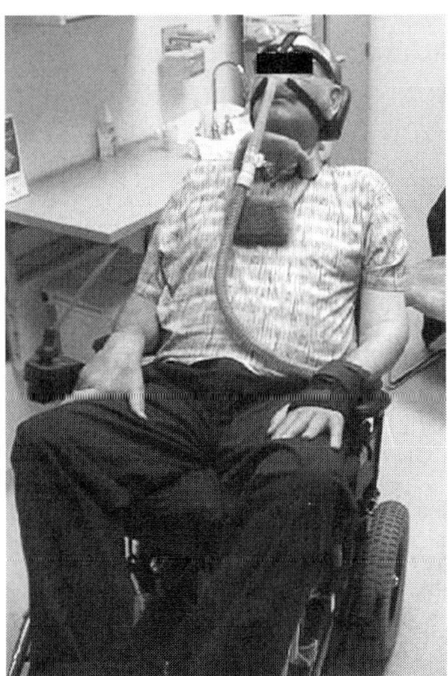

Fig. 4. Application of mask NPPV for a patient who is wheelchair bound. Battery pack allows independent function.

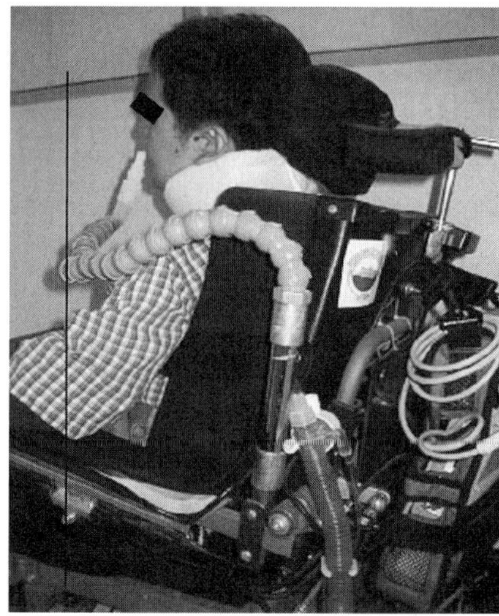

Fig. 5. Portable mouthpiece ventilation system on a power wheelchair.

of the practice parameter) by patients who had ALS showed that usage was low, with only 28% of patients who had dyspnea and 7% of patients who had an FVC of less than 40% using the device. An attractive feature of NPPV is the fact that it does not require a surgical procedure and is easily removed. Unfortunately, NPPV is only a temporizing measure. All patients who have ALS will, at some point, develop bulbar symptoms that are severe enough that patients will be unable to continue use of NPPV without developing aspiration pneumonia, or the device will fail to ventilate the patient effectively despite 24-hour-per-day use. At this point, invasive ventilation becomes the only option for continued survival.

Invasive ventilation involves placement of a tracheostomy and use of a small, usually volume-cycled, home ventilator. This intervention is clearly life prolonging and patient survivals of up to 20 years and more have been reported [40]. Unfortunately, invasive ventilation has no effect on the progression of the disease, and most patients will develop complete paresis of limb muscles. Approximately 10% of patients will develop complete paresis of all muscles, including the extraocular muscles, and will develop a "locked-in" syndrome in which no communication is possible. The costs to patients and families in financial and emotional terms are significant [46]. Family members provide much of the care for these patients at home and may have to relinquish employment outside the home to do so. Despite these costs, many patients who have ALS report a good quality of life while receiving mechanical ventilation [47]. Most patients who undergo invasive mechanical ventilation do so in the setting of emergent hospitalization without having planned in advance for this eventuality.

Cazzolli and Oppenheimer [40] reviewed their experience with 50 patients who had ALS and were on invasive mechanical ventilation. They found that only 4 (8%) of the patients had chosen tracheostomy in advance, before acute respiratory failure and emergent intubation. Few patients who have ALS have advanced directives or living wills in place at the time that respiratory failure occurs. The authors have developed an instructive advanced directive [48] that they have found particularly helpful in assisting discussions of mechanical ventilation and end-of-life issues with patients who have ALS. Few patients in the United States (5%–10%) choose invasive mechanical ventilation as an option [40,49], which may be because of several factors, including patient expectation of reduced quality of life, physicians not offering this as a medical option, the exorbitant costs of mechanical ventilation (estimates of $15,000/month), and unavailability of family members to assist in patient care. The frequency of mechanical ventilation use in ALS varies worldwide, from almost never (United Kingdom) to up to 48% (Japan) [49], which appears to be because of cultural views of ALS and financial and structural differences in health care systems.

Palliative care of the amyotrophic lateral sclerosis patient

ALS is a progressive disease without cure that results in significant patient disability and ultimately death if the option of invasive ventilation is not chosen. The average life span from the time of diagnosis is approximately 3 to 5 years. Few suffering with ALS choose to undergo invasive mechanical ventilation and therefore, a good deal of time is spent caring for the patient who has ALS during a progressive, "terminal" portion of his/her life. Little has been written concerning palliative care of the patient who has ALS. In fact, more attention has focused on the issue of physician-assisted suicide [50] than supportive care of these patients. Fortunately, a good deal can be done to relieve some of the most troubling symptoms in patients who have ALS and to improve the quality of life at the end of life. Several major areas are of particular importance to patients who have ALS: physical needs (eg, wheelchairs, transfer devices, and so forth), pain issues, nutrition, psychologic needs of patient and family, sialorrhea, and dyspnea. No one health care provider can address all these end-of-life issues and the interdisciplinary team approach can result in significant benefit to the patient. The authors have found that an open discussion of the progression and prognosis of the disease, and assiduous symptom management up to, and including, home visits can ease suffering significantly in these individuals. Dyspnea can be managed effectively with NPPV and appropriate narcotics when necessary. Home hospice services are invaluable and should be offered. Perhaps the most important point to keep in mind is that, although no cure is currently available for ALS, excellent medical care can still be provided.

References

[1] Milonas I. Amyotrophic lateral sclerosis: an introduction. J Neurol 1998;245(Suppl 2):S1–3.
[2] Boukaftane Y, Khoris J, Moulard B, et al. Identification of six novel SOD1 gene mutations in familial amyotrophic lateral sclerosis. Can J Neurol Sci 1998;25(3):192–6.
[3] Brown DW. Amyotrophic lateral sclerosis: hypothetical pathogenesis. Med Hypotheses 1994;42(6):393–4.
[4] Rowland LP. Controversies about amyotrophic lateral sclerosis. Neurologia 1996;11 (Suppl 5):S72–4.
[5] Rowland LP. Amyotrophic lateral sclerosis: human challenge for neuroscience. Proc Natl Acad Sci U S A 1995;92(5):1251–3.
[6] Rowland LP. Amyotrophic lateral sclerosis. Curr Opin Neurol 1994;7(4):310–5.
[7] Tidwell J. Pulmonary management of the ALS patient. J Neurosci Nurs 1993;25(6): 337–42.
[8] Miller RG, Rosenberg JA, Gelinas DF, et al. Practice parameter: the care of the patient with amyotrophic lateral sclerosis (an evidence-based review): report of the Quality Standards Subcommittee of the American Academy of Neurology: ALS Practice Parameters Task Force. Neurology 1999;52(7):1311–23.
[9] Kasarskis EJ, Neville HE. Management of ALS: nutritional care. Neurology 1996; 47(4 Suppl 2):S118–20.
[10] Leith DE, Butler JP, Sneddon SL, et al. Cough. In: Fishman AP, editor. Handbook of physiology: the respiratory system. Bethesda (MD): American Physiologic Society; 1990. p. 315–36.
[11] Polkey MI, Lyall RA, Green M, et al. Expiratory muscle function in amyotrophic lateral sclerosis. Am J Respir Crit Care Med 1998;158(3):734–41.
[12] Bach JR. Amyotrophic lateral sclerosis: predictors for prolongation of life by noninvasive respiratory aids. Arch Phys Med Rehabil 1995;76(9):828–32.
[13] Bach JR. Amyotrophic lateral sclerosis. Communication status and survival with ventilatory support [published erratum appears in Am J Phys Med Rehabil 1994 Jun;73(3):218]. Am J Phys Med Rehabil 1993;72(6):343–9.
[14] Kang SW, Bach JR. Maximum insufflation capacity: vital capacity and cough flows in neuromuscular disease. Am J Phys Med Rehabil 2000;79(3):222–7.
[15] Barthlen GM, Lange DJ. Unexpectedly severe sleep and respiratory pathology in patients with amyotrophic lateral sclerosis. Eur J Neurol 2000;7(3):299–302.
[16] Carre PC, Didier AP, Tiberge YM, et al. Amyotrophic lateral sclerosis presenting with sleep hypopnea syndrome. Chest 1988;93(6):1309–12.
[17] de Carvalho M, Matias T, Coelho F, et al. Motor neuron disease presenting with respiratory failure. J Neurol Sci 1996;139(Suppl):117–22.
[18] Fromm GB, Wisdom PJ, Block AJ. Amyotrophic lateral sclerosis presenting with respiratory failure. Diaphragmatic paralysis and dependence on mechanical ventilation in two patients. Chest 1977;71(5):612–4.
[19] Fallat RJ, Norris FH, Holden D, et al. Respiratory monitoring and treatment: objective treatments using non-invasive measurements. Adv Exp Med Biol 1987;209:191–200.
[20] Black LF, Hyatt RE. Maximal static respiratory pressures in generalized neuromuscular disease. Am Rev Respir Dis 1971;103(5):641–50.
[21] Chaudri MB, Liu C, Watson L, et al. Sniff nasal inspiratory pressure as a marker of respiratory function in motor neuron disease. Eur Respir J 2000;15(3):539–42.
[22] Chokroverty S. Sleep and degenerative neurologic disorders. Neurol Clin 1996;14(4):807–26.
[23] Culebras A. Sleep and neuromuscular disorders. Neurol Clin 1996;14(4):791–805.
[24] David WS, Bundlie SR, Mahdavi Z. Polysomnographic studies in amyotrophic lateral sclerosis. J Neurol Sci 1997;152(Suppl 1):S29–35.
[25] Ferguson KA, Strong MJ, Ahmad D, et al. Sleep-disordered breathing in amyotrophic lateral sclerosis. Chest 1996;110(3):664–9.

[26] Hetta J, Jansson I. Sleep in patients with amyotrophic lateral sclerosis. J Neurol 1997; 244(4 Suppl 1):S7–9.

[27] Gay PC, Westbrook PR, Daube JR, et al. Effects of alterations in pulmonary function and sleep variables on survival in patients with amyotrophic lateral sclerosis. Mayo Clin Proc 1991;66(7):686–94.

[28] Bensimon G, Lacomblez L, Meininger V. A controlled trial of riluzole in amyotrophic lateral sclerosis. ALS/Riluzole Study Group. N Engl J Med 1994;330(9):585–91.

[29] Blasco PA, Stansbury JC. Glycopyrrolate treatment of chronic drooling. Arch Pediatr Adolesc Med 1996;150(9):932–5.

[30] Brodtkorb E, Wyzocka-Bakowska MM, Lillevold PE, et al. Transdermal scopolamine in drooling. J Ment Defic Res 1988;32(Pt 3):233–7.

[31] Camp-Bruno JA, Winsberg BG, Green-Parsons AR, et al. Efficacy of benztropine therapy for drooling. Dev Med Child Neurol 1989;31(3):309–19.

[32] Kasarskis EJ, Scarlata D, Hill R, et al. A retrospective study of percutaneous endoscopic gastrostomy in ALS patients during the BDNF and CNTF trials. J Neurol Sci 1999; 169(1–2):118–25.

[33] Mazzini L, Corra T, Zaccala M, et al. Percutaneous endoscopic gastrostomy and enteral nutrition in amyotrophic lateral sclerosis. J Neurol 1995;242(10):695–8.

[34] Boitano LJ, Jordan T, Benditt JO. Noninvasive ventilation allows gastrostomy tube placement in patients with advanced ALS. Neurology 2001;56(3):413–4.

[35] Trebbia G, Lacombe M, Fermanian C, et al. Cough determinants in patients with neuromuscular disease. Respir Physiol Neurobiol 2005;146(2–3):291–300.

[36] Hanayama K, Ishikawa Y, Bach JR. Amyotrophic lateral sclerosis. Successful treatment of mucous plugging by mechanical insufflation-exsufflation. Am J Phys Med Rehabil 1997; 76(4):338–9.

[37] Lechtzin N, Shade D, Clawson L, et al. Supramaximal inflation improves lung compliance in subjects with amyotrophic lateral sclerosis. Chest 2006;129(5):1322–9.

[38] Stambler N, Charatan M, Cedarbaum JM. Prognostic indicators of survival in ALS. ALS CNTF Treatment Study Group. Neurology 1998;50(1):66–72.

[39] Aboussouan LS, Khan SU, Meeker DP, et al. Effect of noninvasive positive-pressure ventilation on survival in amyotrophic lateral sclerosis [see comments]. Ann Intern Med 1997; 127(6):450–3.

[40] Cazzolli PA, Oppenheimer EA. Home mechanical ventilation for amyotrophic lateral sclerosis: nasal compared to tracheostomy-intermittent positive pressure ventilation. J Neurol Sci 1996;139(Suppl):123–8.

[41] Kleopa KA, Sherman M, Neal B, et al. Bipap improves survival and rate of pulmonary function decline in patients with ALS. J Neurol Sci 1999;164(1):82–8.

[42] Lyall RA, Donaldson N, Fleming T, et al. A prospective study of quality of life in ALS patients treated with noninvasive ventilation. Neurology 2001;57(1):153–6.

[43] Pinto AC, Evangelista T, Carvalho M, et al. Respiratory assistance with a non-invasive ventilator (Bipap) in MND/ALS patients: survival rates in a controlled trial. J Neurol Sci 1995; 129(Suppl):19–26.

[44] Bourke SC, Tomlinson M, Williams TL, et al. Effects of non-invasive ventilation on survival and quality of life in patients with amyotrophic lateral sclerosis: a randomised controlled trial. Lancet Neurol 2006;5(2):140–7.

[45] Newsom-Davis IC, Lyall RA, Leigh PN, et al. The effect of non-invasive positive pressure ventilation (NIPPV) on cognitive function in amyotrophic lateral sclerosis (ALS): a prospective study. J Neurol Neurosurg Psychiatry 2001,71(4):482–7, #732.

[46] Oppenheimer EA. Decision-making in the respiratory care of amyotrophic lateral sclerosis: should home mechanical ventilation be used? Palliat Med 1993;7(4):49–64.

[47] Gelinas DF, O'Connor P, Miller RG. Quality of life for ventilator-dependent ALS patients and their caregivers. J Neurol Sci 1998;160(Suppl 1):S134–6.

[48] Benditt J, Smith T, Tonelli MR. Empowering the individual with ALS at the end-of-life: disease-specific advanced care planning. Muscle Nerve 2001;24:1706–9.
[49] Borasio GD, Gelinas DF, Yanagisawa N. Mechanical ventilation in amyotrophic lateral sclerosis: a cross- cultural perspective. J Neurol 1998;245(Suppl 2):S7–12 [discussion: S29].
[50] Ganzini L, Block S. Physician-assisted death–a last resort? N Engl J Med 2002;346(21): 1663–5.

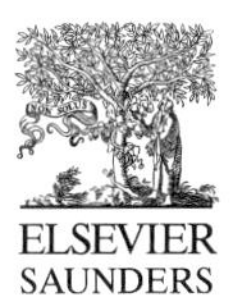

ELSEVIER
SAUNDERS

Phys Med Rehabil Clin N Am
19 (2008) 573–589

PHYSICAL MEDICINE
AND REHABILITATION
CLINICS OF
NORTH AMERICA

Nutrition and Dietary Supplements in Motor Neuron Disease

Jeffrey Rosenfeld, PhD, MD[a,*],
Amy Ellis, MPH, RD, CNSD[b]

[a]*Division of Neurology, University of California San Francisco-Fresno, Fresno, CA, USA*
[b]*Department of Nutrition Science, University of Alabama at Birmingham, Birmingham, AL, USA*

The role of nutrition in motor neuron disease

Compromised nutrition leading to weight loss is a common and significant problem in the amyotrophic lateral sclerosis (ALS) patient population. Malnutrition and consequent weight loss are significant negative prognostic indices to survival [1–3]. The benefit of aggressive and early nutritional therapy can profoundly influence the disease course, quality of life, and survival.

This article reviews the role of nutrition, both as sustenance and treatment for patients who have ALS. Self-medication with dietary supplements has become increasingly popular within this patient population. Despite their popularity, the efficacy of these compounds has been largely unsupported by formal clinical trials. Available data will be highlighted to provide a basis upon which to advise patients requesting guidance.

The etiology of impaired nutrition leading to weight loss is multifactorial including: dysphagia; weakness in the extremities; difficulty with mastication; and the possibility of a hypermetabolic state resulting from enhanced energy expenditure [4–7]. Interventions to maintain adequate nutritional intake may include altering food consistency, feeding assistance (eg, hand braces, altered utensils, mobile arm supports, modified plates, bowls, and cups) and high calorie nutritional supplements.

Percutaneous endoscopic gastrostomy

Placement of a percutaneous endoscopic gastrostomy (PEG) tube is one of the most effective means of proactive intervention to maintain body

* Corresponding author. 1011 Jericho Lane, Charlotte, NC 28270.
E-mail address: jrosenfeld@carolina.rr.com (J. Rosenfeld).

doi:10.1016/j.pmr.2008.03.001 ***pmr.theclinics.com***

weight and hydration [8]. Optimally, the PEG tube should be introduced early to supplement oral intake and reduce the stress of maintaining all nutritional needs by mouth. Patient acceptance of the PEG tube can be greatly improved by educating the patient that they may still enjoy favorite foods by mouth. Moreover, use of the PEG to meet the increased caloric requirements of the disease can conserve time and energy for both patient and caregiver. The patient's autonomy, confidence, and quality of life are enhanced by knowing that they can aggressively affect their disease course by the use of a PEG tube, while minimizing their fear of choking and the caregiver's burden.

The timing of PEG tube placement varies widely among practitioners; however, the American Academy of Neurology recommends PEG placement before the patient's forced vital capacity falls below 50% predicted [9]. This timing is to avoid risk of respiratory compromise during the procedure. This recommendation is based on available outcomes data from studies meeting the qualifications for the guidelines. General consensus among practitioners suggests that adopting the tube early in the course of progressive dysphagia, even before significant weight loss, is well accepted and allows the patient the choice of incrementally using the PEG for their nutritional needs [5]. Alternative protocols for feeding tube placement, including insertion of the tube with radiographic guidance (RIG) have been endorsed as means of lessening the risk of aspiration [10]. Recently an alternative Bi-level positive airway pressure mask was introduced allowing for continuous noninvasive ventilatory support during PEG placement reducing risk of respiratory compromise and improving patient comfort even when forced vital capacity falls much below 50% [11].

Nutrition and survival

The consequences of malnutrition in patients with ALS are well known. Inadequate dietary intake can exacerbate catabolism and atrophy of respiratory muscles, weaken the immune system, and contribute to infection [12,13]. Weight loss and below-normal body mass index (BMI) resulting from deficient energy intake among ALS patients are correlated with shortened survival [14]. Several more recent studies confirm the observation that weight loss (and/or malnutrition), defined as BMI $\leq$ 18.5 kg/m^2, is an independent, negative, prognostic indicator for survival [2,3,15]. In at least nine studies, evaluating a total of 469 ALS patients receiving enteral nutrition via PEG, a consistent benefit of either weight stabilization or weight gain was determined [3,15–20].

The magnitude of the survival advantage from improved nutrition can even be greater than the magnitude of the treatment effects being targeted in current clinical drug trials. A population-based study from Italy, found a greater than three-fold improved survival with patients using PEG compared with patients with oral intake [21,22].

Despite these published reports, some controversy remains as to the magnitude of the survival benefit following PEG placement. These dissenting opinions have, however, followed retrospective and population-based studies [5,8].

Nutraceuticals, functional foods, and dietary supplements

"Nutraceuticals," "functional foods" and "dietary supplements" are terms used to describe chemical components of foods that may display unique, disease-fighting pharmacokinetics and pharmacodynamics when ingested in amounts above that of one's typical diet [23]. The emergence of nutraceutical use within the patient population has defined a growing and substantial treatment modality. Often such dietary supplements are self-prescribed based on theoretic benefits or anecdotal reports, addressing proposed mechanisms leading to motor neuron death. A sense of autonomy and self-determination, along with the reality of advancing disability and the ease of availability for many supplements, combine to make the practice of supplementation attractive to patients. Most dietary supplements are easily obtained in retail outlets or via the Internet. Despite the absence of documented benefits in controlled trials, these supplements are conservatively estimated to be used by at least 75% of the patient population [24] based solely on the potential of efficacy.

The etiology of motor neuron cell death is multifactorial. Oxidative injury, calcium dysregulation, inflammation, excitotoxicity, mitochondrial dysfunction, and cytoskeletal abnormalities are all hypotheses supported by substantial evidence from both animal models and patient samples [25,26]. Most dietary supplements that are directed to patients who have ALS are touted as having relevance to mechanisms with substantial preclinical data in motor neuron cell death. Study and evaluation of dietary supplement use in the ALS patient population is also complicated as most patients take several supplements simultaneously, hoping to address synergistic or complementary pathways [27]. The use of such combination or "cocktail" therapy is appealing to patients and intuitive to physicians, but currently such use not supported with data from blinded clinical trials. Regardless, it is a common practice with potential adverse health implications as well as benefits.

The authors' current approach toward the use of nutraceuticals as nutritional supplements is to remain aware of known adverse effects, as well as unfounded or unrealistic claims. The role of the practitioner has been largely to offer advice or caution as patients explore their own therapeutic combinations. Since the passage of the Dietary Supplement Health and Education Act in 1994, entry to the market of dietary supplements has been faster, often without any regulation or oversight common in prescription medications.

Rationale for the use of dietary supplements in ALS

Oxidative injury

Oxidative damage is thought to be a major contributing factor in the death of motor neurons [28]. Oxidative injury can have both a primary role and a secondary role triggered by other mechanisms mentioned below. Reactive oxygen species (ROS) include superoxide, hydrogen peroxide (H_2O_2), hydroxyl free radicals (OH), and nitric oxide (NO). ROS readily react with lipids, proteins, and DNA to induce cellular damage [29–31]. The high metabolic activity of neurons leads to considerable ROS formation in these cells [32]. The high content of lipids and iron in the nervous system may make it particularly sensitive to ROS damage [29]. Glutathione peroxidase, catalase, and superoxide dismutase (SOD) are all endogenous antioxidants that counteract ROS damage. Toxicity resulting from mutated SOD has been directly implicated in the pathophysiology in familial ALS. Further support for the ROS hypothesis comes from elevated levels of protein carbonyls and 8-hydroxy-2-deoxyguanosine (8-OHdG), both markers of oxidative damage, in the motor cortex of sporadic ALS patients [33]. In addition, elevated plasma levels of 8-OHdG [34] and thiobarbituric acid reactive substances (TBARS) [35] have been identified in sporadic ALS patients compared with healthy controls. Possible benefit from exogenous nutraceuticals may result from their direct antioxidant activity and/or effects on endogenous enzyme pathways [36].

Excitotoxicity

Glutamate is a primary excitatory neurotransmitter in CNS. Dysfunction in synaptic uptake of glutamate may lead to prolonged opening of glutamate-dependent Ca^{+2} channels in neuron, which may, in turn, generate free radicals and directly damage intracellular organelles (ie, mitochondria). Glutamate release and reuptake is usually tightly regulated; however, increased glutamate in cerebrospinal fluid was found in sporadic ALS patients. Riluzole, the only FDA-approved drug with indication for ALS, acts by blocking the presynaptic release of glutamate [37,38]. Supplements that likewise act to block glutamate release, enhance reuptake, or protect cells against the damaging effects of excessive glutamate may aid in the medicinal management of ALS.

Mitochondrial dysfunction

Strong evidence exists for mitochondrial dysfunction in motor neuron disease. Morphologic changes in mitochondria have been identified in SOD-1 mice [39] and in sporadic ALS patients without SOD-1 mutations [40]. Structural abnormalities within the electron transport chain and mutations within mitochondrial DNA have been implicated in the pathogenesis of ALS [39]. The primary role of mitochondria in cells is energy production by oxidative phosphorylation. Given the high metabolic demand of neurons, energy supply and use is critical and is reflected in the large number of neuronal mitochondria. Mitochondrial damage may be due to, or result in, increased free radical activity, increased intracellular free Ca^{+2} [41,42], defective electron transport enzymes (complexes I-IV), or coenzymes [43,44]. Dysfunctional mitochondria lead to the overproduction of ROS; abnormalities in the mitochondrial transition pore may activate a caspase cascade resulting in further oxidative damage [39].

Mitochondrial activity and the underlying physiology in neurons may also differ from the brain and spinal cord [45,46]. These differences may ultimately provide essential insights into disease heterogeneity in upper versus lower motor neuron clinical presentations.

Nutritional supplements that prevent free radical damage, stabilize mitochondrial membranes, or stimulate electron transport chain complexes may be of value.

Dietary supplements commonly used in the ALS patient population: fact versus fiction

Vitamin E

Reports of alpha-tocopherol, an isomer of vitamin E, as a trial therapy for ALS date back to the 1940s when Lou Gehrig received weekly intramuscular injections as putative therapy [47]. Despite the absence of documented clinical benefit in controlled trials, vitamin E continues to be among the most popular of the dietary supplements. This is likely the result of preclinical data, the association of vitamin E and motor neuron disease from other species, and the ease of availability with few or no documented side effects.

Preclinical data

In the G93A/SOD1 mouse model of ALS, vitamin E supplementation had no effect on survival; however, it did significantly delay symptom onset and slow disease progression as assessed by wheel activity [32]. The mutant SOD-1 mouse model is associated with an increase of hydrogen peroxide production, yielding an increase in hydroxyl free radicals [48]. Because alpha-tocopherol can directly neutralize hydroxyl radicals and some effect on disease progression has been demonstrated, alpha-tocopherol is commonly implicated as an ideal candidate for neuroprotection in ALS [49].

In the equine population, vitamin E deficiency has also been closely linked to motor neuron disease with implications to human disease [50]. In an inherited canine motor neuron disease, vitamin E levels were found to be lower than in controls, which suggests a potential role for supplementation [51]. Furthermore, experimentally-induced vitamin E deficiency has been reported to affect nerve regeneration and perhaps to affect the axonal integrity of healthy motor neurons [52].

Clinical data

The hypothesis that patients with motor neuron disease suffer from a deficiency of vitamin E is unfounded in data from at least three studies comparing both serum and or CSF levels in patients who have ALS and healthy, matched controls [35,53,54].

Presymptomatic use of vitamin E has also been implicated in the patient population as a source of neuroprotection in vulnerable motor neurons in patients showing early signs. No direct studies have been reported testing this hypothesis; however, a large epidemiologic evaluation of 957,740 adults participating in the American Cancer Society's Cancer Prevention Study II was collected in 1982. Information about the use of vitamins A, C, E, (all antioxidants) and multivitamins revealed that respondents categorized as "regular users of vitamin E for 10 or more years" demonstrated a significantly improved mortality related to ALS. The risk of death in this group was 62% lower than non-users of vitamin E. The study was limited (eg, observational design, use of other supplements, patient assessed at only time, no detail on dose); however, these data have helped propagate speculation leading to ongoing use [55]. In a separate case-control study, food-frequency questionnaires were administered to 132 patients who had ALS and 220 age and sex-matched controls. Comparing highest to lowest tertiles, individuals with highest polyunsaturated fat intake and highest vitamin E intake demonstrated 60% and 50% lower risk of developing ALS, respectively [56]. These data revealed significant reductions in the odds ratio for vitamin E and polyunsaturated acids together, suggesting a synergistic benefit.

Considering all of the population data collectively, available studies suggest that higher intakes of vitamin E may have a positive, protective effect on developing ALS. Nevertheless, data from formal clinical trials in the patient population is less convincing. The first such trial randomized 289 ALS patients in France to receive either alpha-tocopherol 1000 mg daily or placebo for 12 months. The primary outcome was function as assessed by the Norris Limb score, a validated four-point rating scale of physical function. Secondary outcomes included survival and biological markers of oxidative stress. Although supplementation did significantly decrease plasma concentration of TBARS and increase plasma concentrations of plasma glutathione peroxidase compared with placebo, there were no significant effects on the functional rating scale or survival [57]. In a separate open, randomized clinical trial assessing the same outcomes of survival and functional status, 35 Polish patients were randomized to receive vitamin E (600 IU/day) and selegiline (10 mg/day) for 18 months, while 32 patients received only symptomatic treatment. Again, there were no significant differences between groups [58]. Another study examined vitamin E in conjunction with riluzole. The participants were 160 ALS patients from Germany who were all receiving riluzole at the standard dosage. They were randomized to receive either 5000 mg of vitamin E or placebo daily for 18 months. The primary outcome was survival, and secondary outcomes were Norris function scale score, spasticity scale score, manual muscle testing, and the score of a validated quality-of-life scale. Again, no treatment effect for vitamin E was seen for any of the outcomes measured [59]. A separate observational study also confirmed no differences in quality-of-life scores between patients either taking or not taking vitamin E supplements at a dosage of 600 mg/day [60]. A current randomized, double-blind, placebo-controlled, crossover study to evaluate vitamin E for the treatment of muscular cramps is currently underway.

In summary, although vitamin E appeared promising in population studies and in the transgenic mouse model, clinical trials have thus far failed to show benefits for outcomes of survival, functional status, or quality of life.

B vitamins (folic acid, B6, B12)

Use of the B vitamins, particularly folic acid and methylcombalamin, have been largely driven by the observation that patients who have ALS may have elevated plasma homocysteine levels [61]. In the transgenic SOD-1 mouse model similar elevation of plasma homocysteine was found [62]. Vitamin B12 and folate are involved in reactions that convert homocysteine to methionine, thereby potentially reducing homocysteine levels. Furthermore, vitamin B6 functions in an alternative pathway to convert homocysteine to sulfur amino acids [63].

In 1998, a double-blind, randomized clinical trial examined the effects of megadose methylcobalamin, an analog of vitamin B12, on averaged compound muscle action potential amplitudes (CMAPs) in ALS patients. Twenty-four ALS patients with similar CMAPs at baseline were randomly assigned to two groups. Group 1 received 25 mg of methylcobalamin daily by intramuscular injection for 28 days. Group 2 received a lower dose (0.5 mg/day) for 28 days. CMAPs of selected muscle groups were measured at baseline, day 14, and day 28. The low-dose methylcobalamin group showed no significant changes in CMAPs from baseline, while the eight patients in the higher-dose group showed significantly higher CMAPs at 28 days compared with baseline. The investigators classified these eight subjects as "responders" and the remaining four subjects as "non responders." Based on these data, it was concluded that among certain ALS patients, high-dose methylcobalamin enhances neuronal functioning.

Despite the small sample size, the absence of a placebo group, and the absence of any documented improvement in clinical function, this study has contributed to speculation that such therapy may be of benefit [64]. The study does raise the important possibility that the ALS patient population may be quite heterogeneous, consisting of responders and nonresponders to a certain supplement or medication. If the disease pathophysiology is accepted as multifactorial, then the possibility emerges that there may be a subgroup of responders to selected treatments. Such possibilities have propagated the use of B complex vitamins, in part due to their availability and low side effect profile [64].

Zinc

Zinc is implicated as a supplement with potential benefit due to its integral role in the function of SOD-1. Mutant forms of SOD-1, as found in the transgenic model of ALS, have impaired ability to bind zinc and are toxic [65]. Zinc supplementation has been shown to up-regulate metallothioneins, and facilitate antioxidant function [66]. Zinc has therefore been implicated especially in patients possessing a mutated SOD-1 protein (ie, familial ALS patients).

Two experiments examining this hypothesis in the transgenic mouse model have yielded contrasting results. In the first experiment, three groups (11 transgenic mice per group) were given 75 mg/kg zinc, 375 mg/kg zinc, or no zinc in their drinking water. Contrary to their hypothesis that zinc would be protective, supplementation actually decreased survival in a dose-dependent manner. Zinc had no effect on symptom onset or on motor neuron numbers. These results suggested that zinc supplementation may actually accelerate motor neuron loss [66].

In a second study, more moderate dosages of zinc (12 mg/kg) delayed death in G93A-mutant SOD mice by 11 days compared with mice on a zinc-deficient diet [67]. Slightly higher doses (approximately 18 mg/kg) significantly shortened survival and this effect was blocked by concurrent supplementation with copper, which may have been displaced by the higher zinc dose. These data highlight the importance of dosage in supplementing zinc and the synergistic interaction of copper and zinc in predicting the toxic or neuroprotective effects [67].

Careful attention to the daily dosage of zinc, often found in compounded nutraceutical supplements, in the patient population is advised. It may be most prudent to simply assure adequate intake of zinc to meet the recommended dietary allowance.

Genistein

Genistein is a phytoestrogen that has been implicated in oxidative insult resulting from cerebral ischemia. Estrogen compounds have also been implicated as neuroprotective agents promoting survival of motor neurons. Survival differences between males and female SOD-1 transgenic mice have been attributed to the role of estrogen. This hypothesis was tested using genistein (16 mg/kg, twice daily) in that model. Genistein significantly delayed symptom onset and prolonged survival in male animals, but not in female animals. The study concludes that phytoestrogens in genistein pose gender-specific neuroprotection, likely by the same mechanism of endogenous estrogen. This provides support that the estrogenic effects of genistein may be neuroprotective but not at levels above normal, endogenous estrogen [63]. Clinical trials using genestein have not been reported.

Melatonin

Melatonin displays a wide array of antioxidant activities, including activation of glutathione peroxidase and inhibition of nitric oxide synthase [68]. Treatment with melatonin resulted in a significant, dose-dependent attenuation of glutamate-induced cell death in vitro using a motor neuron cell line. In transgenic mice, melatonin has been tested by administration before symptom onset or on the day of symptom onset. Symptom onset was delayed and survival prolonged when administered before symptom onset, however, not when administered after symptom onset.

In the ALS population, 31 ALS patients were given high-dose melatonin (300 mg/day) by rectal suppository for 24 months and compared with healthy, matched controls. The extent of oxidative injury was accessed by measurement of protein carbonyl levels in serum. At baseline, ALS patients displayed significant elevations of serum protein carbonyl groups. After four months of treatment with melatonin, serum protein carbonyl levels were the same in ALS patients as in healthy controls, indicating that melatonin attenuated oxidative damage. No report on symptom modification or alteration in disease course has been made [69].

Creatine

Creatine has received much attention within the patient population based largely on preclinical data and anecdotal patient reports. The use of creatine in combination with other agents has also been encouraging, albeit unproven in clinical trials. Creatine monohydrate displays many pharmacokinetic properties relevant to mechanisms of motor neuron loss in ALS. Enhancing energy production within mitochondria and possibly limiting the uptake of glutamate into cells have been proposed as putative neuroprotective effects [62]. The compound also displays antioxidant properties by acting as a mitochondrial membrane stabilizer [70].

In the transgenic SOD-1 model of ALS, creatine supplementation resulted in a dose-dependent increase in survival and motor performance as well as dose-dependent decreases in motor neuron loss and biomarkers of oxidative damage [71]. Another study reported that supplementation significantly attenuated chemically-induced increases in glutamate, delay in symptom onset and prolonged survival [72]. By contrast, a third study examining the effects of creatine on muscle function and muscle metabolism showed no improvements in rotorod performance, grip strength, ATP concentrations, or glycogen concentrations [73].

Combination therapies using creatine have been tested in several forms. The effects of riluzole, creatine, or the combination of both yielded delay in symptom onset and prolonged survival compared with control mice; however, no significant differences between treatment groups were observed [74]. The combination appeared to have additive, synergistic effects on these outcome measures compared with the control group or either agent alone [75]. Celecoxib and rofecoxib (both COX-2 inhibitors) were also tested alone and in combination with creatine; this combination resulted in significantly improved motor performance, reduced motor neuron loss, and extended survival. In combination with creatine, the effects on survival were significantly additive [76].

Despite such promising results from these animal studies, clinical trials have failed to show any significant effects of creatine for any outcomes examined. To date, three large clinical trials of creatine have been completed in the ALS population. All three studies concluded no efficacy in the primary endpoints [77–79]. While the studies differed somewhat in either dose and/or design, the conclusion followed that creatine, by itself, using available clinical outcomes, did not help. An interesting trend in improved survival in the creatine treatment groups from two of the studies has prompted a meta-analysis. A significant trend of improved survival was noted when the two trials recently completed in North America were combined. This benefit was more modest (not significant) when the third European trial was also included. The implication followed that larger study of survival in the patient population may be warranted.

Coenzyme Q10

Coenzyme Q10 (CoQ10) is a critical component of the electron transport chain of mitochondria. It also exhibits antioxidant properties [80]. Although serum levels of CoQ10 do not differ between sporadic ALS patients and healthy controls [81], sporadic ALS patients do display significantly higher levels of oxidized CoQ10 [40,82]. Oxidized CoQ10 can generate superoxide and hydrogen peroxide. Hydrogen peroxide can then react with iron-rich cytochromes to form hydroxyl free radicals [31].

In an open-label dose escalation study, 31 ALS patients received CoQ10, formulated with 300 IU of vitamin E, on a monthly dosage escalation scale (1200–3000 mg/day). CoQ10 was found to be safe and well-tolerated at the maximum dosage. When compared with a placebo group from a previous clinical trial, no differences between CoQ10 and historical placebo groups were observed in strength, grip, forced vital capacity, or ALS functional rating scale scores [83]. These pilot data have yielded a follow-up randomized, double-blind, placebo-controlled multicenter trial now in progress [84].

Alpha-lipoic acid

Alpha-lipoic acid is an antioxidant and also a cofactor for mitochondrial enzymes. In a study with G93A/SOD-1 mice, alpha-lipoic acid (0.05% in food) beginning at 4 weeks of age showed a significant delay in onset of impaired motor performance, increased survival, and attenuated weight loss in treated mice compared with controls [85].

L-carnitine

L-carnitine is an essential cofactor for the beta-oxidation of long-chain fatty acids in mitochondria. It has also been shown to inhibit mitochondrial damage and apoptosis in vitro and in vivo. Early oral administration of L-carnitine significantly delayed symptom onset, prolonged motor function as assessed by rotorod, and extended survival in SOD-1 transgenic mice. In a second experiment, 20 transgenic mice were injected with L-carnitine every two days after symptom onset. Survival of these mice was compared with that of 20 transgenic mice not receiving injections. Treatment with subcutaneous L-carnitine increased survival [86].

Glutathione, N-acetyl-cysteine, and pro-cysteine

Glutathione peroxidase activity has been shown to be lower in plasma and cerebrospinal fluid of patients who have ALS [87]. This observation has led to an open-crossover study, which failed to demonstrate any benefit in measures of manual muscle testing, Norris functional scale ratings, or forced vital capacity [87].

Cysteine supplementation has been hypothesized to increase intracellular concentrations of glutathione; however, neither intravenous nor oral pro-cysteine had any effect on cerebrospinal concentrations of glutathione with 29 days of treatment [88]. Likewise, in a randomized, double-blind, placebo-controlled clinical trial of acetylcysteine in ALS patients, no significant differences were seen in survival and disease progression between the two groups [89].

Studies of N-acetylcysteine (NAC) in transgenic mice models have produced conflicting results. In at least one study, transgenic mice given NAC (1% concentration) in drinking water beginning 4–5 weeks of age, showed significantly improved survival and delayed symptom [90]. An earlier study, with similar dosages given after symptom onset, showed no benefit [91].

Herbs and L-carnosine

In vitro experiments with ginseng suggest that it may act to decrease calcium flux into neurons. In the SOD-1 transgenic mice, Panax quiquefolium ginseng (100 μg, 200 μg versus control) was added to drinking water. Ginseng treated mice had significantly delayed symptom onset and prolonged survival [92]. Similar controlled trials have not been done in the patient population.

EGb761 is a standardized extract of Ginkgo biloba that has shown antioxidant properties in vitro. When tested in the same G93A/SOD-1 transgenic mice, EGb761 (0.022% or 0.045% via diet) significantly prolonged survival and decreased loss of motor neurons in the spinal cords of male transgenic mice but not in female mice. This gender-specific protection, while provocative, is currently unexplained [93].

Functional foods

Red wine is known to be rich in antioxidant compounds. Lyphilized red wine was dissolved in the drinking water of eight transgenic mice. Supplemented mice were compared with a control group of seven control transgenic mice not receiving treatment. The treatment group displayed significantly prolonged survival [94].

Epigallocatechin gallate (EGCG) is a major catechin in green tea. It has been shown to display antioxidant, anti-inflammatory, and iron-chelating properties in vitro. Eleven transgenic mice and six wild-type mice received EGCG by intraoral injection (10 mg/kg). Eleven transgenic mice serving as controls did not receive the injections. ECGC significantly delayed symptom onset and prolonged survival. The compound also significantly decreased markers of neuroinflammation and oxidative stress [95].

In another study of transgenic mice receiving intraoral injections of one of three different dosages of EGCG or control vehicle, dosages of 2.9 mcg/g and 5.8 mcg/g of EGCG also significantly delayed symptom onset and prolonged survival. Treatment was also associated with protective effects on markers of cell signaling associated with cell death and cell survival [96].

Summary

The benefits of aggressive nutritional support in affecting disease course and survival are well documented. Enteral nutrition is best thought of as an early adjunctive therapy, rather than as a late palliative therapy. The patient population has embraced the use of dietary supplements in the form of vitamins, nutraceuticals, and functional foods, often despite the absence of documented efficacy. The axiom that "the absence of proof does not equate to the proof of absence" [97] has fueled speculation among patients that these compounds should be tried even if the benefits are solely theoretic. The role of practitioners is to provide oversight into potential adverse consequences from especially high doses or drug interactions. The concept of combining compounds or drugs is currently empiric, although controlled trials are needed to address this logical treatment approach. The multifactorial pathophysiology of ALS has resulted in hypotheses that there may be subgroups of patients, eventually defined by a specific underlying etiology or clinical presentation, which selectively respond to a particular treatment. Future research endeavors exploring nutritional management and drug therapy will need to address this possibility.

References

[1] Hardiman O. Symptomatic treatment of respiratory and nutritional failure in amyotrophic lateral sclerosis. J Neurol 2000;247(4):245–51.

[2] Desport JC, Preux PM, Truong TC, et al. Nutritional status is a prognostic factor for survival in ALS patients. Neurology 1999;53(5):1059–63.

[3] Mazzini L, Corra T, Zaccala M, et al. Percutaneous endoscopic gastrostomy and enteral nutrition in amyotrophic lateral sclerosis. J Neurol 1995;242(10):695–8.

[4] Desport JC, Preux PM, Magy L, et al. Factors correlated with hypermetabolism in patients with amyotrophic lateral sclerosis. Am J Clin Nutr 2001;74(3):328–34.

[5] Ludolph AC. 135th ENMC International Workshop: nutrition in amyotrophic lateral sclerosis 18-20 of March 2005, Naarden, The Netherlands. Neuromuscul Disord 2006; 16(8):530–8.

[6] Desport JC, Torny F, Lacoste M, et al. Hypermetabolism in ALS: correlations with clinical and paraclinical parameters. Neurodegener Dis 2005;2(3–4):202–7.

[7] Sherman M, Pillai A, Jackson A, et al. Standard equations are not accurate in assessing resting energy expenditure in patients with amyotrophic lateral sclerosis. JPEN J Parenter Enteral Nutr 2004;28(6):442–6.

[8] Heffernan C, Jenkinson C, Holmes T, et al. Nutritional management in MND/ALS patients: an evidence based review. Amyotroph Lateral Scler Other Motor Neuron Disord 2004;5(2): 72–83.

[9] Miller RG, Rosenberg JA, Gelinas DF, et al. Practice parameter: the care of the patient with amyotrophic lateral sclerosis (an evidence-based review): report of the Quality Standards Subcommittee of the American Academy of Neurology: ALS Practice Parameters Task Force. Neurology 1999;52(7):1311–23.

[10] Desport JC, Mabrouk T, Bouillet P, et al. Complications and survival following radiologically and endoscopically-guided gastrostomy in patients with amyotrophic lateral sclerosis. Amyotroph Lateral Scler Other Motor Neuron Disord 2005;6(2):88–93.

[11] Pacicco TJ, Lindblom S, Rosenfeld J. Enhancing PEG tube placement: a new device to maintain respiratory function during endoscopy in ALS patients. Paper presented at: International Motor Neuron Disease Symposium. Dublin, Ireland, December, 2005.

[12] Aldrich TK. Nutritional factors in the pathogenesis and therapy of respiratory insufficiency in neuromuscular diseases. Monaldi Arch Chest Dis 1993;48(4):327–30.

[13] Cameron A, Rosenfeld J. Nutritional issues and supplements in amyotrophic lateral sclerosis and other neurodegenerative disorders. Curr Opin Clin Nutr Metab Care 2002;5(6): 631–43.

[14] Kasarskis EJ, Berryman S, Vanderleest JG, et al. Nutritional status of patients with amyotrophic lateral sclerosis: relation to the proximity of death. Am J Clin Nutr 1996;63(1): 130–7.

[15] Chio A, Finocchiaro E, Meineri P, et al. Safety and factors related to survival after percutaneous endoscopic gastrostomy in ALS. ALS Percutaneous Endoscopic Gastrostomy Study Group. Neurology 1999;53(5):1123–5.

[16] Kasarskis EJ, Scarlata D, Hill R, et al. A retrospective study of percutaneous endoscopic gastrostomy in ALS patients during the BDNF and CNTF trials. J Neurol Sci 1999; 169(1–2):118–25.

[17] Chio A, Galletti R, Finocchiaro C, et al. Percutaneous radiological gastrostomy: a safe and effective method of nutritional tube placement in advanced ALS. J Neurol Neurosurg Psychiatry 2004;75(4):645–7.

[18] Desport JC, Preux PM, Truong CT, et al. Nutritional assessment and survival in ALS patients. Amyotroph Lateral Scler Other Motor Neuron Disord 2000;1(2):91–6.

[19] Mitsumoto H, Davidson M, Moore D, et al. Percutaneous endoscopic gastrostomy (PEG) in patients with ALS and bulbar dysfunction. Amyotroph Lateral Scler Other Motor Neuron Disord 2003;4(3):177–85.

[20] Miller RG, Jackson CE, Kasarskis EJ, et al. Practice parameter update: the care of the patient with amyotrophic lateral sclerosis (an evidence-based review): report of the quality standards subcommittee of the american academy of neurology. Neurology, in press.
[21] Chio A, Mora G, Leone M, et al. Early symptom progression rate is related to ALS outcome: a prospective population-based study. Neurology 2002;59(1):99–103.
[22] Shaw AS, Ampong MA, Rio A, et al. Survival of patients with ALS following institution of enteral feeding is related to pre-procedure oximetry: a retrospective review of 98 patients in a single centre. Amyotroph Lateral Scler 2006;7(1):16–21.
[23] Costello RB, Coates P. In the midst of confusion lies opportunity: fostering quality science in dietary supplement research. J Am Coll Nutr 2001;20(1):21–5.
[24] Bradley WG, Anderson F, Gowda N, et al. Changes in the management of ALS since the publication of the AAN ALS practice parameter 1999. Amyotroph Lateral Scler Other Motor Neuron Disord 2004;5:240–4.
[25] Pasinelli P, Brown RH. Molecular biology of amyotrophic lateral sclerosis: insights from genetics. Nat Rev Neurosci 2006;7(9):710–23.
[26] Strong M, Rosenfeld J. Amyotrophic lateral sclerosis: a review of current concepts. Amyotroph Lateral Scler Other Motor Neuron Disord 2003;4(3):136–43.
[27] Vardeny O, Bromberg MB. The use of herbal supplements and alternative therapies by patients with amyotrophic lateral sclerosis (ALS). J Herb Pharmacother 2005;5(3): 23–31.
[28] Beal MF, Lang AE, Ludolph AC. Neurodegenerative diseases: neurobiology, pathogenesis, and therapeutics. New York: Cambridge University Press; 2005.
[29] Singh RP, Sharad KS, Suman K. Free radicals and oxidative stress in neurodegenerative diseases: relevance of dietary antioxidants. Journal of the Indian Academy of Clinical Medicine 2004;5:218–25.
[30] Esposito E, Rotilio D, Di Matteo V, et al. A review of specific dietary antioxidants and the effects on biochemical mechanisms related to neurodegenerative processes. Neurobiol Aging 2002;23(5):719–35.
[31] Halliwell B. Role of free radicals in the neurodegenerative diseases: therapeutic implications for antioxidant treatment. Drugs Aging 2001;18(9):685–716.
[32] Gurney ME, Cutting FB, Zhai P, et al. Benefit of vitamin E, riluzole, and gabapentin in a transgenic model of familial amyotrophic lateral sclerosis [see comments]. Ann Neurol 1996;39(2):147–57.
[33] Ferrante RJ, Browne SE, Shinobu LA, et al. Evidence of increased oxidative damage in both sporadic and familial amyotrophic lateral sclerosis. J Neurochem 1997;69(5): 2064–74.
[34] Bogdanov M, Brown RH, Matson W, et al. Increased oxidative damage to DNA in ALS patients. Free Radic Biol Med 2000;29(7):652–8.
[35] Bonnefont-Rousselot D, Lacomblez L, Jaudon M, et al. Blood oxidative stress in amyotrophic lateral sclerosis. J Neurol Sci 2000;178(1):57–62.
[36] Orrell RW, Lane JM, Ross MA. Antioxidant treatment for amyotrophic lateral sclerosis/ motor neuron disease. Cochrane Database Syst Rev 2005;(1):CD002829.
[37] Doble A. The role of excitotoxicity in neurodegenerative disease: implications for therapy. Pharmacol Ther 1999;81(3):163–221.
[38] Shaw PJ, Ince PG. Glutamate, excitotoxicity and amyotrophic lateral sclerosis. J Neurol 1997;244(Suppl 2):S3–14.
[39] Menzies FM, Ince PG, Shaw PJ. Mitochondrial involvement in amyotrophic lateral sclerosis. Neurochem Int 2002;40(6):543–51.
[40] Murata T, Ohtsuka C, Terayama Y. Increased mitochondrial oxidative damage in patients with sporadic amyotrophic lateral sclerosis. J Neurol Sci 2008;267(1–2):66–9.
[41] Cassarino DS, Bennett JP Jr. An evaluation of the role of mitochondria in neurodegenerative diseases: mitochondrial mutations and oxidative pathology, protective nuclear responses, and cell death in neurodegeneration. Brain Res Brain Res Rev 1999;29(1):1–25.

[42] Shaw PJ, Eggett CJ. Molecular factors underlying selective vulnerability of motor neurons to neurodegeneration in amyotrophic lateral sclerosis. J Neurol 2000;247(Suppl 1):I17–27.

[43] Fosslien E. Mitochondrial medicine–molecular pathology of defective oxidative phosphorylation. Ann Clin Lab Sci 2001;31(1):25–67.

[44] Bolanos JP, Heales SJ, Land JM, et al. Effect of peroxynitrite on the mitochondrial respiratory chain: differential susceptibility of neurones and astrocytes in primary culture. J Neurochem 1995;64(5):1965–72.

[45] Sullivan PG, Rabchevsky AG, Keller JN, et al. Intrinsic differences in brain and spinal cord mitochondria: Implication for therapeutic interventions. J Comp Neurol 2004;474(4): 524–34.

[46] Panov A, Rosenfeld J. Glutamate enhances mitochondrial ATP production and ROS generation in nonsynaptic brain and spinal cord mitochondria of the wild type and SOD1 mutant rats. Paper presented at: International Symposium on Motor Neuron Disease. Toronto, Canada, 2007.

[47] Reider CR, Paulson GW. Lou Gehrig and amyotrophic lateral sclerosis. Is vitamin E to be revisited? Arch Neurol 1997;54(5):527–8.

[48] Butterfield DA, Castegna A, Drake J, et al. Vitamin E and neurodegenerative disorders associated with oxidative stress. Nutr Neurosci 2002;5(4):229–39.

[49] Ricciarelli R, Argellati F, Pronzato M, et al. D. Vitamin E and neurodegenerative diseases. Mol Aspects Med 2007;28:591–606.

[50] Mohammed HO, Divers TJ, Summers BA, et al. Vitamin E deficiency and risk of equine motor neuron disease. Acta Vet Scand 2007;49(1):17.

[51] Green SL, Bouley DM, Pinter MJ, et al. Canine motor neuron disease: clinicopathologic features and selected indicators of oxidative stress. J Vet Intern Med 2001;15(2):112–9.

[52] Enrione EB, Weeks OI, Kranz S, et al. A vitamin E-deficient diet affects nerve regeneration in rats. Nutrition 1999;15(2):140–4.

[53] de Bustos F, Jimenez-Jimenez FJ, Molina JA, et al. Cerebrospinal fluid levels of alpha-tocopherol in amyotrophic lateral sclerosis. J Neural Transm 1998;105(6–7):703–8.

[54] Iwasaki Y, Ikeda K, Kinoshita M, et al. E levels are normal in amyotrophic lateral sclerosis. J Neurol Sci 1995;132(2):193–4.

[55] Ascherio A, Weisskopf MG, O'Reilly EJ, et al. Vitamin E intake and risk of amyotrophic lateral sclerosis. Ann Neurol 2005;57(1):104–10.

[56] Veldink JH, Kalmijn S, Groeneveld GJ, et al. Intake of polyunsaturated fatty acids and vitamin E reduces the risk of developing amyotrophic lateral sclerosis [erratum appears in J Neurol Neurosurg Psychiatry. 2007 Jul;78(7):779]. 2007;78(4):367–71.

[57] Desnuelle C, Dib M, Garrel C, et al. A double-blind, placebo-controlled randomized clinical trial of alpha-tocopherol (vitamin E) in the treatment of amyotrophic lateral sclerosis. ALS riluzole-tocopherol Study Group. Amyotroph Lateral Scler Other Motor Neuron Disord 2001;2(1):9–18.

[58] Kwiecinski H, Janik P, Jamrozik Z, et al. [The effect of selegiline and vitamin E in the treatment of ALS: an open randomized clinical trials]. Neurol Neurochir Pol 2001;35(Suppl 1): 101–6 [in Polish].

[59] Graf M, Ecker D, Horowski R, et al. High dose vitamin E therapy in amyotrophic lateral sclerosis as add-on therapy to riluzole: results of a placebo-controlled double-blind study. J Neural Transm 2005;112(5):649–60.

[60] Galbussera A, Tremolizzo L, Brighina L, et al. Vitamin E intake and quality of life in amyotrophic lateral sclerosis patients: a follow-up case series study. Neurol Sci 2006;27(3): 190–3.

[61] Zoccolella S, Simone IL, Lamberti P, et al. Elevated plasma homocysteine levels in patients with amytrophic lateral sclerosis. Neurology 2008;70(3):222–5.

[62] Xu CJ, Klunk WE, Kanfer JN, et al. Phosphocreatine-dependent glutamate uptake by synaptic vesicles. A comparison with atp-dependent glutamate uptake. J Biol Chem 1996; 271(23):13435–40.

[63] Trieu VN, Uckun FM. Genistein is neuroprotective in murine models of familial amyotrophic lateral sclerosis and stroke. Biochem Biophys Res Commun 1999;258(3):685–8.
[64] Izumi Y, Kaji R. [Clinical trials of ultra-high-dose methylcobalamin in ALS]. Brain Nerve 2007;59(10):1141–7 [in Japanese].
[65] Smith AP, Lee NM. Role of zinc in ALS. Amyotroph Lateral Scler Other Motor Neuron Disord 2007;8(3):131–43.
[66] Groeneveld GJ, de Leeuw van Weenen J, van Muiswinkel FL, et al. Zinc amplifies mSOD1-mediated toxicity in a transgenic mouse model of amyotrophic lateral sclerosis. Neurosci Lett 2003;352(3):175–8.
[67] Ermilova IP, Ermilov VB, Levy M, et al. Protection by dietary zinc in ALS mutant G93A SOD transgenic mice. Neurosci Lett 2005;379(1):42–6.
[68] Jacob S, Poeggeler B, Weishaupt JH, et al. Melatonin as a candidate compound for neuroprotection in amyotrophic lateral sclerosis (ALS): high tolerability of daily oral melatonin administration in ALS patients. J Pineal Res 2002;33(3):186–7.
[69] Weishaupt JH, Bartels C, Polking E, et al. Reduced oxidative damage in ALS by high-dose enteral melatonin treatment. J Pineal Res 2006;41(4):313–23.
[70] Strong MJ, Pattee GL. Creatine and coenzyme Q10 in the treatment of ALS. Amyotroph Lateral Scler Other Motor Neuron Disord. 2000;1(Suppl 4):17–20.
[71] Klivenyi P, Ferrante RJ, Matthews RT, et al. Neuroprotective effects of creatine in a transgenic animal model of amyotrophic lateral sclerosis. Nat Med 1999;5(3):347–50.
[72] Andreassen OA, Jenkins BG, Dedeoglu A, et al. Increases in cortical glutamate concentrations in transgenic amyotrophic lateral sclerosis mice are attenuated by creatine supplementation. J Neurochem 2001;77(2):383–90.
[73] Derave W, Van Den Bosch L, Lemmens G, et al. Skeletal muscle properties in a transgenic mouse model for amyotrophic lateral sclerosis: effects of creatine treatment. Neurobiol Dis 2003;13(3):264–72.
[74] Snow RJ, Turnbull J, da Silva S, et al. Creatine supplementation and riluzole treatment provide similar beneficial effects in copper, zinc superoxide dismutase (G93A) transgenic mice. Neuroscience 2003;119(3):661–7.
[75] Zhang W, Narayanan M, Friedlander RM. Additive neuroprotective effects of minocycline with creatine in a mouse model of ALS [comment]. Ann Neurol 2003;53(2):267–70.
[76] Klivenyi P, Kiaei M, Gardian G, et al. Additive neuroprotective effects of creatine and cyclooxygenase 2 inhibitors in a transgenic mouse model of amyotrophic lateral sclerosis. J Neurochem 2004;88(3):576–82.
[77] Groeneveld G, Veldink J, Tweel I, et al. A randomized sequential trial of creatine in amyotrophic lateral sclerosis. Ann Neurol 2003;43:437–45.
[78] Shefner JM, Cudkowicz ME, Schoenfeld D, et al. A clinical trial of creatine in ALS. Neurology 2004;63(9):1656–61.
[79] Rosenfeld J, King R, Jackson C, et al. Creatine monohydrate in ALS: Effects on strength, fatigue, respiratory status and ALSFRS. Amyotroph Lateral Scler Other Motor Neuron Disord, in press.
[80] Galpern WR, Cudkowicz ME. Coenzyme Q treatment of neurodegenerative diseases of aging. Mitochondrion 2007;7(Suppl):S146–53.
[81] Molina JA, de Bustos F, Jimenez-Jimenez FJ, et al. Serum levels of coenzyme Q10 in patients with amyotrophic lateral sclerosis. J Neural Transm 2000;107(8–9):1021–6.
[82] Sohmiya M, Tanaka M, Suzuki Y, et al. An increase of oxidized coenzyme Q-10 occurs in the plasma of sporadic ALS patients. J Neurol Sci 2005;228(1):49–53.
[83] Ferrante KL, Shefner J, Zhang H, et al. Tolerance of high-dose (3,000 mg/day) coenzyme Q10 in ALS. Neurology 2005;65(11):1834–6.
[84] Levy G, Kaufmann P, Buchsbaum R, et al. A two-stage design for a phase II clinical trial of coenzyme Q10 in ALS [see comment]. Neurology 2006;66(5):660–3.

[85] Andreassen OA, Dedeoglu A, Friedlich A, et al. Effects of an inhibitor of poly(ADP-ribose) polymerase, desmethylselegiline, trientine, and lipoic acid in transgenic ALS mice. Exp Neurol 2001;168(2):419–24.

[86] Kira Y, Nishikawa M, Ochi A, et al. L-carnitine suppresses the onset of neuromuscular degeneration and increases the life span of mice with familial amyotrophic lateral sclerosis. Brain Res 2006;1070(1):206–14.

[87] Chio A, Cucatto A, Terreni AA, et al. Reduced glutathione in amyotrophic lateral sclerosis: an open, crossover, randomized trial. Ital J Neurol Sci 1998;19(6):363–6.

[88] Cudkowicz ME, Sexton PM, Ellis T, et al. The pharmacokinetics and pharmaco-dynamics of Procysteine in amyotrophic lateral sclerosis. Neurology 1999;52(7):1492–4.

[89] Louwerse ES, Weverling GJ, Bossuyt PM, et al. Randomized, double-blind, controlled trial of acetylcysteine in amyotrophic lateral sclerosis. Arch Neurol 1995;52(6):559–64.

[90] Andreassen OA, Dedeoglu A, Klivenyi P, et al. N-acetyl L-cysteine improves survival and preserves motor performance in an animal model of familial amyotrophic lateral sclerosis. Neuroreport 2000;11(11):2491–3.

[91] Jaarsma D, Guchelaar HJ, Haasdijk E, et al. The antioxidant N-acetylcysteine does not delay disease onset and death in a transgenic mouse model of amyotrophic lateral sclerosis. Ann Neurol 1998;44(2):293.

[92] Jiang F, DeSilva S, Turnbull J. Beneficial effect of ginseng root in SOD-1 (G93A) transgenic mice. J Neurol Sci 2000;180(1–2):52–4.

[93] Ferrante RJ, Klein AM, Dedeoglu A, et al. Therapeutic efficacy of EGb761 (Gingko biloba extract) in a transgenic mouse model of amyotrophic lateral sclerosis. J Mol Neurosci 2001; 17(1):89–96.

[94] Esposito E, Rossi C, Amodio R, et al. Lyophilized red wine administration prolongs survival in an animal model of amyotrophic lateral sclerosis. Ann Neurol 2000;48(4):686–7.

[95] Xu Z, Chen S, Li X, et al. Neuroprotective effects of (-)-epigallocatechin-3-gallate in a transgenic mouse model of amyotrophic lateral sclerosis. Neurochem Res 2006;31(10): 1263–9.

[96] Koh SH, Lee SM, Kim HY, et al. The effect of epigallocatechin gallate on suppressing disease progression of ALS model mice. Neurosci Lett 2006;395(2):103–7.

[97] Cowper W. (English poet 1731–1800).

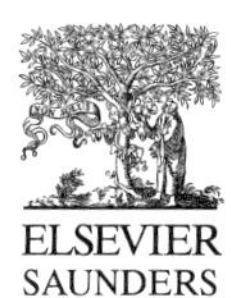
ELSEVIER
SAUNDERS

Phys Med Rehabil Clin N Am
19 (2008) 591–605

PHYSICAL MEDICINE
AND REHABILITATION
CLINICS OF
NORTH AMERICA

Quality of Life in Amyotrophic Lateral Sclerosis

Mark B. Bromberg, MD, PhD

Clinical Neurosciences Center, Department of Neurology, 175 North Medical Drive, Salt Lake City, UT 84132, USA

Amyotrophic lateral sclerosis (ALS) is characterized by relentless progression of weakness causing loss of physical independence for the patient and also for the caregiver and family. There is no effective therapy to slow progression, and ALS is uniformly fatal with median survival of 2 to 4 years after diagnosis. At the time of diagnosis and explanation of the nature of the disease, patients express concern for their quality of life. Their perceptions can influence decisions on drug treatment (riluzole) and interventions (noninvasive ventilation and gastric feeding tube). Thus, it is important that health care providers for patients who have ALS be knowledgeable about quality of life when addressing patients' and families' concerns and questions. It perhaps is surprising that, when measured formally, patients who have ALS usually rate their quality of life to be relatively good. Although this finding may be counterintuitive to the newly diagnosed patient, it is important to convey this finding to the patient and his or her family. To assist health care providers, this article reviews definitions of quality of life, how it is measured, data from numerous studies, and how quality of life can be influenced. Consideration is given to both the patient and the caregiver.

Defining quality of life

It is difficult to provide a concise definition of quality of life. Many factors and different vantage points should be considered. Obvious factors include the patient's background (ethnic, cultural, past experiences), expectations, current support (family, friends), and spiritual beliefs (organized religion or beliefs). The World Health Organization states that quality of life

E-mail address: mbromberg@hsc.utah.edu

doi:10.1016/j.pmr.2008.02.005

"is a broad ranging concept affected in a complex way by the person's physical health, psychologic state, level of independence, social relationships, personal beliefs and their relationship to salient features of their environment." From a patient's vantage point, especially when there is a serious illness such as ALS, physical health looms large and can influence the interpretation of quality of life and outlook for the future. The progression of weakness and loss of physical independence with no cure emphasizes the negative aspects of the illness, including fears about dying and concerns for the caregiver and family. There are, however, positive aspects for the patient and caregiver that may not be appreciated at time of diagnosis. It is important to consider all these factors when helping the patient view his or her quality of life and to review these factors as they change over time.

Measuring quality of life

Questionnaires or instruments addressing issues related to quality of life can be divided into three broad groups: those that cover general health status, those that focus on a specific factor or issue that may be influential in quality of life, and those that specifically address overall quality of life (Box 1). Within these groups, questionnaires can be simple (a single question) or complex (multiple sections, each with many questions). This article focuses on questionnaires and instruments that specifically address quality of life with limited reference to the other two groups.

Box 1. Questionnaires and instruments frequently used in assessing quality of life in amyotrophic lateral sclerosis[a]

General health-related status

- Sickness Impact Profile (SIP)
- Short Form-36 (SF-36)

Specific for quality of life in general of for other diseases

- Single question
- McGill Quality of Life Questionnaire (MQOL)
- Schedule of the Evaluation of Individual Quality of Life-Direct Weigh (SEIQoL-DW)

Specific for quality of life in ALS

- Amyotrophic Lateral Sclerosis Assessment Questionnaire (ALSAQ-40)
- ALS-Specific Quality Of Life (ALSSQOL)

[a] See text for full descriptions.

Instrument development

Formal methods are used to design, refine, and validate complex questionnaires.

Questionnaires or instruments are designed to address specific elements or areas that, from prior ground work, are thought to be factors affecting quality of life. Responses to the elements or areas result in subscores for the various sections in addition to a summation score that gives an overall measure of quality of life. Complex quality-of-life questionnaires are developed and validated by a rigorous multistep process. The areas or elements of interest frequently are identified from interviews with the groups of interest (patients and caregivers). Specific questions are formulated to address issues and concerns brought out from the interviews. An initial version of the questionnaire is tested in the designated group. The validity of the various elements or areas is assessed by having subjects simultaneously complete other focused questionnaires that previously have been established as good measures of the particular element or area. Comparisons then are made to determine how the new questions capture the specific information. To reduce the number of questions to a minimum while retaining full information, answers to each question are compared with each other to determine which questions are answered similarly and thus can be dropped. The final, shortened version then is retested to see if it retains overall sensitivity and specificity to the original version.

Quality-of-life questionnaires developed for one patient population (eg, patients who have cancer) can be used for another population (eg, patients who have ALS) but should be assessed formally for consistency and validity in the new patient population. When an existing questionnaire developed for one population is modified for another population, questions frequently are changed, added, or dropped to meet specific perceived needs of the new population. The modified questionnaire should be reassessed in the new population to ensure validity. When translating a questionnaire or instrument to another language, the document should be translated to the new language and then back to the original language and then validated for consistency.

Questionnaires related to general health status

Questionnaires related to general health status cover a broad spectrum of perceived contributors to health and can be used for a variety of medical conditions; comparisons can be made between conditions. Such a questionnaire includes sections that assess emotional and mental well-being and sections that assess functional activities. In ALS, muscle strength and the ability to perform activities of daily living inexorably decline. Thus, functional element subscores fall over time and may drive or influence the total score [1].

Although questionnaires related to health status are considered also to assess quality of life, quality of life encompasses a broader array of life's experiences than those related to health status [2]. Despite these limitations, health-related quality-of-life scales have been used in ALS as a measure of quality of life. Specific instruments include the Sickness Impact Profile (SIP) [3] and especially the Short Form-36 (SF-36) [4]. One concern is that these questionnaires can be long and tiring for patients who have ALS, especially the SIP, which consists of 136 questions [5]. Shorter versions have been developed, such as a 19-question version of the SIP (SIP/ALS-19) [6], and a 12-question version of the SF-36 (SF-12) [7].

An offshoot of the functional subscales in these instruments is linkage to patient strength. There are strong correlations between loss of muscle strength measured quantitatively by the Tufts Quantitative Neurologic Examination (TQNE) [8] and the SF-36 [9]. The set of questions related to function from the SIP were selected and incorporated in the shorter SIP/ALS-19, which is offered as a proxy for quantitative strength testing [6].

Single-question instruments

The simplest assessment instrument is a single question asking patients to rate their own quality of life over a specific time frame, such as currently, during the past week, in the past month, since an event, and so forth. The answer can be marked on a visual analogue scale from 0 to 10 cm, and the mark can be measured in metric units. This scale gives a general or global indication of quality of life. Despite its simplicity, there is merit in letting patients reach their own conclusions in a single score. The scale, however, does not provide insight into factors that affect quality of life.

Open instruments

Open quality-of-life instruments impose no specific questions and allow the subject to decide what elements make up their quality of life [10]. In addition to the single global question discussed earlier, a more informative instrument has been developed in the Schedule of the Evaluation of Individual Quality of Life (SEIQoL) and a shorter direct weight version (SEIQoL-DW) [11]. The procedure has three steps. In the first, the subject is asked to list five areas that make up his or her quality of life at the current time. In the second, the subject is asked to rate the current status of each area using a visual analogue scale. In the third, the patient is asked to rank the relative importance of each area using a pie chart. The data available for analysis include the five areas, the patient's evaluation of each area, the areas' relative importance, and a combined index score. These instruments have been validated with patients who have ALS and with patients who have a number of other diseases [12]. An advantage of open questionnaires is that the same questionnaire can be used to assess quality of life for the patient and for the caregiver, among patients who have different diseases, and in healthy individuals.

Questionnaires specific to amyotrophic lateral sclerosis

ALS-specific quality-of-life questionnaires have been developed from the ground up based on interviews with patients and caregivers and with formal verification and statistical analysis to yield a validated instrument. Such questionnaires are the 40-question Amyotrophic Lateral Sclerosis Assessment Questionnaire (ALSAQ-40) and a shorter version, the five-question ALSAQ-5 [13]. The ALSAQ-40 includes five dimensions: physical mobility, activities of daily living/independence, eating and drinking, communication, and emotional functioning, leading to subscores and a total score. It was developed in the United Kingdom, and a Dutch-language translation has been verified [14].

Another approach is to modify for ALS an existing quality-of-life questionnaire originally validated for another disorder. The McGill Quality of Life Questionnaire originally was designed for patients who have cancer or HIV [15]. It is attractive for ALS because it is not heavily weighted toward physical function and includes an existential element (perception of purpose, meaning in life, and capacity for personal growth). The existential element is thought to be as important for patients who have ALS, as it is for patients who have cancer. A modified version of the McGill questionnaire for patients who have ALS has been validated as the ALS-Specific Quality of Life (ALSSQOL) questionnaire [16]. Changes for the ALS population include reformatting for ease of administration and incorporating nondominant physical function, psychologic support, and existential elements and a broad spiritual element. Included is an open question asking the patient to list things that had the greatest effect on his or her quality of life over the past seven days. In an effort to include issues pertinent to the patient, a section was added asking the patient to identify troublesome symptoms from a list of 10.

Quality of life in amyotrophic lateral sclerosis

When able-bodied people are asked to imagine the quality of life for a person who has impaired function, a poor rating is predicted [17]. In contrast, the data support a relatively good quality of life for people who have impaired function of all types. Following are data from a large selection of studies assessing quality of life in ALS. With the variety of instruments and questionnaires available and their use in various combinations, some differences are observed between studies, but the overall conclusions seem to hold true across the majority of studies.

Perceived quality of life in amyotrophic lateral sclerosis

At the time of diagnosis and explanation of the features of ALS, despair is high and perceived quality of life in the future is low. The extreme is predicting a quality of life with ALS that is so poor that it is not felt to be worth living, leading to the patient's wish to end his or her life through suicide or assisted death. To assess this feeling, a survey of patients who had ALS in the state of Oregon, which at the time of the survey had approved but had not enacted an assisted-suicide initiative, posed the question: "Under some circumstances would you consider taking a prescription for a medicine whose sole purpose was to end your life?" Fifty-six percent answered in the affirmative [18]. A feeling of hopelessness, but not depression, was a factor in giving an affirmative response; strong religious belief was a factor in giving a negative response. A subset of caregivers interviewed after patients who had ALS had died reported that 33% of these patients had discussed with their caregiver an interest in assisted suicide in the last month of life [19]. In a companion study by the same authors, correlates of suffering by patients who had ALS were assessed, and although approximately 20% of patients reported suffering in the form of pain, there were no correlations between ratings of pain, suffering, quality of life, and interest in physician-assisted suicide [20]. In similar study, nearly 20% of patients who had terminal-stage ALS expressed a wish to die, but only 6% hastened dying [21]. Among the 20% expressing a wish to die, depression was not more marked than in the remaining 80%, but a feeling of hopelessness was a factor. It is likely that there are differences between "considering" suicide, "expressing a wish" for assisted suicide, and "taking specific actions." The initial thoughts of despair at living through ALS seem to be reduced for many patients during the course of the disease. Among the group of patients in Oregon, political discussion of assisted suicide may have raised awareness.

Quality of life for the patient

A large number of studies have been administered to patients who have ALS assessing quality of life between the extremes of time of diagnosis and time of death. They consistently show that when assessed either at a single point in time or at multiple points, quality of life remains relatively high even though strength and functional abilities to carry out activities of daily life decline. A lesser number of studies show a low or declining quality of life, but these studies are based on data from health-related questionnaires [22].

Cross-sectional studies using ALS-specific questionnaires or open instruments show both a generally good quality of life and absence of depression in patients who have ALS [23–28]. Further, these studies show no correlations with general health status questionnaires or functional rating scales [24,26]. The open SEIQoL-DW instrument was rated by patients who had ALS as having greater validity for them than other questionnaires such as the SIP and SF-36 [5]. It is of interest that although "health" is frequently mentioned with the SEIQoL-DW as one of the five factors important in quality of life, this factor is not mentioned more frequently as disease progresses [5,26].

Longitudinal studies show a relatively stable assessment of quality of life in the setting of declining physical function and no increase in depression [5,23,29–32]. There may be cultural differences in perceived quality of life issues, and global generalities about specific issues must be made with caution [33].

These studies have limitations. Within a study, not every patient describes a good quality of life; there are extremes at both ends of the spectrum, with some patients describing a poor quality of life and others describing a clear improvement as they refocus their lives. Cross-sectional studies are based on patients at a midpoint in their disease course. Longitudinal studies are based on sample sizes ranging from 17 to 80 patients with assessments made every 2 to 3 months for a total of three to five visits. Patients in longitudinal studies also are in the midpoint of their disease, and there are few data on quality of life over the total duration of the disease or at the end of life. It is possible that there is a change to a lower quality of life, especially at late stages.

Response shift

An important question is "Why do many people with serious and persistent disability report that they experience good or excellent quality of life when to most external observes these people seem to live an undesirable daily existence?" [34]. Further, in ALS, there is a progression of weakness and greater disability without a cure. The answer is given in terms of a "response shift," defined as a recalibration of an individual's internal standards and values [35,36]. The response shift follows a poorly understood process that probably includes a catalyst (such as the disease) modified by a variety of factors and pre-existing components (including sociodemographics, personality, expectations, spirituality) and adaptive components (including coping mechanisms, social support, goal reformatting) leading to the response shift and the perceived quality of life [35]. It can be argued that response shifts are normal adaptive psychologic mechanisms for coping with a wide range of life's disturbances, including normal aging with unfulfilled hopes and plans and reduced functioning abilities.

A striking example of a response shift in ALS comes from a study using the SEQoL-DW in a German patient who listed football (soccer) as one of the five important elements in his quality of life [5]. Over time, as he became weaker, he shifted from actively playing football to watching football. Despite this shift in type of involvement, football remained high as a source of satisfaction, and its relative contribution to quality of life remained unchanged.

Although the response shift can be viewed as a natural process with aging, it may not go well with everyone, especially when faced with a severe disease. When shifts do not go well, an individual may experience variable degrees of stress and a lower quality of life [36]. Perhaps it is these patients who deserve specific attention to help them.

Factors affecting quality of life

It is valuable to identify specific factors that influence quality of life in ALS. Positive factors include strong social support and a prominent role of religion and spirituality [28,37–40]. Spirituality was shown to be a positive factor with respect to thoughts of suicide, and those who were more likely to consider suicide were less likely to be religious [18]. Religiousness is a factor (higher correlations) with quality of life over the course of the disease [38,40]. Hope also is important but is difficult to discuss in the setting of no clinically effective therapy. The act of discussing hope on an individual basis can be helpful to the patients [41].

Negative factors include hopelessness, which is composed of a variety of factors that probably are different for individual patients, including loss of control, severity of illness, social support, satisfaction, and the role of spiritual beliefs in coping [42]. Depression is not common and when present is of mild-to-moderate severity and rarely severe [30,43], but negatively affects quality of life [44]. Of note, rates of depression tested in the same population vary depending on which instrument is used [43]. Physical factors that can have a negative impact are general in type and include increased physical fatigue, loss of speech, impaired respiratory function, and inadequate nutrition (from dysphagia) [37,44–48]. Of note, several physical factors (dysarthria, dysphagia, and respiratory failure) can be addressed and are amenable to interventions (communication aids, noninvasive ventilation, and gastric feeding tubes) that may improve quality of life. Sexual function is rarely considered in ALS, but there is a greater frequency of problems with disease progression [49]. It is worthwhile to discuss this element in quality of life for the patient and caregiver.

A number of clinical interventions, including noninvasive ventilation and nutritional support, have been shown to have a positive impact on the patient's quality of life. Noninvasive ventilation is recommended when respiratory function reaches 50% of predicted [50]. The overall number of patients using noninvasive ventilation is approximately 21% (Anderson F, personal communication, ALS Care Database, 2007), and some refuse this intervention when respiratory function is reduced because of concerns about a poor quality of life. A number of studies, however, show prolonged survival [51] and improvement in sleep-related problems and quality of life [47,52]. The extreme form of respiratory support is tracheal ventilation. Tracheal ventilation can prolong survival indefinitely, but few patients who have ALS chose this intervention, expressing concern for a poor quality of life and burden on their family. Several studies, however, indicate a reasonable quality of life for patients who have ALS on a ventilator [53–55].

Inadequate nutrition and impaired mechanics of eating caused by upper extremity weakness in the setting of marked dysphagia can affect quality of life. For the patient there is the effort and fatigue of eating, and for the family there is the pressure of offering food and the time spent to complete a meal. Approximately 21% of patients use a feeding tube (Anderson F, personal communication, ALS Care Database, 2007). Some refuse this intervention, despite progressive weight loss, for a variety of reasons, including fear that it signals a negative change in the course of the disease. A gastric feeding tube, however, can lead to improvements in quality of life for the patient and the caregiver who must officiate during long meals [56].

Patients who have ALS who are cared for in multidisciplinary clinics score higher on social functioning and mental health subscores and receive more interventional aids than patients cared for in the setting of a general medical practice [57]. An intensive study of a small number of patients emphasized the role of professional services in their sense of well-being [40]. A positive effect on patient survival for those enrolled in a multidisciplinary clinic has been described [58]. The effects of these clinics may be attributed to interventional aids related to efforts to adhere to American Academy of Neurology ALS Practice Parameters [50] and to sensitivity to psychologic distress.

Quality of death for the patient who has amyotrophic lateral sclerosis

In addition to the term "quality of life," it is appropriate to consider the term "quality of death." Patients and their caregivers are concerned about death. Many say they are not afraid to die. It is likely that all patients want to ask, "How am I going to die?" Overall, death from ALS occurs peacefully, which can be defined as the manner of death one would chose if there were a choice [59]. There are issues that must be managed to help ensure such a death. These issues include poor ability to communicate, shortness of breath, difficulty sleeping, and pain [19]. Communication devices can help and should be offered early, when dysarthria is mild. The other symptoms can be managed with the help of hospice services [60].

Returning to the issue of patients' wishing to hasten death, it has been found that toward the end of life a number of patients (43%) entertained thoughts about ending their lives, a lesser number (19%) expressed an interest doing so, and a small number (6%) probably acted on that desire [21]. Although these numbers are not unique to ALS and are similar to the numbers for cancer and AIDS, it is important to explore specific factors. In patients who have ALS, depression does not increase with progression of the disease [21,30]. Patients who entertained thoughts about ending their lives, and in particular those who did hasten death, frequently lost pleasure and expressed the thought that they would be better off dead. An alternative view of the negative feelings at time of death and the wish to die is related to a broader syndrome of "end-of-life despair." Thoughts of and the means to hasten death can represent retention of a degree of control and an element of dignity at the end of life [21]. It is to be noted that none of the patients who acted to hasten death expressed an interest in noninvasive ventilation, perhaps supporting an early feeling of despair. Finally, although religion is a positive aspect of life for many patients who have ALS [38], it was not an important factor for patients who expressed a wish to die [21].

Another point raised is whether the outlook of some patients might be affected by frontotemporal dementia, which was noted in nearly half the patients who had ALS and who were formally tested [61]. Euphoria, lack of insight, and denial are features of frontotemporal dementia, and it is possible that these features mask depression or give the appearance of satisfaction with the current situation [62].

Quality of life for the caregiver of the patient who has amyotrophic lateral sclerosis

With disease progression, patients who have ALS become weaker, lose independence, and need greater care. This burden usually falls to the caregiver, and as patients lose independence, so do caregivers. Thus, it is important to consider the caregiver's quality of life [63]. As caregivers spend greater numbers of hours giving care, questionnaires given to them reveal feelings of physical and psychologic ill health, including greater depression [32,64,65]. The caregiver's sense of burden increases with worsening of the patient's disability [65,66]. This burden falls disproportionately on women caregivers, and outside help with caregiving did not reduce the perceived burden [65]. The SEIQoL-DW allows the same instrument to be given to both the patient and caregiver. One study showed lower scores for the caregiver than for the patient [25], and another study showed low scores for both [67]. There are positive factors for the caregiver, however, including finding a fulfilling role in providing care to the patient. Negative issues are stress, loss of independence, financial consequences, and poor coping skills [23].

Some interventions that improve quality of life for the patient impose a greater burden on the caregiver. Specifically, noninvasive ventilation and tracheal ventilation prolong survival in the setting of a good quality of life for the patient who has ALS but reduce quality of life for the caregiver [52,54,55]. A gastric feeding tube, on the other hand, can improve the quality of life for the caregiver by reducing the burden of feeding. Uncertainty about how these interventions will affect patient and caregiver is reflected in more caregivers than patients opposing their use during the deliberation period before receiving the interventions [27].

Hospice and quality of life

Hospice can contribute to the quality of life and death for the patient and caregiver. Hospice services include home aids for assistance in personal hygiene and dressing, nursing evaluation to assist in patient management, drugs for management of discomfort, and social and spiritual support. Most patients who have ALS meet hospice criteria for progression of disability during the last 12 months of life, but fewer than two thirds of patients who have ALS use hospice services at all [60]. What is most unfortunate is that, although hospice is set to provide care during the final 6 months of life, most patients who have ALS use it for less than the final month of life. Reasons for patients' not embracing hospice are probably many and likely include the feeling that the end is near [68]. In practice, however, it is difficult to predict a time course accurately, and patients who have ALS frequently remain on hospice care longer than 6 months, so long as they fulfill the criterion of progression of weakness.

Quality of life and bereavement

Quality of life for the caregiver and family should also be considered after the death of the patient. Issues for the caregiver, in particular, are a feeling of being burned-out from providing care, repercussions from forced changes in living arrangements to accommodate the patient's progressive weakness, and financial hardships, which may extend for some time (years after the death) [69]. Bereavement in ALS is an area that has not received sufficient attention [70,71]. Acknowledging these issues and efforts after the patient's death may help the caregiver feel that his or her efforts are valued. A personal telephone call and a letter of condolence are appreciated and are important means for closure for both family and health care provider [72].

Summary

ALS has a marked impact on the patient, caregiver, and family. There are major challenges during the course of the disease and after. Helping manage these challenges should be the major goal of the health care provider. With only minimally effective drugs and interventions available at this time, it is very important that providers, aided by a multidisciplinary team, work with the patient, caregiver, and family members to maintain quality of life for each. The challenge of maintaining a reasonable quality of life, at least for the patient, is aided by the natural response shift. Added burdens for the caregiver and family make the task harder. There is the final challenge of helping ensure a good death.

A number of issues should be kept in mind and reviewed or enquired about:

1. Explain to the patient and family that patients who have ALS judge their quality of life to be good. Emphasize that actual challenges are dealt with more easily than concern about challenges that might occur in the future.

2. Keep in mind that depression, although not common or of marked degree, should be sought out, because it is treatable.
3. Ask about fears of dying and explain that the end of life is manageable and that patients die a peaceful death.
4. Keep in mind that caregivers shoulder a major burden, and their physical and mental health should be reviewed.
5. Approach the idea of hospice as an organization that can provide physical and emotional help to both patient and caregiver; hospice care should be offered early.
6. Finally, bereavement is important, and a letter of condolence is important for closure.

References

[1] Jenkinson C, Hobart J, Chandola T, et al. Use of the short form health survey (SF-36) in patients with amyotrophic lateral sclerosis: tests of data quality, score reliability, response rate and scaling assumptions. J Neurol 2002;249(2):178–83.

[2] Schwartz CE, Andresen EM, Nosek MA, et al. Response shift theory: important implications for measuring quality of life in people with disability. Arch Phys Med Rehabil 2007; 88(4):529–36.

[3] Bergner M, Bobbitt R, Carter R, et al. The sickness impact profile: development and final revision of a health status measure. Med Care 1981;19:787–805.

[4] Ware J, Sherbourne C. The MOS 36-item short-form survey (SF-36). I. Conceptual framework and item selection. Med Care 1992;30:473–83.

[5] Neudert C, Wasner M, Borasio GD. Patients' assessment of quality of life instruments: a randomised study of SIP, SF-36 and SEIQoL-DW in patients with amyotrophic lateral sclerosis. J Neurol Sci 2001;191(1–2):103–9.

[6] McGuire D, Garrison L, Armon C, et al. A brief quality-of-life measure for ALS clinical trials based on a subset of items from the sickness impact profile. J Neurol Sci 1997;152:S18–22.

[7] Ware J, Kosinski M, Keller S. A 12-item short-form health survey. Med Care 1996;34: 220–33.

[8] Andres P, Hedlund W, Finison L, et al. Quantitative motor assessment in amyotrophic lateral sclerosis. Neurology 1986;36:937–41.

[9] Shields RK, Ruhland JL, Ross MA, et al. Analysis of health-related quality of life and muscle impairment in individuals with amyotrophic lateral sclerosis using the medical outcome survey and the Tufts Quantitative Neuromuscular Exam. Arch Phys Med Rehabil 1998; 79(7):855–62.

[10] O'Boyle C, McGee H, Joyce C. Quality of life: assessing the individual. In: Albrecth G, Fitzpatrick R, editors. Quality of life in health care. Advances in medical sociology, vol. 5. Greenwich (CT): JAI Press Inc.; 1994. p. 159–80.

[11] Hickey A, Bury G, O'Boyle C, et al. A new short form individual quality of life measure (SEIQoL-DW): application in a cohort of individuals with HIV/AIDS. BMJ 1996;313:29–33.

[12] Clarke S, Hickey A, O'Boyle C, et al. Assessing individual quality of life in amyotrophic lateral sclerosis. Qual Life Res 2001;10(2):149–58.

[13] Jenkinson C, Fitzpatrick R, Brennan C, et al. Development and validation of a short measure of health status for individuals with amyotrophic lateral sclerosis/motor neurone disease: The ALSAQ-40. J Neurol 1999;246(Suppl 3):III/16–21.

[14] Maessen M, Post MW, Maille R, et al. Validity of the Dutch version of the Amyotrophic Lateral Sclerosis Assessment Questionnaire, ALSAQ-40, ALSAQ-5. Amyotroph Lateral Scler 2007;8(2):96–100.

[15] Cohen S, Mount B, Strobel M, et al. The McGill Quality of Life Questionnaire: a measure of quality of life appropriate for people with advanced disease. A preliminary study of validity and acceptability. Palliat Med 1995;9:207–19.
[16] Simmons Z, Felgoise S, Bremer B, et al. The ALSSQOL: balancing physical and nonphysical factors in assessing quality of life in ALS. Neurology 2006;67:1659–64.
[17] Bach JR, Campagnolo DI, Hoeman S. Life satisfaction of individuals with Duchenne muscular dystrophy using long-term mechanical ventilatory support. Am J Phys Med Rehabil 1991;70(3):129–35.
[18] Ganzini L, Johnston WS, McFarland BH, et al. Attitudes of patients with amyotrophic lateral sclerosis and their care givers toward assisted suicide. N Engl J Med 1998;339(14): 967–73.
[19] Ganzini L, Johnston WS, Silveira MJ. The final month of life in patients with ALS. Neurology 2002;59(3):428–31.
[20] Ganzini L, Johnston W, Hoffman W. Correlates of suffering in amyotrophic lateral sclerosis. Neurology 1999;52:1434–40.
[21] Albert SM, Rabkin JG, Del Bene ML, et al. Wish to die in end-stage ALS. Neurology 2005; 65(1):68–74.
[22] Kiebert GM, Green C, Murphy C, et al. Patients' health-related quality of life and utilities associated with different stages of amyotrophic lateral sclerosis. J Neurol Sci 2001; 191(1–2):87–93.
[23] Rabkin J, Wagner G, Del Bene M. Resilience and distress among amyotrophic lateral sclerosis patients and caregivers. Psychosom Med 2000;62:271–9.
[24] Simmons Z, Bremer B, Robbins R, et al. Quality of life in ALS depends on factors other than strength and physical function. Neurology 2000;55:388–92.
[25] Bromberg M, Forshew D. Comparison of instruments addressing quality of life in patients with ALS and their caregivers. Neurology 2002;58:320–2.
[26] Goldstein LH, Atkins L, Leigh PN. Correlates of quality of life in people with motor neuron disease (MND). Amyotroph Lateral Scler Other Motor Neuron Disord 2002;3(3):123–9.
[27] Trail M, Nelson ND, Van JN, et al. A study comparing patients with amyotrophic lateral sclerosis and their caregivers on measures of quality of life, depression, and their attitudes toward treatment options. J Neurol Sci 2003;209(1–2):79–85.
[28] Chio A, Gauthier A, Montuschi A, et al. A cross sectional study on determinants of quality of life in ALS. J Neurol Neurosurg Psychiatry 2004;75(11):1597–601.
[29] Robbins R, Simmons Z, Bremer B, et al. Quality of life in ALS is maintained as physical function declines. Neurology 2001;56:442–4.
[30] Rabkin JG, Albert SM, Del Bene ML, et al. Prevalence of depressive disorders and change over time in late-stage ALS. Neurology 2005;65(1):62–7.
[31] Nygren I, Askmark H. Self-reported quality of life in amyotrophic lateral sclerosis. J Palliat Med 2006;9(2):304–8.
[32] Gauthier A, Vignola A, Calvo A, et al. A longitudinal study on quality of life and depression in ALS patient-caregiver couples. Neurology 2007;68(12):923–6.
[33] Albert SM, Wasner M, Tider T, et al. Cross-cultural variation in mental health at end of life in patients with ALS. Neurology 2007;68(13):1058–61.
[34] Albrecht GL, Devlieger PJ. The disability paradox: high quality of life against all odds. Soc Sci Med 1999;48(8):977–88.
[35] Sprangers MA, Schwartz CE. Integrating response shift into health-related quality of life research: a theoretical model. Soc Sci Med 1999;48(11):1507–15.
[36] Wilson I. Clinical understanding and clinical implications of response shift. Soc Sci Med 1999;45:1577–88.
[37] Hecht M, Hillemacher T, Grasel E, et al. Subjective experience and coping in ALS. Amyotroph Lateral Scler Other Motor Neuron Disord 2002;3(4):225–31.
[38] Walsh SM, Bremer BA, Felgoise SH, et al. Religiousness is related to quality of life in patients with ALS. Neurology 2003;60(9):1527–9.

[39] Trail M, Nelson N, Van J, et al. Major stressors facing patients with amyotrophic lateral sclerosis (ALS): a survey to identify their concerns and to compare with those of their caregivers. Amyotrophic Lateral Scler 2004;5:40–5.
[40] Foley G, O'Mahony P, Hardiman O. Perceptions of quality of life in people with ALS: effects of coping and health care. Amyotroph Lateral Scler 2007;8(3):164–9.
[41] Vitale A, Genge A. Codman Award 2006: the experience of hope in ALS patients. Axone 2007;28(2):27–35.
[42] Plahuta JM, McCulloch BJ, Kasarskis EJ, et al. Amyotrophic lateral sclerosis and hopelessness: psychosocial factors. Soc Sci Med 2002;55(12):2131–40.
[43] Wicks P, Abrahams S, Masi D, et al. Prevalence of depression in a 12-month consecutive sample of patients with ALS. Eur J Neurol 2007;14(9):993–1001.
[44] Lou JS, Reeves A, Benice T, et al. Fatigue and depression are associated with poor quality of life in ALS. Neurology 2003;60(1):122–3.
[45] Max M, Lynch S, Muir J, et al. Effects of desipramine, amitriptyline, and fluoxetine on pain in diabetic neuropathy. N Engl J Med 1992;326:1250–6.
[46] Bourke SC, Shaw PJ, Gibson GJ. Respiratory function vs sleep-disordered breathing as predictors of QOL in ALS. Neurology 2001;57(11):2040–4.
[47] Bourke SC, Bullock RE, Williams TL, et al. Noninvasive ventilation in ALS: indications and effect on quality of life. Neurology 2003;61(2):171–7.
[48] Ramirez C, Piemonte ME, Callegaro D, et al. Fatigue in amyotrophic lateral sclerosis: frequency and associated factors. Amyotroph Lateral Scler 2007;1–6.
[49] Wasner M, Bold U, Vollmer TC, et al. Sexuality in patients with amyotrophic lateral sclerosis and their partners. J Neurol 2004;251(4):445–8.
[50] Miller R, Rosenberg J, Gelinas D, et al. Practice parameter: the care of the patient with amyotrophic lateral sclerosis (an evidence-based review). Neurology 1999;52:1311–23.
[51] Piepers S, van den Berg JP, Kalmijn S, et al. Effect of non-invasive ventilation on survival, quality of life, respiratory function and cognition: a review of the literature. Amyotroph Lateral Scler 2006;7(4):195–200.
[52] Mustfa N, Walsh E, Bryant V, et al. The effect of noninvasive ventilation on ALS patients and their caregivers. Neurology 2006;66(8):1211–7.
[53] Bromberg M, Forshew D, Iaderosa S, et al. Ventilator dependency in ALS; management, disease progression, and issues of coping. J Neurol Rehabil 1996;10:195–216.
[54] Gelinas DF, O'Connor P, Miller RG. Quality of life for ventilator-dependent ALS patients and their caregivers. J Neurol Sci 1998;160(Suppl 1):S134–6.
[55] Kaub-Wittemer D, Steinbuchel N, Wasner M, et al. Quality of life and psychosocial issues in ventilated patients with amyotrophic lateral sclerosis and their caregivers. J Pain Symptom Manage 2003;26(4):890–6.
[56] Mazzini L, Corrà T, Zaccala M, et al. Percutaneous endoscopic gastrostomy and enteral nutrition in amyolateral sclerosis. J Neurol 1995;242:695–8.
[57] Van den Berg JP, Kalmijn S, Lindeman E, et al. Multidisciplinary ALS care improves quality of life in patients with ALS. Neurology 2005;65(8):1264–7.
[58] Traynor BJ, Alexander M, Corr B, et al. Effect of a multidisciplinary amyotrophic lateral sclerosis (ALS) clinic on ALS survival: a population based study, 1996–2000. J Neurol Neurosurg Psychiatry 2003;74(9):1258–61.
[59] Neudert C, Oliver D, Wasner M, et al. The course of the terminal phase in patients with amyotrophic lateral sclerosis. J Neurol 2001;248:612–6.
[60] Mandler R, Anderson F, Miller R, et al. The ALS patient care database: insights into end-of-life care in ALS. ALS 2001;2:203–8.
[61] Lomen-Hoerth C, Murphy J, Langmore S, et al. Are amyotrophic lateral sclerosis patients cognitively normal? Neurology 2003;60(7):1094–7.
[62] Olney RK, Lomen-Hoerth C. Exit strategies in ALS: an influence of depression or despair? Neurology 2005;65(1):9–10.

[63] Mitsumoto H. Caregiver assessment: summary. Amyotroph Lateral Scler Other Motor Neuron Disord 2002;(3 Suppl 1):S31–4.
[64] Krivickas LS, Shockley L, Mitsumoto H. Home care of patients with amyotrophic lateral sclerosis (ALS). J Neurol Sci 1997;152(Suppl 1):S82–9.
[65] Hecht MJ, Graesel E, Tigges S, et al. Burden of care in amyotrophic lateral sclerosis. Palliat Med 2003;17(4):327–33.
[66] Chio A, Gauthier A, Calvo A, et al. Caregiver burden and patients' perception of being a burden in ALS. Neurology 2005;64(10):1780–2.
[67] Lo Coco G, Lo Coco D, Cicero V, et al. Individual and health-related quality of life assessment in amyotrophic lateral sclerosis patients and their caregivers. J Neurol Sci 2005; 238(1–2):11–7.
[68] Carter GT, Bednar-Butler LM, Abresch RT, et al. Expanding the role of hospice care in amyotrophic lateral sclerosis. Am J Hosp Palliat Care 1999;16(6):707–10.
[69] Martin J, Turnbull J. Lasting impact in families after death from ALS. Amyotroph Lateral Scler Other Motor Neuron Disord 2001;2(4):181–7.
[70] Mitsumoto H, Bromberg M, Johnston W, et al. Promoting excellence in end-of-life care in ALS. Amyotroph Lateral Scler Other Motor Neuron Disord 2005;6(3):145–54.
[71] Hebert RS, Lacomis D, Easter C, et al. Grief support for informal caregivers of patients with ALS: a national survey. Neurology 2005;64(1):137–8.
[72] Bedell SE, Cadenhead K, Graboys TB. The doctor's letter of condolence. N Engl J Med 2001;344(15):1162–4.

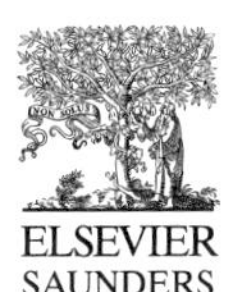
ELSEVIER
SAUNDERS

Phys Med Rehabil Clin N Am 19 (2008) 607–617

PHYSICAL MEDICINE AND REHABILITATION CLINICS OF NORTH AMERICA

Cognitive and Behavioral Impairment in Amyotrophic Lateral Sclerosis

Susan C. Woolley, PhD*, Jonathan S. Katz, MD

Forbes Norris MDA/ALS Rsearch Center, California Pacific Medical Center, 2324 Sacramento Street, Suite 111, San Francisco, CA 94115, USA

Overview

The study of cognition and behavior as a feature of amyotrophic lateral sclerosis (ALS) is an evolving field that still lacks consensus on terminology, diagnostic criteria, and the clinical significance of any detected abnormalities. Currently, fairly marked discrepancies remain regarding the incidence of abnormalities and characteristics of the impairments that define the disease. Although substantial pathologic and genetic evidence shows an overlap between ALS and frontotemporal dementia (FTD), cognitive and behavioral syndromes also occur among patients who have ALS that cannot be characterized as frank FTD.

The terms *ALSci* (ALS with cognitive impairment), *ALSbi* (ALS with behavioral impairment), and *ALS-FTD* are developing concepts that aim to capture the key differences between various phenotypes. Whether these conditions fall into a single disease spectrum or represent distinct clinical syndromes is still debated.

Cognitive impairment in amyotrophic lateral sclerosis

Most patients who have ALS diagnosed with a cognitive disorder are characterized as having ALSci. The impairment reflects frontal lobe dysfunction [1–6] but is not considered synonymous with the more severe and disabling dementia associated with FTD. Numerous studies show that the primary deficits in ALSci occur in the domains of attention [7], cognitive flexibility [7,8], word generation, and retrieval (Box 1) [5,9].

* Corresponding author.
E-mail address: woolles@sutterhealth.org (S.C. Woolley).

doi:10.1016/j.pmr.2008.04.002 *pmr.theclinics.com*

Box 1. Cognitive deficits that have been identified in amyotrophic lateral sclerosis

Cognitive domain
Attention and concentration [1,7,11]
Working memory [8]
Cognitive flexibility [8]
Response inhibition [7]
Planning/problem solving/abstract reasoning [8,52]
Visual-perceptual skills [8,9]
Memory [8]
Intrinsic response generation (ie, fluency) [9,10]

Many studies have identified impaired intrinsic response generation and particularly abnormalities in verbal fluency [1,4–7,9–11]. Consistent with a frontal syndrome, visuospatial functions, praxis, and memory storage are typically spared [1,5,11], whereas reports suggesting that impaired memory may be found probably reflect deficiencies in retrieval processes associated with frontal lobe dysfunction [12] rather than an amnestic process.

Estimates of the prevalence of cognitive impairment in patients who have ALS range from 10% [13] to 75% [7]. This wide range probably reflects differences in the selection of patients and methods used for diagnosis.

Where neuropsychological testing is the gold standard for diagnosis, reports have used varied cognitive tests and different cutoffs for distinguishing normal from abnormal, resulting in different conclusions about the nature of the disease. A single consensus on diagnostic criteria for ALSci has not been reached, but an increasingly common threshold used in the field requires the presence of two or more neuropsychological scores at or below the fifth percentile compared with a normative group. This requirement assumes the tests are part of a comprehensive battery including measures that are distinct and sensitive to executive functioning and language processing. With this methodology, the incidence of ALSci within a typical multidisciplinary clinic seems to be approximately 50% [10,11].

Whether a specific clinical presentation predicts ALSci is not entirely clear. Several studies have indicated an association of ALSci with bulbar involvement [1,4,8]. Studies suggesting a correlation between dysarthria and higher levels of distractibility [14] or between pseudobulbar affect and cognitive impairment [15] reflect similar conclusions.

The authors have identified a distinct clinical syndrome marked by ocular apraxia and upper motor neuron bulbar involvement in a group of patients who have relatively obvious cognitive deficits [16]. Pathologic studies have also found that patients who have bulbar palsy may have a degenerative process that extends beyond the motor cortex into frontotemporal lobar regions [2]. The relationship is not entirely clear, however, as other studies have failed to find strong correlations between ALSci and bulbar involvement [1,7,11,17]. Any discrepancies across studies may reflect the measures used for diagnosis of impairment, and depend on whether bulbar onset versus bulbar involvement was used for the comparison.

Frontotemporal dementia in amyotrophic lateral sclerosis

Frontotemporal lobar degeneration (FTLD) describes a group of disorders caused by frontal and temporal lobe degeneration sharing common pathologic features. FTD, also known as the frontal or behavioral variant FTLD, tends to be caused by bilateral or right-sided degeneration and manifests primarily as a behavior disorder. Left-sided involvement leads to disorders of language that include progressive nonfluent aphasia (PNFA) and semantic dementia.

Outside of ALS, the Neary criteria are most commonly used for diagnosing FTD [18]. These criteria use a behavioral rather than cognitive approach, defining FTD through an insidious onset and gradual progression, altered social conduct, impaired regulation of personal conduct, emotional blunting, and loss of insight. All five core features are required for the diagnosis, whereas secondary findings may include disinhibition; restlessness; reduced empathy or lack of concern for others; lack of foresight; impulsiveness; social withdrawal; verbal stereotypes or echolalia; verbal or motor perseveration; or sexual hyperactivity [18]. A diagnostic approach that relies solely on cognitive testing may fail to detect patients who have early or mild ALS-FTD, in whom these behavioral abnormalities can occur in the context of intact cognition [2].

The literature reflects varied frequencies of FTLD subtypes within the ALS population. Again, these discrepancies likely reflect biases introduced by the methodology used for diagnosis and subjectivity in behavioral assessment. Similarly, discrepancies can be found in the estimates of the FTLD subtypes frequencies. In one study that used a combination of cognitive testing and the Neary criteria [4], 65% of patients who where diagnosed with ALS-FTLD had the behavioral (frontal) variant, characterized by apathy, disinhibition, and poor social monitoring. In contrast, a subsequent study [11] found that 63% of patients who had ALS and dementia had a language variant of FTLD, more consistent with PNFA or semantic dementia.

A population based sample of patients who had ALS estimated that 17% had frank dementia and 11% had clear aphasia [19], whereas in tertiary care clinics, the prevalence of impairment meeting criteria for frank dementia has ranged from 15% [11] to 41% [4]. Rippon and colleagues [20] reported dementia in 23% of their ALS cohort but used *Diagnostic and Statistical Manual of Mental Disorders, Fourth Edition* (DSM-IV) criteria, which uses memory impairment as the defining feature of dementia.

In the authors' experience, only a small subset of patients, perhaps as low as approximately 5%, presents to a multidisciplinary clinic with clear FTD. These patients differ dramatically from those who have ALSci because of vast behavioral alterations, which usually begin before motor weakness becomes apparent. Many of these patients present initially to centers that focus on cognition, and they may be underrepresented in a center focusing specifically on ALS.

In contrast to ALSci, FTD symptoms typically occur before ALS symptoms. For example, a recent study of 24 patients who had motor neuron disease–FTD (MND-FTD) [21] showed that 58% experienced the onset of FTD more than 3 years before MND, whereas 38% reported simultaneous onset. A prospective study of patients who had ALS found that those who met criteria for a dementia exhibited cognitive or behavioral decline an average of 7 years and 7 months before motor symptoms [6].

Although the incidence of clinical or EMG abnormalities suggestive of motor neuron disease within an FTD clinic was approximately 15% [22], no clear reports exist of patients in ALS centers developing frank FTD during the course of motor degeneration. Some experts hypothesize that patients who have ALS die before cognitive or behavioral impairments become apparent, in contrast to patients who develop FTD and have years to develop ALS. The loss of speech and movement in ALS may also mask the cognitive and behavioral degradation if it occurs. An alternative explanation would be that patients who have typical ALS rarely develop FTD.

Reports have suggested that FTD reflects one end of a disease continuum, with ALSci as the more benign, initial manifestation. However, the argument is difficult to support when considering temporal data. Prospective studies have failed to detect significant progression of ALSci over time [5,23–25]. Only Robinson and colleagues [26] reported declines in cognitive test scores, defined by a 1 SD change, but they did not specify whether performances declined to levels consistent with clinical impairment (ie, below the fifth percentile).

Strong and colleagues [8] documented cognitive changes over 6 months in a small cohort of patients who had bulbar-onset but experienced no progression to typical FTD. In contrast, patients who present to ALS clinics with frank FTD show clear progression of dementia along with motor decline. A report by Moretti and colleagues [25] found that among a cohort of patients documented at baseline to have varying degrees of cognitive and behavioral impairment, progression was only evident in those initially diagnosed with FTD.

Behavioral changes in amyotrophic lateral sclerosis

The term *ALSbi* describes behavioral impairment that does not meet diagnostic criteria for FTD, yet reflects a mood-independent change since

ALS onset. Estimates of the prevalence of ALSbi vary depending on methodology and diagnostic criteria.

One feature consistent across several studies is the presence of marked apathy that can occur despite whether significant cognitive impairments are present (Fig. 1) [6,27]. One multicenter study found abnormal levels of apathy in 55% of patients who had ALS [27]. The apathy correlated with deficits in verbal fluency but not depression, disease duration, forced vital capacity, or ALS-FRS scores. Similar to cognitive impairment in ALS, no current evidence shows that ALSbi progresses to ALS-FTD or that it is part of a continuum. However, disinhibition, which is a common feature in FTD, is not seen with high frequency as a behavioral manifestation of ALS.

Why the incidence of apathy is so high is also not entirely apparent. Although apathy could develop on an organic basis, it is also known to be a manifestation of fatigue, respiratory weakness, impaired sleep, anxiety, or medication side effects. Two large placebo-controlled studies of riluzole have documented higher rates of asthenia in treatment groups compared with placebo controls. Apathy may also reflect a psychologic coping mechanism for patients who have terminal illness or paralysis. Although apathy is

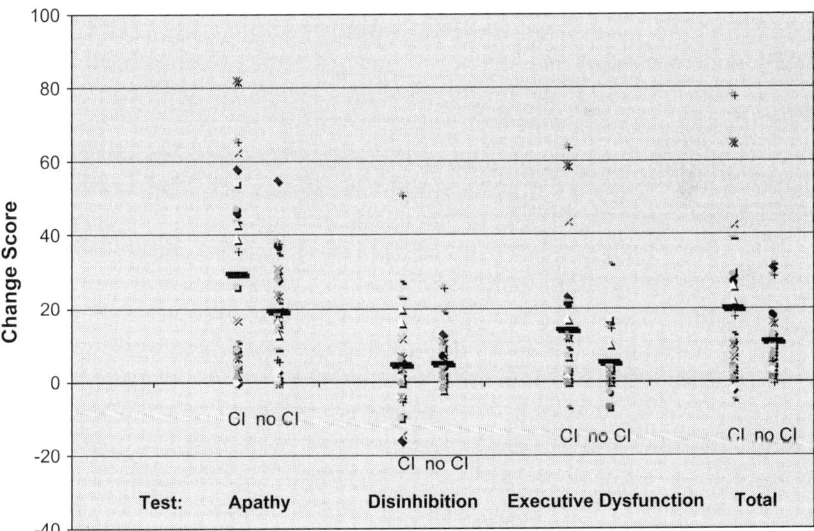

Fig. 1. Changes in behavior since the onset of amyotrophic lateral sclerosis according to the Frontal Systems Behavioral Scale. One figure is used to represent each of the four categories for the same patient. Apathy shows marked changes in patients who have cognitive impairment and those who do not (mean, 2.4 SD for those who have cognitive impairment; 2.0 SD for those who do not have cognitive impairment). In contrast, disinhibition is uncommon, whereas executive dysfunction is slightly greater in patients who are cognitively impaired. Change score of 20 represents 2 SD worsening of the behavior since disease onset. CI, cognitive impairment.

often associated with depression, it occurs with a much higher frequency in ALS than depression, which occurs in only 10% [28] to 26% [29] of patients.

Behavior is typically assessed through caregiver interview as opposed to direct patient questioning, primarily because patients who have behavioral changes may lack insight. Standardized measures for assessment include the Frontal Behavioral Inventory [30], Frontal Systems Behavioral Scale [31], and the Neuropsychiatric Inventory [32]. Diagnostic criteria that have been proposed for ALSbi include frontal-lobe type behavioral impairment in two or more areas measured using one of these standardized caregiver interviews [33].

Neuroimaging

Numerous imaging studies have described abnormalities outside the motor cortex in patients who have ALS compared with normal controls, and differences between patients who have ALS and neuropsychological abnormalities and those who are cognitively normal [2,6,9,10,14,21,34–36]. Patients who have ALS have significantly lower frontal and overall cortical metabolism [10,34,35,37] compared with controls, whereas regional cerebral blood flow to nonmotor areas is reduced in patients who have ALS regardless of whether they have cognitive impairment [36,38].

Patients who have ALS have larger ventricles compared with age-matched controls [7], and show changes in frontal lobe white matter [38,39] and prefrontal and temporal gray matter, suggesting atrophy [40]. Frontotemporal white matter changes have also been described in cognitively normal patients who have ALS, although the changes were greater when cognitive impairment was present [39]. These findings have been used to support the notion of a continuum between ALS and FTD [39,41].

A specific cause of ALSci can be gathered from various imaging studies that have attempted to localize abnormalities in verbal fluency, because this finding tends to correlate the highest with this cognitive syndrome.

These studies have resulted in various findings. One study using positron emission tomography (PET) found that activity in the dorsolateral prefrontal cortex is decreased in patients who have ALS with cognitive impairment compared with those who are unimpaired and controls [14]. Impairments in verbal fluency have also been correlated with decreased activation in the limbo-thalamo-cortical pathways [38] and have been associated with impaired activation of the middle and inferior frontal gyri, anterior cingulate, and regions of the parietal and temporal lobes [42]. A subset of patients who had bulbar-onset who were shown to have progressive neuropsychological deficits over a 6-month interval were found to have structural changes localized to the anterior cingulate gyrus [8].

The imaging correlates of patients who have definite ALS-FTD, however, seem to be more consistent with those of FTD in general. Voxel-based morphometry showed that frontal volume loss patterns were similar between

ALS and ALS-FTLD cohorts [40]. However, volume reductions in patients who had ALS-FTLD were greater, particularly in the left hemisphere, than in patients who had ALS and no dementia.

In contrast, another study found right temporal lobe volume loss was most predictive of classification in a frontotemporal dysfunction group [6]. A single photon emission CT study [21] compared patients who had FTD and MND-FTD to age- and gender-matched controls. Clinically, all patients had frontal variant FTD, and patients who had FTD and MND-FTD had the same pattern of asymmetric anterior hypoperfusion involving frontal, temporal, cingular, and insular cortices. Bilateral hypoperfusion of the thalamus and striatum was also noted.

Neuropathology

A specific correlation appears to exist between ALS frontal pathology and the presence of cognitive impairment within this population. Abe and colleagues [41] found greater frontal neuropathology in patients who had ALSci compared with patients who had ALS who were cognitively normal, supporting an organic basis for inattention and executive dysfunction. Intraneuronal ubiquitin-positive inclusions and dystrophic neuritis, which are found in degenerating motor neurons in ALS, are increased and can be found in a greater distribution of cortical regions in patients who have ALS who have cognitive impairment [43]. ALSci has been associated with superficial linear spongiosis, which is a pathologic feature common to several forms of FTD and hypothesized to be the most reliable pathologic marker of ALSci [8].

Frontal neuropathology shows numerous similarities between ALS and FTD. As in ALS, ubiquinated inclusions are a pathologic marker of FTD and, in particular, ubiquitin-positive, tau-negative, alpha-synuclein-negative (MND-type) inclusions are present in both diseases [44].

The recently discovered protein TDP-43 is also a significant component of neuronal ubiquinated inclusions in ALS and FTD [45]. Although its function remains unknown, the presence of similar pathologic features has been used to support the disease continuum between ALS with or without cognitive impairment and FTD.

Frontal dysfunction and respiratory compromise

A multitude of disease-related factors that impact ALS may have cognitive or behavioral consequences. Respiratory compromise, for example, has direct effects on brain functioning. Kim and colleagues [46] grouped patients who had ALS based on FVC and found that the lower FVC group had significantly lower scores in memory retention, retrieval efficiency, and verbal fluency. The ALS-FTD group in another study [4] had significantly lower mean FVCs (66%) compared with the normal ALS cohort (mean FVC, 99%).

It can be argued that the low FVCs may be a consequence of poor bulbar function in some cases, rather than respiratory compromise, and that the poor cognitive results in these studies reflect cognitive changes that are especially likely to occur in patients who have bulbar impairment. However, noninvasive ventilation has resulted in significant cognitive improvement over 6 weeks in patients who had ALS experiencing reduced respiratory muscle strength and nocturnal hypoventilation [47].

Some abnormalities on imaging studies could also be explained potentially by hypoventilation. Frontal-type cognitive decline associated with worsening of hypoxia [48] in chronic obstructive pulmonary disease (COPD) may appear similar to the impairments seen in ALS. Imaging studies also show that patients who have COPD who show cognitive impairment have significantly altered frontal and parietal cerebral perfusion [48,49].

Management of patients who have amyotrophic lateral sclerosis with cognitive or behavioral impairment

A cohort of patients who had frontotemporal dysfunction, presumably including a combination of ALS-FTD and ALSci, had higher rates of noncompliance with recommendations for using percutaneous endoscopic gastrostomy (72%) and noninvasive ventilation (75%) compared with patients who had normal ALS, and median survival was shorter in the frontotemporal group by 11 months [50]. However, because ALSci was not distinguished from ALS-FTD, the extent to which poor outcomes relate to dementia versus cognitive impairment is difficult to determine. No studies have evaluated pharmacologic treatment for cognitive or behavioral impairment in ALS or ALS-FTD.

Future directions

To ensure consistency in diagnosis and research, specific criteria for ALSci, ALSbi, and ALS-FTD are needed. A common language would help evaluate the prevalence and characterization of behavioral impairments in ALS, whereas longitudinal studies assessing the evolution of cognitive and behavioral impairment in ALS would shed more light on specific outcomes and risks. Screening tests for all three conditions are currently being developed [51], which would enable more consistent testing and make assessment practical in centers that do not have the time or resources to perform extensive neuropsychological batteries over time.

References

[1] Massman PJ, Sims J, Cooke N, et al. Prevalence and correlates of neurocognitive deficits in amyotrophic lateral sclerosis. J Neurol Neurosurg Psychiatry 1996;61:450–5.

[2] Neary D, Snowden JS, Mann DMA. Cognitive change in motor neuron disease/amyotrophic lateral sclerosis. J Neurol Sci 2000;180:15–20.
[3] Evdokimidis I, Constantinidis TS, Gourtzelidis P, et al. Frontal lobe dysfunction in amyotrophic lateral sclerosis. J Neurol Sci 2002;195:25–33.
[4] Lomen-Hoerth C, Murphy J, Langmore S, et al. Are amyotrophic lateral sclerosis patients cognitively normal? Neurology 2003;60(7):1094–7.
[5] Abrahams S, Leigh PN, Goldstein LH. Cognitive change in ALS: a prospective study. Neurology 2005;64:1222–6.
[6] Murphy JM, Henry RG, Langmore S, et al. Continuum of frontal lobe impairment in amyotrophic lateral sclerosis. Arch Neurol 2007;64:530–4.
[7] Frank B, Haas J, Heinze H, et al. Relation of neurocognitive and magnetic resonance findings in amyotrophic lateral sclerosis: evidence for subgroups. Clin Neurol Neurosurg 1997; 99:79–86.
[8] Strong MJ, Grace GM, Orange JB, et al. A prospective study of cognitive impairment in ALS. Neurology 1999;53:1665–70.
[9] Abrahams S, Leigh PN, Harvey A, et al. Verbal fluency and executive dysfunction in amyotrophic lateral sclerosis. Neuropsychologia 2000;38:734–47.
[10] Ludolf AC, Langen KJ, Regard M, et al. Frontal lobe function in amyotrophic lateral sclerosis: a neurocognitive and positron emission tomography study. Acta Neurol Scand 1992; 85:81–9.
[11] Ringholz GM, Appel SH, Bradshaw M, et al. Prevalence and patterns of cognitive impairment in sporadic ALS. Neurology 2005;65(4):586–90.
[12] Mantovan MC, Baggio L, Barba G, et al. Memory deficits and retrieval processes in ALS. Eur J Neurol 2003;10(3):221–7.
[13] Poloni M, Capitani E, Mazzini L, et al. Neuropsychological measures in amyotrophic lateral sclerosis and their relationship with CT scan-assessed cerebral atrophy. Acta Neurol Scand 1986;74(4):257–60.
[14] Abrahams S, Goldstein LH, Kew JJM, et al. Frontal lobe dysfunction in amyotrophic lateral sclerosis: a PET Study. Brain 1996;119:2105–20.
[15] McCullagh S, Moore M, Gawel M, et al. Pathological laughing and crying in amyotrophic lateral sclerosis: an association with prefrontal cognitive dysfunction. J Neurol Sci 1999;169: 43–8.
[16] Katz JS, Woolley-Levine S. Ocular apraxia and cognitive impairment in ALS. Amyotroph Lateral Scler 2006;7(1):95.
[17] Portet F, Cadilhac C, Touchon J, et al. Cognitive impairment in motor neuron disease with bulbar onset. Amyotroph Lateral Scler Other Motor Neuron Disord 2001;2(1): 23–9.
[18] Neary D, Snowden JS, Gustafson L, et al. Frontotemporal lobar degeneration: a consensus on clinical diagnostic criteria. Neurology 1998;51:1546–54.
[19] Rakowicz WP, Hodges JR. Dementia and aphasia in motor neuron disease: an underrecognised association? J Neurol Neurosurg Psychiatry 1998;65(6):881–9.
[20] Rippon GA, Scarmeas N, Gordon PH, et al. An observational study of cognitive impairment in amyotrophic lateral sclerosis. Arch Neurol 2006;63:345–52.
[21] Guedj E, Ber I, Lacomblez L, et al. Brain spect perfusion of frontotemporal dementia associated with motor neuron disease. Neurology 2007;69(5):488–90.
[22] Lomen-Hoerth C, Anderson T, Miller B. The overlap of amyotrophic lateral sclerosis and frontotemporal dementia. Neurology 2002;59(7):1077–9.
[23] Kilani M, Micallef J, Soubrouillard C, et al. A longitudinal study of the evolution of cognitive function and affective state in patients with amyotrophic lateral sclerosis. Amyotroph Lateral Scler Other Motor Neuron Disord 2004;5(1):46–54.
[24] Schreiber H, Gaigalat T, Wiedemuth-Catrinescu U, et al. Cognitive function in bulbar- and spinal-onset amyotrophic lateral sclerosis. A longitudinal study in 52 patients. J Neurol 2005; 252(7):772–81.

[25] Moretti R, Torre P, Antonello RM, et al. Complex cognitive disruption in motor neuron disease. Dement Geriatr Cogn Disord 2002;14(3):141–50.
[26] Robinson KM, Lacey SC, Grugan P, et al. Cognitive functioning in sporadic amyotrophic lateral sclerosis: a six month longitudinal study. J Neurol Neurosurg Psychiatry 2006; 77(5):668–70.
[27] Grossman AB, Woolley-Levine S, Bradley WG, et al. Detecting neurobehavioral changes in amyotrophic lateral sclerosis. Amyotroph Lateral Scler 2007;8:56–61.
[28] Patten SB, Svenson LW, White CM, et al. Affective disorders in motor neuron disease: a population-based study. Neuro-epidemiology 2007;28:1–7.
[29] Wicks P, Abrahams S, Masi D, et al. Prevalence of depression in a 12-month consecutive sample of patients with ALS. Eur J Neurol 2007;14(9):993–1001.
[30] Kertesz A, Davidson W, Fox H. Frontal behavioural inventory: diagnostic criteria for frontal lobe dementia. Can J Neurol Sci 1997;24(1):29–36.
[31] Grace J, Malloy PF. Frontal systems behavior scale professional manual. Lutz (FL): Psychological Assessment Resources, Inc.; 2001.
[32] Cummings JL, Mega M, Gray K, et al. The neuropsychiatric inventory: comprehensive assessment of psychopathology in dementia. Neurology 1994;44:2308–14.
[33] Murphy JM, Henry RG, Lomen-Hoerth C. Establishing subtypes of the continuum of frontal lobe impairment in amyotrophic lateral sclerosis. Arch Neurol 2007;64: 330–4.
[34] Hatazawa J, Brooks RA, Dalakas MC, et al. Cortical motorsensory hypometabolism in amyotrophic lateral sclerosis: a PET study. J Comput Assist Tomogr 1988;12: 630–6.
[35] Ohnishi T, Hoshi H, Jinnouchi S, et al. The utility of cerebral blood flow imaging in patients with the unique syndrome of progressive dementia with motor neuron disease. J Nucl Med 1990;31:688–91.
[36] Lloyd CM, Richardson MP, Brooks DJ, et al. Extramotor involvement in ALS: pet studies with the GABA(A) ligand [(11)C]flumazenil. Brain 2000;123(11):2289–96.
[37] Dalakas MC, Hatazawa J, Brooks RA, et al. Lowered cerebral glucose utilization in amyotrophic lateral sclerosis. Ann Neurol 1987;22:471–4.
[38] Kew JJM, Goldstein LH, Leigh PN, et al. The relationship between abnormalities of cognitive function and cerebral activation in amyotrophic lateral sclerosis: a neurocognitive and positron emission tomography study. Brain 1993;116:1399–423.
[39] Abrahams S, Goldstein LH, Suckling J, et al. Frontotemporal white matter changes in amyotrophic lateral sclerosis. J Neurol 2005;252(3):321–31.
[40] Chang JL, Lomen-Hoerth C, Murphy J, et al. A voxel-based morphometry study of patterns of brain atrophy in ALS and ALS/FTLD. Neurology 2005;65:75–80.
[41] Abe K, Fujimura H, Toyooka K, et al. Cognitive function in amyotrophic lateral sclerosis. J Neurol Sci 1997;148(1):95–100.
[42] Abrahams S, Goldstein LH, Simmons A, et al. Word retrieval in amyotrophic lateral sclerosis: a functional magnetic resonance imaging study. Brain 2004;127(7):1507–17.
[43] Wilson CM, Grace GM, Munoz DG, et al. Cognitive impairment in sporadic ALS: a pathologic continuum underlying a multisystem disorder. Neurology 2001;57:651–7.
[44] Lipton AM, White CL, Bigio EH. Frontotemporal lobar degeneration with motor-neuron disease-type inclusions predominate in 76 cases of frontotemporal degeneration. Acta Neuropathol 2004;108:379–85.
[45] Neumann M, Sampathu DM, Kwong LK, et al. Ubiquinated TDP-43 in frontotemporal lobar degeneration and amyotrophic lateral sclerosis. Science 2006;314:130–3.
[46] Kim S, Lee K, Hong Y, et al. Relation between cognitive dysfunction and reduced vital capacity in ALS. J Neurol Neurosurg Psychiatry 2007;78(12):1387–9.
[47] Newsom-Davis IC, Lyall RA, Leigh PN, et al. The effect of non-invasive positive pressure ventilation (NIPPV) on cognitive function in amyotrophic lateral sclerosis (ALS): a prospective study. J Neurol Neurosurg Psychiatry 2001;71(4):482–7.

[48] Antonelli Incalzi R, Marra C, Giordano A, et al. Cognitive impairment in chronic obstructive pulmonary disease: a neuropsychological and spect study. J Neurol 2003; 250(3):325–32.
[49] Ortapamuk H, Naldoken S. Brain perfusion abnormalities in chronic obstructive pulmonary disease: comparison with cognitive impairment. Ann Nucl Med 2006;20(2):99–106.
[50] Olney RK, Murphy J, Forshew D, et al. The effects of executive and behavioral dysfunction on the course of ALS. Neurology 2005;65(11):1774–7.
[51] Woolley-Levine S, York M, Haring K, et al. Development of a cognitive behavioral screen for use with ALS patients: preliminary data. Amyotroph Lateral Scler 2007;8(1):102.
[52] Flaherty-Craig C, Eslinger P, Stephens B, et al. A rapid screening battery to identify frontal dysfunction in patients with ALS. Neurology 2006;67:2070–2.

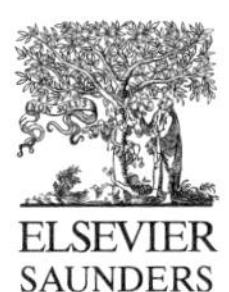

ELSEVIER
SAUNDERS

Phys Med Rehabil Clin N Am
19 (2008) 619–631

PHYSICAL MEDICINE
AND REHABILITATION
CLINICS OF
NORTH AMERICA

The Amyotrophic Lateral Sclerosis Center: A Model of Multidisciplinary Management

Angeli S. Mayadev, MD[a], Michael D. Weiss, MD[b], B. Jane Distad, MD[b], Lisa S. Krivickas, MD[c], Gregory T. Carter, MD, MS[a,*]

[a]*Department of Physical Medicine and Rehabilitation, University of Washington Medical Center, 1959 NE Pacific Street, Seattle, WA 98195, USA*

[b]*Department of Neurology, University of Washington Medical Center, 1959 NE Pacific Street, Seattle, WA 98195, USA*

[c]*Harvard Medical School, Spaulding Rehabilitation Hospital, 125 Nashua Street, Boston, MA 02114, USA*

Although most everyone knows that Lou Gehrig, the great "Iron Horse" of baseball, died of amyotrophic lateral sclerosis (ALS), it was his wife Eleanor who played a major role in the establishment of formal ALS centers. After Gehrig was diagnosed with ALS and retired from the New York Yankees, Eleanor became his chauffeur, nurse, nutritionist, and constant companion. In 1950, Eleanor heard that a new organization called the Muscular Dystrophy Association (MDA) was being formed to combat neuromuscular diseases. With Eleanor's help, MDA was to become and remain the world's leading private research organization and service provider for those who have ALS. Eleanor served as MDA's national campaign chairman during crucial formative years in the 1950s and 1960s. Today, at Columbia Presbyterian Medical Center, Eleanor and Lou Gehrig's names are enshrined at The Eleanor and Lou Gehrig MDA/ALS Center, the first of the now many MDA centers dedicated to ALS research and care.

Currently two major funding agencies sponsor formal ALS Centers: the MDA, which is the largest, and the ALS Association. These centers have now become the standard of care for the evaluation and management of ALS. A multidisciplinary approach to patient care is associated with a higher

* Corresponding author. 1800 Cooks Hill Road, Suite E, Centralia, WA 98531.
E-mail address: gtcarter@u.washington.edu (G.T. Carter).

1047-9651/08/$ - see front matter
doi:10.1016/j.pmr.2008.04.004

percentage of patients who have adequate aids and appliances compared with those patients not involved in an ALS center (93.1% versus 81.3%) and higher mental quality-of-life scores on the Short Form Health Survey (SF-36) [1]. A prospective population-based study using the Ireland ALS data registry showed that patients enrolled in a multidisciplinary ALS clinic had a decreased 1-year mortality of 30% compared with the general neurology clinic-based cohort [2].

An ALS center can serve as the comprehensive center for care and research. The initial diagnostic evaluation is generally confirmed by a second opinion, often sought because of the gravity of the diagnosis. Once the diagnosis is confirmed, the rehabilitation team can manage clinical problems and the patient can be enrolled in any ongoing research trials. Rehabilitative care is directed by a neurologist or physiatrist, and, in some centers, facilitated by a neuromuscular nurse practitioner. A pulmonologist who has experience in ALS should be involved early on, as should physical and occupational therapists, speech-language pathologists, and social workers.

Rehabilitation management of amyotrophic lateral sclerosis

At the initial clinic visit, it is important to thoroughly educate the patient about the diagnosis, the expected outcome, and the issues to be encountered. The visit should also allow adequate time for questions by the patient and family. The patient should have a clinic contact should further questions arise subsequent to the initial visit. Efforts should be made to educate that patient about all available options so that the patient can make informed decisions about the plan of care. In the next several visits, it is crucial for the physician to assess the patient's goals and orchestrate a rehabilitative and ultimately a palliative program that matches those goals. In ALS, palliative care should be aimed at maximizing a patient's comfort and quality of life but not necessarily extending life. Throughout the follow-up, enrollment in experimental drug trials, when they become available and appropriate, should be encouraged and facilitated. This participation not only furthers our knowledge about ALS but also provides some hope for the patient.

Impaired mobility and activities of daily living

A properly fitted wheelchair not only improves a patient's mobility but also prevents complications. Wheelchairs should have adequate lumbar support and appropriate cushioning to prevent pressure ulcers. A survey given to 42 patients who had ALS who used wheelchairs found that the most desirable wheelchair features provide extra comfort (supports for the head, neck, trunk, extremities) and improved maneuverability (lightweight frame, smaller wheelbase) [3]. A power wheelchair, although expensive, can be justified because it helps prolong independent mobility for the patient and thus markedly improves quality of life [4]. Pressure relief and proper positioning in bed are also important. An air or dense foam mattress is often necessary to provide good pressure relief. Foam wedges for proper positioning in bed can help to prevent pressure ulcers and contractures. Regular passive and active-assisted range of motion is critical in maintaining mobility and patient functional independence as long as possible. Ankle-foot orthoses with the ankle at neutral position may prolong ambulation and help avoid injury if there is unilateral or bilateral foot drop. Wheeled walkers or quad canes may also help, depending on the pattern of weakness.

Useful equipment to improve a patient's functional independence includes hand-held showers, bathtub benches, grab bars, raised toilet seats, a hospital bed, commode chairs, activities of daily living aids, such as sock aid and grabbers, and wheelchair ramps. An occupational therapist can help define which, if any, of these devices will be useful to the patient. During an in-home evaluation, the occupational therapist can also help with coordinating architectural and in-home modifications to maximize a patient's mobility and improve safety. Modifications may involve moving the patient's bedroom to the ground floor, removing any rugs or floor coverings, relocating furniture, installing grab bars, or covering slippery floors.

Bowel and bladder management

Sphincter function is generally spared in ALS, thus incontinence is usually not a significant problem [5]. When incontinence is an issue, it is most commonly because of immobility rather than lack of sphincter control. Urinary urgency may also be the result of the lack of frontal inhibition over micturition centers [6]. Drinking large amounts of fluids after dinner or before bed should be avoided. If the problem persists, condom catheters (for men) and absorbent undergarments are other options that may be used. Pseudoephedrine, a sympathomimetic agent, may help increase urinary outlet sphincter tone. Increased blood pressure and urinary retention can result, however, and should be monitored when using this medication, especially in men who have prostate enlargement or use anticholinergic agents. For patients who have urgency, oxybutynin may be of value to help patients regain continence. Indwelling urinary catheters should be avoided because of risk for urinary tract infection but may be necessary later in the course of the disease when mobility becomes a significant problem. In a recent study, 9 of 14 patients who had ALS showed markedly delayed colonic transit times compared with healthy controls.

The colonic transit in ALS patients was significantly delayed, which could be a result of inadequate fluid intake or denervation of the colonic nervous system [7]. Patients should maintain a regular bowel program with intake of fiber/bulking agents and adequate fluids. Suppositories, stool softeners, and mini-enemas may be used as needed.

Strengthening

Skeletal muscle weakness is the most prominent clinical feature of adult motor neuron disease, including ALS. It is also the ultimate cause of most clinical problems associated with these diseases. Patients who have ALS present with weakness in the following distribution: legs (41%), arms (34%), bulbar muscles (24%), generalized weakness (1%), respiratory muscles: 1 of 613 patients [8]. The most common presenting complaint of patients is focal weakness (60%). Rarely, patients present with generalized weakness or cramps, and rarely generalized fasciculations or respiratory failure [9]. Head drop is a manifestation of muscle weakness commonly seen in ALS, although not usually at presentation. Although it can be seen in other neuromuscular disorders, ALS and myasthenia gravis are the two most common causes of head drop, as a result of cervical paraspinal extensor muscular weakness. A hard Philadelphia or Headmaster-type cervical collar may be helpful to maintain posture and control pain.

There are no well-controlled studies examining the efficacy of exercise in this population. Aitkens and colleagues [10] showed that in slowly progressive neuromuscular diseases, a 12-week moderate-resistance (30% of maximum isometric force) exercise program resulted in strength gains ranging from 4% to 20% without any notable deleterious effects. In the same population, however, a 12-week high-resistance (training at the maximum weight a subject could lift 12 times) exercise program did not show any additional benefit compared with the moderate-resistance program and there was evidence of overwork weakness in some of the subjects [11]. A recent study by Dal Bello-Haas and colleagues [12] randomized 27 patients who had ALS into a resistance exercise group verses a usual care group who completed a daily stretching routine. After 6 months, the resistance exercise group performed better on the ALS Functional Rating Scale and physical function subscale of the SF-36. Although there are no conclusive data to support it, ALS patients are advised to refrain from exercising too vigorously or to the point of exhaustion, for fear of overwork weakness and further muscle damage and dysfunction [13]. Patients participating in an exercise program should be cautioned of the warning signs of overwork weakness, which include feeling weaker rather than stronger within 30 minutes postexercise or excessive muscle soreness 24 to 48 hours following exercise. Other warning signs include severe muscle cramping, heaviness in the extremities, and prolonged shortness of breath [13].

Early intervention with gentle, low-impact aerobic exercise, such as walking, swimming/pool exercise, and stationary bicycling, not only improves cardiovascular performance but also increases muscle efficiency to help fight fatigue [14]. Fatigue in ALS is multifactorial and is believed to be due in part to impaired muscular activation [15,16]. Other contributing factors include generalized deconditioning resulting from immobility and depression [14]. Benefits of aerobic exercise include not only improved physical function but also an improved sense of well-being and pain tolerance.

Managing clinical symptoms

Spasticity

Neurologic examination in patients suspected of having ALS is focused on searching for evidence of upper motor neuron (UMN) and lower motor neuron (LMN) abnormalities. UMN examination findings include spasticity and hyperreflexia, indicated by abnormal spread of reflexes and clonus. Brisk reflexes despite muscle atrophy can be present and may serve as a clue to LMN loss. UMN pathology can be confirmed by the presence of pathologic reflexes, such as the Babinski sign, Hoffman sign, and brisk jaw jerk. In the case of toe extensor paralysis, visualization of the tensor fascia lata contracting in attempts to elicit a Babinski response is equivalent to great toe extension. Additionally, it has been suggested that the corneomandibular reflex may be a more sensitive and specific indicator of UMN pathology in the bulbar region than the jaw jerk [17]. Gag reflex and jaw jerk should also be assessed to look for UMN dysfunction. Typically, UMN pathology results in spasticity, which produces a loss of dexterity or a feeling of stiffness in the limbs. Patients may also complain of weakness caused by spasticity resulting from disinhibition of brainstem control of the vestibulospinal and reticulospinal tracts, which originate in the motor cortex.

Spasticity is a common feature encountered in ALS and likely results from dysfunction of the motor cortex and the spinal cord. It can significantly complicate the problems created by weakness. Baclofen, a γ-aminobutyric acid (GABA) analog, facilitates motor neuron inhibition at the spinal cord and is the medication of choice. Initial dose is 5 to 10 mg two to three times a day and can be titrated up to 20 mg four times a day. Higher doses, up to 160 mg per day, are necessary at times but side effects of weakness, fatigue, and sedation can be problematic. Tizanidine, a relatively new agent with $\alpha 2$-agonist properties, has also been effective in spasticity management. Its mechanism of action is believed to be through the inhibition of excitatory interneurons. The dosing regimen ranges from 4 to 8 mg three to four times a day, with a similar side effect profile as baclofen. Benzodiazepines can be used but can cause respiratory depression and somnolence. Dantrolene, another drug used in the management of spasticity, acts by blocking Ca^{++} release in the sarcoplasmic reticulum. It is an effective medication to reduce muscle tone but its side effect of generalized weakness makes it a less desirable option in ALS. If patients continue to have a significant amount of spasticity, especially of the lower extremities, an intrathecal baclofen pump is useful in reducing spasticity and pain [18]. A combination of positional splinting and slow, frequent, sustained stretching of particularly symptomatic muscle groups, such as the gastrocnemius, can be effective in helping to reduce spasticity.

Muscle cramps

Muscle cramps may occur anywhere in the body, including the thighs, arms, and abdomen. Cramping of abdominal or other trunk muscles is unusual in other conditions and a diagnosis of ALS must be considered in these cases. Quinine sulfate taken orally can be helpful for symptomatic relief in addition to a daily stretching program that would lengthen the shortened, cramping muscle.

Dysphagia and dysarthria

Signs and symptoms suggesting bulbar muscle weakness include dysarthria, dysphagia, drooling, and aspiration. The drooling represents inability to manage secretions secondary to dysphagia. These signs and symptoms may be caused by UMN or LMN dysfunction involving the bulbar muscles. Patients who have ALS may have a mixed spastic-flaccid form of dysarthria. Signs of spastic dysarthria, indicating UMN pathology, include a strained and strangled quality of speech, with reduced rate, low pitch, imprecise consonant pronunciation, vowel distortion, and breaks in pitch. LMN dysfunction creates a flaccid dysarthria in which speech has a nasal or wet quality; pitch and intensity are monotone, phrases are abnormally short, and inspiration is audible. Complaints of difficulty chewing and swallowing and nasal regurgitation or coughing when drinking liquids indicate dysphagia.

Clinical signs and symptoms of dysarthria and dysphagia in a patient who has motor neuron disease may closely parallel one another [19]. Dysarthria in ALS is difficult to treat. Conventional articulation training is ineffective; however, some adaptive strategies taught by a speech-language therapist may be useful [14,20]. These include slowing the speech rate, increasing the precision of speech production, and decreasing background noise.

As the disease progresses, various communicative aids may play an ever-increasing role. Communication through an alphabet or word board works well early on when patients still have reasonable arm function. Binary command and yes/no systems using eye gaze can be particularly useful for a patient using mechanical ventilation. With advances in microprocessor technologies and computer programming, much improvement has been gained in speech synthesizers or multipurpose, multiaccess, computer-based augmentative communication systems. Caregivers of patients report that augmentative and alternative communication devices are helpful to stay connected, respond to patients' needs, and discuss complex important issues, including medical information [21]. Although expensive, these devices can greatly enhance the patient's ability to communicate when they can no longer phonate or write. These types of devices may often be either borrowed or rented from Assistive Technology Centers. For those patients who have no voluntary motor control for communication, brain–computer interfaces are being researched. These interfaces use EEG signals in which patients produce positive or negative shifts in cortical potentials that are sent to a communication device [22].

In addition, patients who have ALS and bulbar symptoms often have difficulty managing their oral secretions. Medications with strong anticholinergic effects, including some of the tricyclic antidepressants and glycopyrrolate, can be effective at drying up secretions. Transdermal scopolamine patches may also be effective in this setting. In severe cases, a transtympanic neurectomy (blocking the parasympathetic innervation of the salivary glands) or Stensen duct ligation may be tried but these procedures have had limited success. Radiation or botulinum toxins delivered to the salivary glands are other options that may be helpful, but are hampered by complications [14].

Changes in voice patterns and persistent coughing after swallowing liquids are two early signs of dysphagia in ALS. A speech-language pathologist should be consulted early for clinical swallowing evaluations and recommendations on dietary modifications. These modifications include thickening liquids and preparing food that forms easily into a bolus. A modified barium swallow or fiberoptic endoscopic examination of swallowing safety is needed when a patient has a history of having more difficulty with solids as opposed to liquids. These examinations are useful not only for accurately determining the presence of aspiration but also for providing a guide as to which food texture is safe for the patient. A thorough history and physical examination can give the clinician enough information to assess risk for aspiration and determine the type of study needed [23]. Cricopharyngeal myotomy may be helpful in a select group of patients who have dysfunction of this particular muscle, but most are unlikely to benefit [14].

Mood symptoms

Pseudobulbar affect

Pseudobulbar affect, also called emotional incontinence, is a symptom of pseudobulbar palsy that refers to an UMN syndrome caused by motor neuron loss in the corticobulbar tracts rather than the medulla. Patients experience inappropriate, uncontrolled laughter or crying that is not concordant with their mood and can be embarrassing. It is postulated that disinhibition of limbic motor control produces pseudobulbar affect, which is more common in the bulbar form of ALS. A recent study showed benefit of the use of dextromethorphan/quinidine (30 mg of each drug) in a multicenter trial in which primary outcomes were a change from baseline on the Center for Neurologic Study–Lability Scale, decrease in laughing/crying episode rates, and improvement in quality of life. There were a significant number of adverse reactions (24%) in the quinidine sulfate group, all of which resolved without significant sequelae [24]. In other neurologic diseases, such as multiple sclerosis and stroke, selective serotonin reuptake inhibitor (SSRI) medications have been helpful to decrease the symptoms associated with pseudobulbar affect [25].

Reactive depression

Reactive clinical depression is common in ALS [26]. Using the *Diagnostic and Statistical Manual of Mental Disorders, Fourth Edition* depression criteria, the rate of depression in ALS is 9% to 11%. Rates of depression do not increase during the later stages of the disease [27]. A supportive surrounding that includes close family, social, and religious support systems, and participation in support groups are all helpful for patients dealing with depression [4,26,28]. Once the diagnosis is confirmed, the patient should be counseled regarding the prognosis. The patient should be supported but allowed time for grieving, anger, and ultimately acceptance of his or her fate, which is important for the mental well-being of the patient and the family [28]. Antidepressant medication may assist with mood elevation, appetite stimulation, and sleep, and should be offered to every patient. In addition to the antidepressant effects the tricyclic medications with anticholinergic activity also assist in reducing oral secretions and minimizing drooling. These medications may also help control the symptoms of pseudobulbar affect in ALS. The European Federation on Neurologic Societies task force stated that amitriptyline may be a good initial choice and can be started at a dose of 25 mg 1 hour before bed and increased to 300 mg per day. SSRI medications are another choice for treatment of depressive symptoms with fewer anticholinergic side effects. Families of patients who have ALS with emotional lability should be reassured that the underlying mood state may be normal. A referral to a psychiatrist or clinical psychologist experienced in treating depression associated with terminal disease may be required. Depression in the spouse or significant other, family, or friends should also be carefully monitored, and when necessary group or family counseling may be helpful.

Anxiety

Measuring anxiety in patients who have ALS is particularly difficult because many somatic symptoms, such as muscle cramps and restlessness, can be confounded as anxiety. The rates of generalized anxiety disorder in ALS increase near the terminal stages of the disease [27]. The medications that are commonly used for treatment of anxiety include the benzodiazepines, which may have sedative side effects, or SSRI medications.

Pain

Pain is not often thought of as a major component of ALS. Most patients experience significant pain in the course of the disease process, however, and effective management can greatly improve a patient's quality of life. Most pain is believed to be a consequence of immobility, with the possibility of adhesive capsulitis, mechanical back pain, pressure areas on the skin, and more rarely, neuropathic pain [14]. Cannabis use has been shown in an anonymous survey of patients who had ALS to be helpful in reducing pain for about 1 hour [29].

Pharmacologic management of pain in ALS includes the use of nonsteroidal anti-inflammatory (NSAID) medications, acetaminophen, or a combination of both. NSAIDs are particularly useful if evidence of an active inflammatory process, such as tenosynovitis or arthritis, is present. For pain with a neuropathic component, tricyclic antidepressants and antiepileptic drugs, such as gabapentin, can sometimes be helpful. Gabapentin may also act to reduce spasticity. Narcotic medications should be reserved for refractory pain and used adequately and on a regular dosing regimen to achieve comfort [30]. Although the exact mechanism is unknown, concomitant use of hydroxyzine (an antiemetic and antihistamine medication) can enhance the effectiveness of narcotic pain medications. It is likely that hydroxyzine's direct muscle relaxant and analgesic properties potentiate the analgesic effect [30]. For easy administration, combination elixirs can be prepared by the pharmacy. The oral or sublingual form of morphine is effective for rapid-onset comfort care. Controlled-release narcotic medication, such as MS Contin, may be effective by providing a steady level of pain relief throughout the day.

Intramuscular delivery of medications should be avoided in ALS because of muscle wasting. Fentanyl or morphine patches are convenient delivery methods, but inconsistent dosing can be a problem, particularly with excessive perspiration. A patient-controlled analgesia is not feasible in advanced stages of ALS because of the patient's inability to control the delivery mechanism and these devices are generally not used in this setting.

The main problems of narcotic medication are respiratory depression and constipation. These side effects may be acceptable in the final phases of life when respiratory insufficiency with dyspnea or severe pain requires increased doses of morphine and lorazepam. It is essential for the patients and caregivers to be continually informed of the rationale for a particular medication and of potential side effects.

End-of-life decision making and palliative care

Although ALS is a fatal condition, it may take many years before a patient who has ALS succumbs to its effects. Poor prognostic factors include older age at onset of symptoms, earlier bulbar or pulmonary dysfunction, short time lag from symptom onset to diagnosis, and predominance of LMN findings at the time of diagnosis [8,31–33]. More women present with bulbar symptoms and they also seem to have a more rapid progression [34,35]. Although young men who have ALS may have a longer life expectancy, the overall life expectancy following diagnosis remains poor. Median 50% survival is 2.5 years for limb-onset and 1 year for bulbar-onset ALS.

The expected survival rates may vary depending on the patient's decision regarding the use of mechanical ventilation and feeding tubes. The overall survival rate remains low, however, and is only 28% by 5 years postdiagnosis [8,31,32]. In the process, ALS contributes to more and more debility for the patient and leads to important ethical and humanitarian issues. Patients who have ALS may have a great deal of time to think of their impending death and also the various decisions they need to make at different stages of their disease.

It is imperative that a social worker is involved early following the diagnosis to aid in the various decisions facing the patient. One such important choice is the decision regarding durable power of attorney. A living will may also be drafted in regard to the patient's wishes for the extent of medical intervention [36]. As a patient enters hospice-level care these issues take on a greater importance. Even though a patient may have accepted the eventual death resulting from ALS, it is often difficult for a patient to accept hospice care, because this implies that the disease has entered its terminal stage [37]. Medicare guidelines for entry into hospice include rapid progression of ALS and one of the following: critically impaired breathing capacity, critical nutritional impairment, or at least one life-threatening complication. These include recurrent aspiration pneumonia, decubitus ulcers, or recurrent fever after antibiotics [38]. It is therefore especially important at these times to not only be sensitive to a patient's needs but also assist the patient in making practical decisions. It is also important for patients to be referred to a support group early through the MDA and the ALS associations. The importance of support groups should not be underestimated because they can provide not only psychologic support but also further education and serve as a resource for problem solving and recycling of equipment, such as modified beds, lift devices, and communication equipment, among other things.

Modern medicine is continually advancing and has numerous interventions that can prolong life by artificial means. Although there are many medical interventions that can be provided, the physician should be sensitive to the possibility that a patient who has advanced ALS may reject such interventions. It is the patient, and not the physician, who determines whether to initiate life-sustaining therapy, artificial devices, or interventions that compensate for the failing organ or system to prevent death [39–41]. Mechanical ventilation, artificial hydration, and nutritional supports are probably the most obvious examples. Both legally and ethically, a competent patient has the right to refuse any prescribed intervention or treatment.

The physician and nurse's role is to thoroughly explain the consequences of the patient's decision and to foster and respect the patient's autonomy. This does not extend to the practice of physician-assisted suicide, however. It is an illegal act raising severe ethical concerns, which in itself deserves volumes, and cannot be adequately discussed in this article. According to a recent study, approximately 56% of patients who had ALS surveyed in Washington and Oregon would consider this alternative [15]. In the

Netherlands, 20% of patients who had ALS chose to end their lives through euthanasia or physician-assisted suicide [42]. The stunning number of patients who would consider physician-assisted suicide is perhaps an indication that the quality of care in the final stages of ALS may be inadequate.

Studies indicate that a lack of effective communication between a physician and a patient, and poor quality of life for the patient as perceived by the physician, may have a negative impact on the patient's quality of life [4]. It takes a great deal of time to explain end-of-life issues, including available treatment options and choices. Without this investment of time by the physician, a patient may be unaware of the available services and choices. An appropriate level of care for ALS patients may change frequently and thus necessitates a close follow-up.

Even in the advanced stages of ALS, optimizing in-home care with hospice can maximize the quality of life for the remaining time in these patients. In general, however, in-home care is either underutilized or initiated too late [43]. An effective hospice care plan provides an interdisciplinary team of professionals whose goal is to support the patient and the family through their remaining days together. It can provide invaluable psychologic, emotional, and spiritual support for the patient and the family in a familiar and comforting setting. The National Hospice Organization has provided guidelines for early entry into hospice for patients who have ALS [44]. These guidelines require physicians to make an estimate of life expectancy for the patient, which is often difficult for patients who have ALS who may progress relatively slowly in the dying process. Despite the advantages that hospice care offers, many physicians are not fully aware of the different services it provides [45]. Specific hospice care includes regular home visits by hospice nurses for medication management and delivery, assessment of pain control, skin and bowel care, and providing a progress report to physicians.

Summary

Although there is no cure for ALS at this time, a compassionate and supportive treatment plan for patients who have ALS is important and effective. This planning includes a comprehensive rehabilitative and palliative care plan that aims to maximize functional capacities, prolong or maintain independent mobility, prevent and minimize physical deformity, enhance comfort, and assist with community integration with the goal of improving quality of life.

References

[1] Van den Berg JP, Kalmijn S, Lindeman E, et al. Multidisciplinary ALS care improves quality of life in patients with ALS. Neurology 2005;65:1264–7.

[2] Traynor BJ, Alexander M, Corr B, et al. Effect of a multidisciplinary amyotrophic lateral sclerosis (ALS) clinic on ALS survival: a population based study, 1996–2000. J Neurol Neurosurg Psychiatry 2003;74:1258–61.

[3] Trail M, Nelson N, Van J, et al. Wheelchair use by patients with amyotrophic lateral sclerosis: a survey of user characteristics and selection preferences. Arch Phys Med Rehabil 2001; 82(1):98–102.
[4] Abresch RT, Seyden NK, Wineinger MA. Quality of life: issues for persons with neuromuscular diseases. Phys Med Rehabil Clin N Am 1998;9(1):233–48.
[5] Carvalho M, Schwartz MS, Swash M. Involvement of the external anal sphincter in amyotrophic lateral sclerosis. Muscle Nerve 1995;18:848–53.
[6] Brown RH, Meininger V, Swash M, editors. Amyotrophic lateral sclerosis. London: Martin Duntz Ltd; 2000. p. 412–3.
[7] Toepfer M, Schroeder M. Delayed colonic transit times in amyotrophic later al sclerosis assessed with radio-opaque markers. Eur J Med Res 1997;2(11):473–6.
[8] Norris F, Sheperd R, Denys E, et al. Onset, natural history and outcome in idiopathic adult motor neuron disease. J Neurol Sci 1993;118(1):48–55.
[9] Mitsumoto H, Chad DA, Pioro EP, et al. Amyotrophic lateral sclerosis. Philadelphia: F.A. Davis; 1998.
[10] Aitkens SG, McCrory MA, Kilmer DD, et al. Moderate resistance exercise program: its effects in slowly progressive neuromuscular disease. Arch Phys Med Rehabil 1993;74(7):711–5.
[11] Kilmer DD, McCrory MA, Wright NC, et al. The effect of a high resistance exercise program in slowly progressive neuromuscular disease. Arch Phys Med Rehabil 1994;75(5):560–3.
[12] Dal Bello-Haas V, Florence J, Krivickas LS, et al. A randomized controlled trial of resistance exercise in individuals with ALS. Neurology 2003;68(23):2003–7.
[13] Kilmer DD. The role of exercise in neuromuscular disease. Phys Med Rehabil Clin N Am 1998;9(1):115–25.
[14] Carter GT, Miller RG. Comprehensive management of amyotrophic lateral sclerosis. Phys Med Rehabil Clin N Am 1998;9(1):271–84.
[15] Sharma KR, Kent-Braun JA, Majumdar S, et al. Physiology of fatigue in amyotrophic lateral sclerosis. Neurology 1995;45(4):733–40.
[16] Sharma KR, Miller RG. Electrical and mechanical properties of skeletal muscle underlying increased fatigue in patients with amyotrophic lateral sclerosis. Muscle Nerve 1996;19:1391–400.
[17] Okuda B, Kodama N, Kawabata K, et al. Corneomandibular reflex in ALS. Neurology 1999;52:1699–701.
[18] McClelland S, Bethoux F, Boulis NM, et al. Intrathecal baclofen for spasticity-related pain in amyotrophic lateral sclerosis: efficacy and factors associated with pain relief. Muscle Nerve 2007;37(3):396–8.
[19] Carter GT, Johnson ER, Bonekat HW, et al. Laryngeal diversion in the treatment of intractable aspiration in motor neuron disease. Arch Phys Med Rehabil 1992;73(7):680–2.
[20] Miller RG, Rosenberg JA, Gelinas DF, et al. Practice parameter: the care of patients with amyotrophic lateral sclerosis (an evidence-base review). Muscle Nerve 1999;22:1104–11.
[21] Fried-Oken M, Fox L, Rau MT, et al. Purposes of AAC device use for persons with ALS as reported by caregivers. Augment Altern Commun 2006;22(3):209–21.
[22] Kubler A, Nijboer F, Sidhu M, et al. Patients with ALS can use sensorimotor rhythms to operate a brain–computer interface. Neurology 2005;64:1775–7.
[23] Langmore SE, Schatz MA, Olsen N. Fiberoptic endoscopic examination of swallowing safety: a new procedure. Dysphagia 1988;2:216–9.
[24] Brooks BR, Thisted RA, Appel SH, et al. Treatment of pseudobulbar affect in ALS with dextromethorphan/quinidine: a randomized trial. Neurology 2004;63(8):1364–70.
[25] Rosen HJ, Cummeins J. A real reason for patients with pseudobulbar affect to smile. Ann Neurol 2007;61(2):92–6.
[26] Hunter MD, Robinson IC, Neilson S. The functional and psychological status of patients with amyotrophic lateral sclerosis: some implications for rehabilitation. Disabil Rehabil 1993;15(3):119–26.
[27] Kurt A, Nijboer F. Depression and anxiety in individuals with amyotrophic lateral sclerosis: epidemiology and management. CNS Drugs 2007;21(4):279.

[28] Meininger V. Breaking bad news in amyotrophic lateral sclerosis. Palliat Med 1993; 7(Suppl 4):37–40.
[29] Amtmann D, Weydt P, Johnson KL, et al. Survey of cannabis use in patients with amyotrophic lateral sclerosis. Am J Hosp Palliat Care 2004;21(2):95–104.
[30] Fields HL. Relief of unnecessary suffering. In: Fields HL, Liebeskind JC, editors. Pharmacologic approaches to the treatment of chronic pain: new concepts and critical issues, vol. 1. Seattle (WA): International Association for the Study of Pain Press; 1994. p. 1–11.
[31] Ringel SP, Murphy JR, Alderson MK, et al. The natural history of amyotrophic lateral sclerosis. Neurology 1993;43(7):1316–22.
[32] Chancellor AM, Warlow CP. Adult onset motor neuron disease: worldwide mortality, incidence, and distribution since 1950. J Neurol Neurosurg Psychiatry 1992;55(12):1106–15.
[33] Neilson S, Robinson I, Alperovitch A. Rising amyotrophic lateral sclerosis mortality in France 1968–1990: increased life expectancy and inter-disease competition as an explanation. J Neurol 1994;241(7):448–55.
[34] Nelson LM, McGuire V, Longstreth WT Jr, et al. Population-based case-control study of amyotrophic lateral sclerosis in western Washington State. I. Cigarette smoking and alcohol consumption. Am J Epidemiol 2000;151(2):156–63.
[35] Nelson LM, Matkin C, Longstreth WT Jr, et al. Population-based case-control study of amyotrophic lateral sclerosis in western Washington State. II. Diet. Am J Epidemiol 2000; 151(2):164–73.
[36] Bernat JL. Ethical and legal issues in the management of amyotrophic lateral sclerosis. In: Belsh JM, Schiffman PL, editors. Amyotrophic lateral sclerosis: diagnosis and management for the clinician. Armonk (NY): Futura Publishing Co.; 1996. p. 357–72.
[37] Carter GT, Butler LM, Abresch RT, et al. Expanding the role of hospice in the care of amyotrophic lateral sclerosis. Am J Hosp Palliat Care 1999;16(6):707–10.
[38] Mitsumoto H, Rabkin JG. Palliative care for patients with amyotrophic lateral sclerosis: "prepare for the worst and hope for the best". JAMA 2007;298(2):207–16.
[39] Ganzini L, Johnston WS, McFarland BH, et al. Attitudes of patients with amyotrophic lateral sclerosis and their caregivers toward assisted suicide. N Engl J Med 1998;339(14): 967–73.
[40] Moore MK. Dying at home: a way of maintaining control for the person with ALS/MND. Palliat Med 1993;7(Suppl 4):65–8.
[41] Oppenheimer EA. Decision-making in the respiratory care of amyotrophic lateral sclerosis: should home mechanical ventilation be used? Palliat Med 1993;7(Suppl 4):49–64.
[42] Veldink JH, Wokke JH, van der Wal G, et al. Euthanasia and physician-assisted suicide among patients with amyotrophic lateral sclerosis in the Netherlands. N Engl J Med 2002; 346(21):1638–44.
[43] Krivickas LS, Shockley L, Mitsumoto H. Homecare of patients with amyotrophic lateral sclerosis (ALS). J Neurol Sci 1997;152(Suppl 1):S82–9.
[44] Standards and Accreditation Committee Medical Guidelines Task Force. Medical guidelines for determining prognosis in selected non-cancer diseases. The National Hospice Organization; 1996. p. 24–6.
[45] Enck RE. Hospice: the next step. Am J Hosp Palliat Care 1999;16(2):436–7.

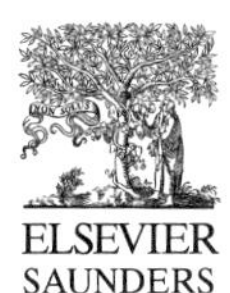
ELSEVIER
SAUNDERS

Phys Med Rehabil Clin N Am
19 (2008) 633–651

PHYSICAL MEDICINE
AND REHABILITATION
CLINICS OF
NORTH AMERICA

Drug Therapy in Amyotrophic Lateral Sclerosis

B. Jane Distad, MD[a,*], Gregg D. Meekins, MD[a], Lee L. Liou, MD, PhD[a], Michael D. Weiss, MD[a], Gregory T. Carter, MD, MS[b], Robert G. Miller, MD[c]

[a]*Department of Neurology, University of Washington Medical Center, 1959 NE Pacific Street, Seattle, WA 98195, USA*

[b]*Department of Physical Medicine and Rehabilitation, University of Washington Medical Center, 1959 NE Pacific Street, Seattle, WA 98195, USA*

[c]*California Pacific Medical Center, Forbes Norris MDA/ALS Research Center, 2324 Sacramento Street #111, San Francisco, CA 94115, USA*

Amyotrophic lateral sclerosis (ALS) is a devastating condition characterized by progressive muscle wasting, inanition, respiratory failure, and death within approximately 2 to 5 years of onset. ALS is among the most common neuromuscular conditions, with an overall prevalence in the world of ~5 to 7 cases/100,000 population [1,2]. The incidence of ALS may be increasing, possibly because of better recognition of the diagnosis and increased life expectancy [3–6]. The disease most commonly afflicts middle-aged individuals between 40 and 60 years of age [7]. Men are more commonly affected than women, with a ratio of ~1.5:1 [8,9]. Epidemiologic studies have identified some potential risk factors for developing ALS, including high dietary glutamate, high dietary fat, and low fiber intake [9]; cigarette smoking [10]; slimness and athleticism [11]; and living in urban areas. Between 5% and 10% of ALS is genetic, with up to 11 genetic loci identified [12]. Although understanding of the pathophysiology of this disease has advanced over the past 60 years, scant progress has been made regarding effective treatment. The authors review the current understanding of the pathogenic mechanisms of ALS and approaches to treating the disease.

* Corresponding author. Department of Neurology, Box 356465, 1959 NE Pacific Street, Seattle, WA 98195.

E-mail address: jdistad@u.washington.edu (B.J. Distad).

doi:10.1016/j.pmr.2008.04.005 *pmr.theclinics.com*

Mechanisms of disease

ALS is a progressive neurodegenerative disease characterized by the selective loss of upper and lower motor neurons present in the motor cortex, brain stem, and spinal cord. The fundamental pathophysiology of ALS is still not understood, but extensive research in this field has identified several potential pathogenic mechanisms. A better understanding of the mechanisms that result in motor neuron death will facilitate the development of methods to treat this devastating illness more effectively.

Genetics

ALS can be divided into two clinically indistinguishable forms: familial (FALS) and sporadic (SALS). FALS is defined by a family history of ALS, and approximately 10% of cases are familial [13]. Of the familial cases, 10% to 20% are associated with mutations in the super oxide dismutase 1 (SOD1) gene on chromosome 21q12.1, inherited as an autosomal dominant trait [14]. This gene codes for Cu, Zn-superoxide dismutase, which catalyzes the conversion of superoxide into hydrogen peroxide and oxygen. Mutations result in a toxic gain of function, which is still not completely understood.

Other genetic factors, which may prove to be susceptibility genes, have been described in SALS and FALS. Haplotypes in the promoter of vascular endothelial growth factor [15], the presence of an apolipoprotein E4 allele [16], and single nucleotide polymorphisms in the paraoxonase genes [17,18] are associated with an increased risk for developing SALS. Mutations in cytoskeletal proteins have been described in patients who have ALS, including neurofilament heavy chain subunit [19,20], peripherin [21], and dynactin [22]. Recently, whole-genome association analysis has been used to search for genes involved in ALS. Three positive studies have identified three leading gene candidates: FLJ10986 [23], inositol 1,4,5-triphosphate receptor 2 [24], and dipeptidyl-peptidase 6 [25]. The contribution of whole-genome association studies to our understanding of ALS is not yet clear.

Excitotoxicity

Excitotoxicity results from the overstimulation of neuronal glutamate receptors, which leads to an excessive influx of calcium into the neuron and can ultimately lead to cell death. Motor neurons are particularly susceptible to excitotoxicity because of a high number of Ca^{2+}-permeable alpha-amino-3-hydroxy-5-methyl-isoxazole-4-propionic acid (AMPA) receptors and a low Ca^{2+}-buffering capacity [26]. MR spectroscopy indicated that glutamate levels were increased in the plasma of patients who had ALS [27] and in the medulla of patients who had ALS [28]. Patients who have ALS have reduced levels of high-affinity glutamate transport in the spinal cord and somatosensory cortex [29] caused by a selective loss of the glial excitatory amino acid glutamate transporter-2 [30]. Cerebrospinal fluid from patients who have ALS is toxic to neuronal cell cultures by activation of AMPA receptors and increased intracellular Ca^{2+} [31,32].

Apoptosis

Apoptosis, or programmed cell death, has been implicated in ALS [33], with decreased levels of Bcl-2 mRNA (an antiapoptotic gene) and increased levels of bax mRNA (a proapoptotic gene) in the spinal cords of patients who have the disease [34]. Caspases are the major effectors of the apoptosis cascade, and activation of caspases is seen in spinal cord tissue from patients who have ALS [35] and in ALS transgenic mice [36]. Localization of mutant SOD1 to the mitochondria induces cell death in a caspase-dependent manner in neuronal cells [37]. A caspase inhibitor, zVAD-fmk, delayed disease onset and mortality in transgenic ALS mice [38].

Oxidative stress and mitochondrial dysfunction

Oxidative stress is the abnormal balance between the production of reactive oxygen species such as superoxide, hydrogen peroxide, and hydroxyl radical, and the removal of reactive oxygen species by the antioxidant system. Studies of postmortem tissue from patients who had ALS have shown accumulation of oxidative damage in proteins, lipids, and DNA [39–41].

In ALS, histologic abnormalities have been observed in the mitochondria in proximal axons [42], spinal cords [43], and dorsal root ganglia [44] of patients. Mitochondria are important in maintaining low cytosolic levels of calcium (Ca^{2+}) by contributing to handling rapid cytosolic Ca^{2+} transients. Mitochondrial Ca^{2+} accumulation seems to play a key role in glutamate excitotoxicity. Thus, mitochondrial dysfunction and Ca^{2+}-mediated excitotoxicity likely contribute to neuronal degeneration in FALS. Also, the Ca^{2+} capacity of mitochondria is impaired in ALS transgenic mice before the onset of motor symptoms [45]. Mutant SOD1 has been found to form aggregates in the mitochondria that can alter the reduction oxidation balance [46], damage mitochondrial proteins [47], and lead to release of cytochrome C [48]. Oxidation of wild-type SOD1 results in acquisition of toxic properties seen in the FALS mutant SOD1 [47], raising the possibility that involvement of SOD1 also occurs in SALS.

Neuroinflammation

Microglia are the resident macrophages of the central nervous system, normally functioning to remove cellular debris, facilitate repair, and enhance neuronal survival by way of production of trophic and anti-inflammatory factors. However, overactivation can be detrimental because of production of cytotoxic factors such as superoxide, nitric oxide, and tumor necrosis factor, and microglia have been implicated in several neurodegenerative diseases [49]. Selective expression of FALS mutant SOD1 in neurons is not sufficient for development of motor neuron disease in mice [50,51]. Microglia show activation in ALS transgenic mice before the development of motor neuron disease [52]. In chimeric mice, motor neurons expressing FALS mutant SOD1 showed prolonged survival when surrounded by wild-type glial cells [53], and transplantation of wild-type microglia into an ALS mouse resulted in slower progression but did not affect onset [54]. Microglia produce NADPH oxidase, which catalyzes the production of reactive oxygen species during inflammation, and is up-regulated in the spinal cords of patients who have ALS and ALS transgenic mice. Deletion of the catalytic subunit lengthens survival [55]. A recent study showed that SOD1 binds to the G-protein Rac1 and modulates its activity as a redox sensor; this process is defective in SOD1 mutants, leading to enhanced activation of NADPH oxidase [56]. Also, treatment of ALS transgenic mice with an inhibitor of NADPH oxidase, apocyanin, slows disease progression and increases lifespan, raising the possibility of a therapeutic target in humans [57].

Protein aggregation

Several neurodegenerative diseases are characterized by the formation of intracellular inclusions, and several inclusions have been described in neuropathologic studies of ALS. These inclusions may contain cystatin C and ubiquitin [58], hyaline, Lewy-body–like hyaline, astrocytic hyaline with immunoreactivity to SOD1 and ubiquitin [59], and phosphorylated neurofilament protein [58]. Mutations in SOD1 appear to cause protein aggregation in vitro and in vivo [60]. The formation of SOD1 aggregates is associated with neurodegeneration in mouse models of ALS, and these aggregates are present in the mitochondria [57,61–64]. The increased aggregation of SOD1 in ALS may disrupt the cellular pathways involved in protein chaperoning and degradation.

Therapeutic trials

The most commonly used model of ALS is the G93A mouse (SOD1G93A). This mouse is genetically engineered to express a mutant form of the human SOD1 gene, and harbors the glycine to alanine mutation at amino acid 93 (hence G93A). Since the development of the SOD1 mouse model of ALS [65], numerous therapeutic trials in SOD1 mice have taken place. The choice of therapeutic agents in many clinical trials of human ALS [66–68] has been dictated, at least in part, by the success of these agents in the SOD1 mouse [69]. Efficacy in human clinical trials has been limited, however, raising doubts about the value of the model in screening therapies for ALS [70].

Riluzole

Despite clinical use for more than 14 years, riluzole, a 2-amino-6-(trifluoromethoxy) benzothiozole, remains the only Food and Drug

Administration–approved medication proved to slow the progression of ALS. Pharmacologic mechanisms of riluzole include interference with N-methyl-D-aspartate (NMDA)-receptor mediated responses, stabilization of the inactivated state of voltage-dependent sodium channels, inhibition of glutamate release from synaptic terminals, and activation of extracellular glutamate uptake. Riluzole has demonstrated neuroprotective effect in motor neuron cultures and SOD1G93A transgenic mice [71–77]. A recent Cochrane Database Review concluded riluzole, 100 mg (total dose per day), prolongs median survival by about 2 to 3 months, based on analysis of four randomized controlled trials [78–82]. Recent studies using large registries suggest a greater benefit, ranging from 4 to 20 months [78]. Although American Academy of Neurology practice guidelines recommend the use of riluzole for nonventilated patients who have ALS, analysis of the ALS CARE Database found that 41% of the cohort was not prescribed this medication, largely because of the expense [83,84]. The drug is generally well tolerated, with asthenia, nausea, and an increase in serum alanine aminotransferase the most common side effects [85]. Liver function should be monitored during therapy.

Growth factors

Growth factors represent a large, heterogeneous group of endogenous polypeptides with varying physiologic activity, including cell signaling, cellular growth and differentiation, angiogenesis, regulation of inflammation, and antiapoptotic effect. Growth factor clinical trials to date have been disappointing. Treatment with subcutaneous recombinant human insulin-like growth factor-1 (rhIGF-1 or myotrophin) for 9 months slowed deterioration on the Appel ALS rating scale in a multicenter, North American trial but not in a similarly designed European study that may have been statistically underpowered [86,87]. A 2007 Cochrane Database Review concluded that available data were insufficient to render definitive assessment of rhIGF-1 as a clinical therapy for treatment of ALS [88]. A third phase III study is currently complete and results are pending. Neurotrophins, including brain-derived neurotrophic factor, ciliary neurotrophic factor, glial cell line-derived neurotrophic factor (GDNF), and oral xaliproden, which has neurotrophic-like activity, have failed to demonstrate benefit in human clinical trials [89–94]. Vascular endothelial growth factor, erythropoietin, and hepatocyte growth factor slow motor neuron deterioration in vitro and prolong survival in transgenic ALS rodent models but, to date, no human trial data have been reported [15,95–104].

Antiexcitotoxic/reducing glutamate

Ceftriaxone

Ceftriaxone increased brain expression of astroglial glutamate transporter 1 and its biochemical and functional activity, and delayed the loss of neurons and muscle strength, associated with increased mouse survival.

Its central nervous system penetration and long half-life are well known, obviating the need for extensive safety trials [105]. Stage I of the clinical trial has now been completed.

Memantine

Memantine is a noncompetitive NMDA receptor antagonist. It has been shown to protect neurons against NMDA- or glutamate-induced toxicity in vitro. Treatment of SOD1G93A mice significantly delayed disease progression and increased life span [106]. Safety studies are completed, and efficacy studies are enrolling patients (Clinicaltrials.gov NCT00409721 & NCT00353665).

N-acetylated alpha-linked acidic dipeptidase

Glutamate carboxypeptidase II (GCP II) N-acetylated alpha-linked acidic dipeptidase (NAALADase) inhibition decreases extracellular excitotoxic glutamate and increases extracellular N-acetylaspartylglutamate, both of which lead to increased neuroprotection [107]. Selective GCP II inhibitors demonstrated efficacy in models of stroke, ALS [108], and neuropathic pain. GCP II inhibition may have benefits over existing glutamate-based neuroprotection strategies, being selective for excitotoxic-induced glutamate release, with potentially fewer side effects. Phase I studies showed GCP II inhibition to be safe and well tolerated by healthy volunteers and patients who had diabetes [107].

ONO-2506

ONO-2506 is an enantiomeric homolog of valproate that restores disturbed astrocyte functions [109]. Subgroup analysis of a phase II trial suggested slowed respiratory deterioration in patients, with shorter duration disease (Public Relations, Ono Pharmaceutical Co., Ltd., August 10, 2005). A phase III trial of valproate has completed enrollment (Clinicaltrials.gov NCT00403104).

Talampanel (8-methyl-7H-1,3-dioxolo(2,3)benzodiazepine)

Talampanel (8-methyl-7H-1,3-dioxolo(2,3)benzodiazepine) is a noncompetitive modulator of AMPA glutamate receptors that crosses the blood–brain barrier and has prolonged SOD1G93A mouse survival. ALS functional rating scale (ALSFRS) and Tufts Quantitative Neuromuscular Examination (TQNE) scores declined at a slower rate in a 9-month phase II study of talampanel in 60 patients who had ALS [110]

Tamoxifen

Tamoxifen inhibits protein kinase C, and may reduce inflammation in the spinal cords of patients who have ALS [111]. Tamoxifen extended survival in a virally induced ALS mouse model [112]. In a phase II study of 60 patients who had ALS, tamoxifen prolonged survival [113].

Antiapoptosis

Minocycline

A tetracycline antibiotic, minocycline inhibits caspase activity by preventing its up-regulation, thereby decreasing motor neuron death. It also reduces glutamate-induced activation of microglia [114]. Minocycline prolonged survival in mouse models of Huntington's disease and FALS [115]. In a controlled trial of minocycline (400 mg/day, n = 412), ALS functional rating scale-revised (ALSFRS-R) declined faster over 9 months in the treatment group. Strength and pulmonary function tended to decline faster, and increased mortality tended to increase [116].

TCH346

TCH346 (dibenz [b,f]oxepin-10-ylmethyl-prop-2-ynyl-amine, hydrogen maleate salt) prevents the apoptotic increases and the nuclear accumulation of the glycolytic enzyme, glyceraldehyde 3-phosphate dehydrogenase. TCH346 (CGP 3466B) slowed disease progression in a murine model [117]. In a controlled study of 554 subjects, TCH346 was evaluated at four different doses, with no significant differences in any outcome measures when compared with placebo [118].

Antioxidants

Arimoclomol

Overexpression of heat shock protein conferred protection from ischemic injury in mammalian brain [119]. Arimoclomol, a coinducer of heat shock proteins, delayed progression of ALS in a mouse model [120]. A dose-ranging phase II study has been completed and a phase III study is planned.

Coenzyme Q10 (CoQ10 or ubiquinone)

Mitochondrial dysfunction in ALS may be aided by coenzyme Q10 (CoQ10 or ubiquinone) [121]. In SOD1G93A transgenic mice, low-dose CoQ10 prolonged median survival by 4.4% [122]. Doses up to 3000 mg per day are safe and well tolerated in patients who have ALS [123]. However, a phase III trial involving 185 people with ALS did not show any benefit over placebo [124].

Edaravone

The efficacy and safety of edaravone (3-methyl-1-phenyl-2-pyrazolin-5-one [MCI-186]), a free radical scavenger previously approved for treatment of acute cerebral infarction, was evaluated in patients who had ALS. Cerebrospinal fluid 3NT, a marker for oxidative stress, was reduced in a phase II trial. Decline in the ALSFRS-R score was significantly less than that in the 6 months before edaravone administration [125].

Melatonin

Melatonin is an amphiphilic molecule with antioxidative effects not conveyed by classic antioxidants. In SOD1G93A transgenic mice, high-dose oral melatonin extended survival. Rectal melatonin, 300 mg/day, was tolerated in a clinical safety study of 31 patients who had SALS [126].

Vitamin E

A study of vitamin E versus placebo in patients on riluzole yielded no difference in survival, although it showed a tendency to remain longer in the milder states of ALS with vitamin E [127]. Five grams per day of vitamin E was well tolerated in a phase III trial. However, no significant difference in survival was noted between treatment groups [128].

Immunomodulatory/anti-inflammatory

Celecoxib

The anti-inflammatory celecoxib, a selective cyclooxygenase-2 inhibitor that demonstrated neuroprotective effects and prolonged longevity in SOD1G93A mice, failed to show benefit on strength measures or survival at 800 mg/day dosing in a large, randomized, placebo-controlled trial [66].

Creatine

Creatine has neuroprotective effects through blockade of the mitochondrial membrane pore and as an antioxidant [129,130], but failed to show benefit in two large, randomized, controlled trials [67,68].

Copaxone

Copolymer-1 (copaxone) induces a neuroprotective T cell-mediated response. ALS mice treated with copolymer-1 experienced delayed disease onset, improved motor function, and extended survival [131]. Phase II trials of daily or biweekly injections demonstrated safety in the ALS population [132].

Thalidomide

Thalidomide reduced tumor necrosis factor–alpha, attenuated weight loss, and increased survival in SOD1 G93A mice [133]. An open-label phase II trial of thalidomide is completed but the results have not been released.

Neurodegeneration

Lithium

Lithium prevents neurodegeneration by promoting autophagy through inhibition of inositol-monophosphatase; it also rescues spinal cord mitochondria and facilitates the clearance of alpha-synuclein, ubiquitin, and SOD1. It delayed disease onset and progression in G93A transgenic mice and increased survival and slowed progression in humans over 15 months, compared with controls [134].

Innovative approaches

Extensive ineffective clinical trials in ALS involving various subcutaneously and orally administered medications have been disappointing, which has led to novel approaches to drug delivery or nonpharmacologic forms of treatment.

Intrathecal delivery

Short half-life compounds, particularly neurotrophic factors, and larger molecules with poor penetration across the blood brain barrier, may not achieve therapeutic concentrations in the brain and spinal cord. For this reason, intrathecal delivery of medications has been attempted in ALS. Intrathecal brain-derived neurotrophic factor in a phase I/II dose escalation study was found to be well tolerated, with spinal fluid levels directly related to dose administration [135]. A small, double-blinded study of rhIGF-1 delivered intrathecally slowed motor deterioration on measures of total and limb Norris scales [136].

Gene therapy

Mechanisms for delivering gene transcripts directly to motor neuron cellular DNA by way of motor axonal retrograde transport include genetically engineered adeno-associated virus (AAV), which may be administered by intramuscular, intraperitoneal, and intravenous injection. The Bcl-xL gene, with antiexcitotoxic properties, incorporated with AAV-2 viral vector, was neuroprotective in a glutamate toxicity model in vitro [137], whereas intramuscularly injected GDNF- and insulin-like growth factor-AAV increased longevity in motor neuron cultures and G93A mice [138–140]. AAV-2, with a coding gene for a small interference RNA to SOD1 and injected intramuscularly into G93A mice, decreased mutant SOD1 load and delayed loss of grip strength [141]. Retrograde transport of intramuscularly injected conjugated recombinant human GDNF linked to neuronal binding fragment of tetanus toxin (tetanus toxin fragment C) produced intense immunostaining in spinal cord motor neurons, but without significant motor neuron preservation, as compared with GDNF in a neonatal rat axonotomy model [142]. A phase I/II clinical trial involving implantation of encapsulated baby hamster kidney cells engineered to release human ciliary neurotrophic factor reported detectable cerebrospinal fluid levels of the neurotrophin in 9 of 12 study subjects, with 2 of these individuals having detectable levels up to 20 weeks postimplantation [143]. No significant side effects were reported.

Stem cell transplant

Feasibility and safety studies of intraspinal cord implantation of autologous mesenchymal stem cells showed no convincing clinical benefits [144,145].

Table 1
Completed phase II/III clinical treatment trials in amyotrophic lateral sclerosis

Medication	Mechanism of action	Number of treated	Number of placebo	Outcome	References
Riluzole	Reduces glutamate	907	503	Prolonged survival 2–3 mo	[79–82] (4 trials)
Talampanel	—	60[a]	—	Slowed decline in ALSFRS and TQNE	[110]
Tamoxifen	—	60[a]	—	Prolonged survival	[113]
BDNF	Growth factor	748	387	No improved survival; slowed rate of respiratory failure	[89]
rhCNTF	—	141	429	No benefit	[91]
rhCNTF	—	485	245	No benefit	[92]
rhIGFI	—	99	42	Slowed deterioration	[86]
rhIGF	—	124	59	No significant difference	[87]
GDNF	—	NA	—	No benefit	[93]
Xaliproden	—	1385	690	No benefit	[94]
Minocycline	Inhibitor of neuronal apoptosis	206	206	Worsened decline on ALSFRS and increased mortality	[116]
TCH346	—	442	111	No benefit	[118]
Edaravone	Antioxidant	20[b]	—	Slowed decline on ALSFRS-R	[124]
Coenzyme Q10	—	185[a]	—	No benefit	[146]
Vitamin E	—	83	77	No change in survival	[128]
Celecoxib	Anti-inflammatory	201	99	No benefit	[66]
Creatine	—	138	141	No benefit	[67,68] (2 trials)
Copaxone	—	20	10	No conclusions about benefit	[132]
Lithium	Prevents neurodegeneration	16	28	Increased survival, slowed progression	[134]

Abbreviations: BDNF, brain-derived neurotrophic factor; GDNF, glial derived neurotrophic factor; NA, not available; rhCNTF, recombinant human ciliary neurotrophic factor; rhIGF, recombinant human insulin-like growth factor; rhIGFI, recombinant insulin derived growth factor.

[a] Only total patient numbers available.

[b] Open trial without a placebo group.

Cannabinoids (marijuana)

Several studies published show a significant benefit from cannabinoids, including delta-9-tetrahydrocannibinol (THC) in the SOD1 mouse model of ALS [147–152]. Administration of delta-9-THC before and after the onset of ALS symptoms slowed disease progression and prolonged survival in animals, compared with untreated controls [152]. Other trials in animal models of ALS have also shown that naturally occurring and synthetic cannabinoids slow down the progression of ALS [148,151]. Another recent study showed that blocking the CB1 cannabinoid receptor extended the life span of mice that had ALS [151], which suggests that some abnormality within our internal cannabinoid system may be part of the underlying disease mechanisms in ALS. The cannabinoids are all 21 carbon terpenes, a chemical structure that is the same as tamoxifen. Similar to tamoxifen, cannabinoids inhibit protein kinase C, and could reduce inflammation in the spinal cord of patients who have ALS, although this remains to be studied.

Therapeutic exercise

Two studies have evaluated exercise, with some favorable response. In one, the decline of ALSFRS slowed [153], and the other showed improved quality of life with a trial of resistance exercise training (Table 1) [154].

Summary

Despite numerous trials, a medication that is effective in arresting or reversing the progression of ALS remains elusive. Multiple pathogenic mechanisms are implicated in ALS and may form a final common pathway. The SOD1 mouse model is directed against only one of these. Therefore, the outcome of preclinical treatment trials in these animals is likely not an accurate determinant of the effect of these drugs on patients who have ALS. Other models of different mechanisms are needed to screen agents more effectively. Genetic engineering and stem cell therapy hold promise in the treatment of this disease but their role in eventually treating ALS is far from certain. The most important issue in finding viable pharmacologic therapies is identifying the earliest (upstream) event or events in ALS.

References

[1] Norris F, Shepherd R, Denys E, et al. Onset, natural history and outcome in idiopathic adult motor neuron disease. J Neurol Sci 1993;118(1):48–55.
[2] Ringel SP, Murphy JR, Alderson MK, et al. The natural history of amyotrophic lateral sclerosis. Neurology 1993;43(7):1316–22.
[3] Neilson S, Robinson I, Alperovitch A. Rising amyotrophic lateral sclerosis mortality in France 1968–1990: increased life expectancy and inter-disease competition as an explanation. J Neurol 1994;241(7):448–55.

[4] Neilson S, Robinson I, Nymoen EH. Longitudinal analysis of amyotrophic lateral sclerosis mortality in Norway, 1966–1989: evidence for a susceptible subpopulation. J Neurol Sci 1994;122(2):148–54.
[5] Eisen A. Amyotrophic lateral sclerosis is a multifactorial disease. Muscle Nerve 1995;18(7): 741–52.
[6] Eisen A, Scultzer M, MacNeil M, et al. Duration of amyotrophic lateral sclerosis is age dependent. Muscle Nerve 1993;16:27–32.
[7] Pradas J, Finison L, Andres PL, et al. The natural history of amyotrophic lateral sclerosis and the use of natural history controls in therapeutic trials. Neurology 1993;43(4):751–5.
[8] Chancellor AM, Warlow CP. Adult onset motor neuron disease: worldwide mortality, incidence, and distribution since 1950. J Neurol Neurosurg Psychiatr 1992;55(12):1106–15.
[9] Nelson LM, Matkin C, Longstreth WT Jr, et al. Population-based case-control study of amyotrophic lateral sclerosis in western Washington State. II. Dict. Am J Epidemiol 2000;151(2):164–73.
[10] Nelson LM, McGuire V, Longstreth WT Jr, et al. Population-based case-control study of amyotrophic lateral sclerosis in western Washington State. I. Cigarette smoking and alcohol consumption. Am J Epidemiol 2000;151(2):156–63.
[11] Scarmeas N, Shih T, Stern Y, et al. Premorbid weight, body mass, and varsity athletics in ALS. Neurology 2002;59(5):773–5.
[12] Goodall EF, Morrison KE. Amyotrophic lateral sclerosis (motor neuron disease): proposed mechanisms and pathways to treatment. Expert Rev Mol Med 2006;8(11):1–22.
[13] Valdmanis PN, Rouleau GA. Genetics of familial amyotrophic lateral sclerosis. Neurology 2008;70(2):144–52.
[14] Rosen DR, Siddique T, Patterson D, et al. Mutations in Cu/Zn superoxide dismutase gene are associated with familial amyotrophic lateral sclerosis. Nature 1993;362:59–62.
[15] Lambrechts D, Storkebaum E, Morimoto M, et al. VEGF is a modifier of amyotrophic lateral sclerosis in mice and humans and protects motoneurons against ischemic death. Nat Genet 2003;34(4):383–94.
[16] Dvory VE, Birnbaum M, Korczyn AD, et al. Association of APOE epsilon4 allele with survival in amyotrophic lateral sclerosis. J Neurol Sci 2001;190:17–20.
[17] Slowik A, Tomik B, Wolkow PP, et al. Paraoxonase gene polymorphisms and sporadic ALS. Neurology 2006;67:766–70.
[18] Saeed M, Siddique N, Hung WY, et al. Paraoxonase cluster polymorphisms are associated with sporadic ALS. Neurology 2006;67:771–6.
[19] Figlewicz DA, Krizus A, Martinoli MG, et al. Variants of the heavy neurofilament subunit are associated with the development of amyotrophic lateral sclerosis. Hum Mol Genet 1994; 3:1757–61.
[20] Al-Chalabi A, Andersen PM, Nilsson P, et al. Deletions of the heavy neurofilament subunit tail in amyotrophic lateral sclerosis. Hum Mol Genet 1999;8:157–64.
[21] Gros-Louis F, Lariviere R, Gowing G, et al. A frameshift deletion in peripherin gene associated with amyotrophic lateral sclerosis. J Biol Chem 2004;279:45951–6.
[22] Munch C, Sedlmeier R, Meyer T, et al. Point mutations of the p150 subunit of dynactin (DCTN1) gene in ALS. Neurology 2004;63:724–6.
[23] Dunckley T, Huentelman MJ, Craig DW, et al. Whole-genome analysis of sporadic amyotrophic lateral sclerosis. N Engl J Med 2007;357(8):775–88.
[24] van Es MA, Van Vught PW, Blauw HM, et al. ITPR2 as a susceptibility gene in sporadic amyotrophic lateral sclerosis: a genome-wide association study. Lancet Neurol 2007;6(10): 869–77.
[25] van Es MA, van Vught PW, Blauw HM, et al. Genetic variation in DPP6 is associated with susceptibility to amyotrophic lateral sclerosis. Nat Genet 2008;40(1):29–31.
[26] Van Den Bosch L, Van Damme P, Bogaert E, et al. The role of excitotoxicity in the pathogenesis of amyotrophic lateral sclerosis. Biochim Biophys Acta 2006;1762(11–12): 1068–82.

[27] Plaitakis A, Constantakakis E. Altered metabolism of excitatory amino acids, N-acetyl-a and N-acetyl-aspartyl-glutamate in amyotrophic lateral sclerosis. Brain Res Bull 1993; 30(3–4):381–6.
[28] Pioro EP, Majors AW, Mitsumoto H, et al. 1H-MRS evidence of neurodegeneration and excess glutamate+glutamine in ALS medulla. Neurology 1999;53:71–9.
[29] Rothstein JD, Martin LJ, Kuncl RW. Decreased glutamate transport by the brain and spinal cord in amyotrophic lateral sclerosis. N Engl J Med 1992;326(22):1464–8.
[30] Rothstein JD, Van Kammen M, Levey AI, et al. Selective loss of glial glutamate transporter GLT-1 in amyotrophic lateral sclerosis. Ann Neurol 1995;38(1):73–84.
[31] Couratier P, Hugon J, Sindou P, et al. Cell culture evidence for neuronal degeneration in amyotrophic lateral sclerosis being linked to glutamate AMPA/kainate receptors. Lancet 1993;341(8840):265–8.
[32] Sen I, Nalini A, Joshi NB, et al. Cerebrospinal fluid from amyotrophic lateral sclerosis patients preferentially elevates intracellular calcium and toxicity in motor neurons via AMPA/kainate receptor. J Neurol Sci 2005;235(1–2):45–54.
[33] Vila M, Przedborski S. Targeting programmed cell death in neurodegenerative diseases. Nat Rev Neurosci 2003;4(5):365–75.
[34] Mu X, He J, Anderson DW, et al. Altered expression of bcl-2 and bax mRNA in amyotrophic lateral sclerosis spinal cord motor neurons. Ann Neurol 1996;40:379–86.
[35] Martin LJ. Neuronal death in amyotrophic lateral sclerosis is apoptosis: possible contribution of a programmed cell death mechanism. J Neuropathol Exp Neurol 1999;58(5): 459–71.
[36] Pasinelli P, Houseweart MK, Brown RH, et al. Caspase-1 and -3 are sequentially activated in motor neuron death in Cu, Zn superoxide dismutase-mediated familial amyotrophic lateral sclerosis. Proc Natl Acad Sci USA 2000;97(25):13901–6.
[37] Takeuchi H, Kobayashi Y, Ishigaki S, et al. Mitochondrial localization of mutant superoxide dismutase 1 triggers caspase-dependent cell death in a cellular model of familial amyotrophic lateral sclerosis. J Biol Chem 2002;277(52):50966–72.
[38] Li M, Ona VO, Guégan C, et al. Functional role of caspase-1 and caspase-3 in an ALS transgenic mouse model. Science 2000;288(5464):335–9.
[39] Ferrante RJ, Browne SE, Shinobu LA, et al. Evidence of increased oxidative damage in both sporadic and familial amyotrophic lateral sclerosis. J Neurochem 1997;69(5):2064–74.
[40] Kikuchi S, Shinpo K, Ogata A, et al. Detection of N epsilon-(carboxymethyl)lysine (CML) and non-CML advanced glycation end-products in the anterior horn of amyotrophic lateral sclerosis spinal cord. Amyotroph Lateral Scler Other Motor Neuron Disord 2002;3(2): 63–8.
[41] Pedersen WA, Fu W, Keller JN, et al. Protein modification by the lipid peroxidation product 4-hydroxynonenal in the spinal cords of amyotrophic lateral sclerosis patients. Ann Neurol 1998;44(5):819–24.
[42] Hirano A, Nakano I, Kurland LT, et al. Fine structural study of neurofibrillary changes in a family with amyotrophic lateral sclerosis. J Neuropathol Exp Neurol 1984;43(5):471–80.
[43] Sasaki S, Iwata M. Mitochondrial alterations in the spinal cord of patients with sporadic amyotrophic lateral sclerosis. J Neuropathol Exp Neurol 2007;66(1):10–6.
[44] Sasaki S, Horie Y, Iwata M. Mitochondrial alterations in dorsal root ganglion cells in sporadic amyotrophic lateral sclerosis. Acta Neuropathol 2007;114(6):633–9.
[45] Damiano M, Starkov AA, Petri S, et al. Neural mitochondrial Ca2+ capacity impairment precedes the onset of motor symptoms in G93A Cu/Zn-superoxide dismutase mutant mice. J Neurochem 2006;96(5):1349–61.
[46] Ferri A, Cozzolino M, Crosio C, et al. Familial ALS-superoxide dismutases associate with mitochondria and shift their redox potentials. Proc Natl Acad Sci USA 2006;103(37): 13860–5.
[47] Liu J, Lillo C, Jonsson PA, et al. Toxicity of familial ALS-linked SOD1 mutants from selective recruitment to spinal mitochondria. Neuron 2004;43(1):5–17.

[48] Kirkinezos IG, Bacman SR, Hernandez D, et al. Cytochrome c association with the inner mitochondrial membrane is impaired in the CNS of G93A-SOD1 mice. J Neurosci 2005; 25(1):164–72.
[49] Block ML, Zecca L, Hong JS. Microglia-mediated neurotoxicity: uncovering the molecular mechanisms. Nat Rev Neurosci 2007;8(1):57–69.
[50] Lino MM, Schneider C, Caroni P. Accumulation of SOD1 mutants in postnatal motoneurons does not cause motoneuron pathology or motoneuron disease. J Neurosci 2002;22(12): 4825–32.
[51] Pramatarova A, Laganière J, Roussel J, et al. Neuron-specific expression of mutant superoxide dismutase 1 in transgenic mice does not lead to motor impairment. J Neurosci 2001; 21(10):3369–74.
[52] Henkel JS, Beers DR, Siklós L, et al. The chemokine MCP-1 and the dendritic and myeloid cells it attracts are increased in the mSOD1 mouse model of ALS. Mol Cell Neurosci 2006; 31(3):427–37.
[53] Clement AM, Nguyen MD, Roberts EA, et al. Wild-type nonneuronal cells extend survival of SOD1 mutant motor neurons in ALS mice. Science 2003;302(5642):113–7.
[54] Beers DR, Henkel JS, Xiao Q, et al. Wild-type microglia extend survival in PU.1 knockout mice with familial amyotrophic lateral sclerosis. Proc Natl Acad Sci USA 2006;103(43): 16021–6.
[55] Wu DC, Ré DB, Nagai M, et al. The inflammatory NADPH oxidase enzyme modulates motor neuron degeneration in amyotrophic lateral sclerosis mice. Proc Natl Acad Sci USA 2006;103(32):12132–7.
[56] Harraz MM, Marden JJ, Zhou W, et al. SOD1 mutations disrupt redox-sensitive Rac regulation of NADPH oxidase in a familial ALS model. J Clin Invest 2008;118(2): 659–70.
[57] Urushitani M, Sik A, Sakurai T, et al. Chromogranin-mediated secretion of mutant superoxide dismutase proteins linked to amyotrophic lateral sclerosis. Nat Neurosci 2006;9(1): 108–18.
[58] Kato S. Amyotrophic lateral sclerosis models and human neuropathology: similarities and differences. Acta Neuropathol 2008;115(1):97–114.
[59] Bruijn LI, Houseweart MK, Kato S, et al. Aggregation and motor neuron toxicity of an ALS-linked SOD1 mutant independent from wild-type SOD1. Science 1998;281(5384): 1851–4.
[60] Shaw BF, Valentine JS. How do ALS-associated mutations in superoxide dismutase 1 promote aggregation of the protein? Trends Biochem Sci 2007;32(2):78–85.
[61] Wang J, Xu G, Gonzales V, et al. Fibrillar inclusions and motor neuron degeneration in transgenic mice expressing superoxide dismutase 1 with a disrupted copper-binding site. Neurobiol Dis 2002;10(2):128–38.
[62] Wang J, Xu G, Borchelt DR. High molecular weight complexes of mutant superoxide dismutase 1: age-dependent and tissue-specific accumulation. Neurobiol Dis 2002;9(2): 139–48.
[63] Deng HX, Shi Y, Furukawa Y, et al. Conversion to the amyotrophic lateral sclerosis phenotype is associated with intermolecular linked insoluble aggregates of SOD1 in mitochondria. Proc Natl Acad Sci USA 2006;103(18):7142–7.
[64] Vijayvergiya C, Beal MF, Buck J, et al. Mutant superoxide dismutase 1 forms aggregates in the brain mitochondrial matrix of amyotrophic lateral sclerosis mice. J Neurosci 2005; 25(10):2463–70.
[65] Gurney ME, Pu H, Chiu AY, et al. Motor neuron degeneration in mice that express a human Cu, Zn superoxide dismutase mutation. Science 1994;264(5166):1772–5.
[66] Cudkowicz ME, Shefner JM, Schoenfeld DA, et al. Trial of celecoxib in amyotrophic lateral sclerosis. Ann Neurol 2006;60(1):22–31.
[67] Groeneveld GJ, Veldink JH, van der Tweel I, et al. A randomized sequential trial of creatine in amyotrophic lateral sclerosis. Ann Neurol 2003;53(4):437–45.

[68] Shefner JM, Cudkowicz ME, Schoenfeld D, et al. A clinical trial of creatine in ALS. Neurology 2004;63(9):1656–61.

[69] Drachman DB, Frank K, Dykes-Hoberg M, et al. Cyclooxygenase 2 inhibition protects motor neurons and prolongs survival in a transgenic mouse model of ALS. Ann Neurol 2002;52(6):771–8.

[70] Benatar M. Lost in translation: treatment trials in the SOD1 mouse and in human ALS. Neurobiol Dis 2007;26(1):1–13.

[71] Hubert JP, Delumeau JC, Glowinski J, et al. Antagonism by riluzole of entry of calcium evoked by NMDA and veratridine in rat cultured granule cells: evidence for a dual mechanism of action. Br J Pharmacol 1994;113(1):261–7.

[72] Boireau A, Meunier M, Doble A. 3-Nitropropionic acid exacerbates [3H]GABA release evoked by glucose deprivation in rat striatal slices. J Pharm Pharmacol 1996;48(1):85–9.

[73] Boireau A, Meunier M, Imperato A. Ouabain-induced increase in dopamine release from mouse striatal slices is antagonized by riluzole. J Pharm Pharmacol 1998;50(11):1293–7.

[74] Martin D, Thompson MA, Nadler JV. The neuroprotective agent riluzole inhibits release of glutamate and aspartate from slices of hippocampal area CA1. Eur J Pharmacol 1993;250(3):473–6.

[75] Fumagalli E, Funicello M, Rauen T, et al. Riluzole enhances the activity of glutamate transporters GLAST, GLT1 and EAAC1. Eur J Pharmacol 2008;578(2–3):171–6.

[76] Estevez AG, Stutzmann JM, Berbeito L. Protective effect of riluzole on excitatory amino acid-mediated neurotoxicity in motoneuron-enriched cultures. Eur J Pharmacol 1995;280(1):47–53.

[77] Gurney ME, Fleck TJ, Himes CS, et al. Riluzole preserves motor function in a transgenic model of familial amyotrophic lateral sclerosis. Neurology 1998;50(1):62–6.

[78] Miller RG, Mitchell JD, Lyon M, et al. Riluzole for amyotrophic lateral sclerosis [ALS]/motor neuron disease [MND]. Cochrane Database Syst Rev 2007;24(1):CD001447.

[79] Bensimon G, Lacomblez L, Meininger V. A controlled trial of riluzole in amyotrophic lateral sclerosis. ALS/Riluzole Study Group. N Engl J Med 1994;330(9):585–91.

[80] Bensimon G, Lacomblez L, Delumeau JC, et al. A study of riluzole in the treatment of advanced stage or elderly patients with amyotrophic lateral sclerosis. J Neurol 2002;249(5):609–15.

[81] Lacomblez L, Bensimon G, Leigh PN, et al. Dose-ranging study of riluzole in amyotrophic lateral sclerosis. Amyotrophic Lateral Sclerosis/Riluzole Study Group II. Lancet 1996;347(9013):1425–31.

[82] Yanagisawa N, Tashiro K, Tohgi H, et al. Efficacy and safety of riluzole in patients with amyotrophic lateral sclerosis: double-blind placebo-controlled study in Japan. Igaku no Ayumi 1997;182:851–66.

[83] Practice advisory on the treatment of amyotrophic lateral sclerosis with riluzole: report of the Quality Standards Subcommittee of the American Academy of Neurology. Neurology 1997;49(3):657–9.

[84] Bradley WG, Anderson F, Gowda N, et al. Changes in the management of ALS since the publication of the AAN ALS practice parameter 1999. Amyotroph Lateral Scler Other Motor Neuron Disord 2004;5(4):240–4.

[85] Bensimon G, Doble A. The tolerability of riluzole in the treatment of patients with amyotrophic lateral sclerosis. Expert Opin Drug Saf 2004;3(6):525–34.

[86] Lange DJ, Felice KJ, Festoff BW, et al. Recombinant human insulin-like growth factor-I in ALS: description of a double-blind, placebo-controlled study. North American ALS/IGF-I Study Group. Neurology 1996;47(4 Suppl 2):S93–5.

[87] Borasio GD, Robberecht W, Leigh PN, et al. A placebo-controlled trial of insulin-like growth factor-I in amyotrophic lateral sclerosis. European ALS/IGF-I Study Group. Neurology 1998;51(2):583–6.

[88] Mitchell JD, Wokke JH, Borasio GD. Recombinant human insulin-like growth factor I [rhIGF-I] for amyotrophic lateral sclerosis/motor neuron disease. Cochrane Database Syst Rev 2007;(4):CD002064.
[89] Bdnf Study GROUP. A controlled trial of recombinant methionyl human BDNF in ALS: The BDNF Study Group [Phase III]. Neurology 1999;52(7):1427–33.
[90] Beck M, Flachenecker P, Magnus T, et al. Autonomic dysfunction in ALS: a preliminary study on the effects of intrathecal BDNF. Amyotroph Lateral Scler Other Motor Neuron Disord 2005;6(2):100–3.
[91] Miller RG, Petajan JH, Bryan WW, et al. A placebo-controlled trial of recombinant human ciliary neurotrophic [rhCNTF] factor in amyotrophic lateral sclerosis. rhCNTF ALS Study Group. Ann Neurol 1996;39(2):256–60.
[92] A double-blind placebo-controlled clinical trial of subcutaneous recombinant human ciliary neurotrophic factor (rHCNTF) in amyotrophic lateral sclerosis. ALS CNTF Treatment Study Group. Neurology 1996;46(5):1244–9.
[93] Available at: http://www.als-mda.org/publications/als/als4_3.html#amgen. 2008. Ref Type: Internet Communication. Accessed May 24, 2008.
[94] Meininger V, Bensimon G, Bradley WR, et al. Efficacy and safety of xaliproden in amyotrophic lateral sclerosis: results of two phase III trials. Amyotroph Lateral Scler Other Motor Neuron Disord 2004;5(2):107–17.
[95] Li B, Xu W, Luo C, et al. VEGF-induced activation of the PI3-K/Akt pathway reduces mutant SOD1-mediated motor neuron cell death. Brain Res Mol Brain Res 2003;111(1–2):155–64.
[96] Zheng C, Nennesmo I, Fadeel B, et al. Vascular endothelial growth factor prolongs survival in a transgenic mouse model of ALS. Ann Neurol 2004;56(4):564–7.
[97] Mennini T, De Paola M, Bigini P, et al. Nonhematopoietic erythropoietin derivatives prevent motoneuron degeneration in vitro and in vivo. Mol Med 2006;12(7–8):153–60.
[98] Koh SH, Kim Y, Kim HY, et al. Recombinant human erythropoietin suppresses symptom onset and progression of G93A-SOD1 mouse model of ALS by preventing motor neuron death and inflammation. Eur J Neurosci 2007;25(7):1923–30.
[99] Turgeon VL, Houenou LJ. Prevention of thrombin-induced motoneuron degeneration with different neurotrophic factors in highly enriched cultures. J Neurobiol 1999;38(4):571–80.
[100] Manabe Y, Nagano I, Gazi MS, et al. Glial cell line-derived neurotrophic factor protein prevents motor neuron loss of transgenic model mice for amyotrophic lateral sclerosis. Neurol Res 2003;25(2):195–200.
[101] Ebens A, Brose K, Leonardo ED, et al. Hepatocyte growth factor/scatter factor is an axonal chemoattractant and a neurotrophic factor for spinal motor neurons. Neuron 1996;17(6):1157–72.
[102] Sun W, Funakoshi H, Nakamura T. Overexpression of HGF retards disease progression and prolongs life span in a transgenic mouse model of ALS. J Neurosci 2002;22(15):6537–48.
[103] Kadoyama K, Funakoshi H, Ohya W, et al. Hepatocyte growth factor [HGF] attenuates gliosis and motoneuronal degeneration in the brainstem motor nuclei of a transgenic mouse model of ALS. Neurosci Res 2007;59(4):446–56.
[104] Ishigaki A, Aoki M, Nagai M, et al. Intrathecal delivery of hepatocyte growth factor from amyotrophic lateral sclerosis onset suppresses disease progression in rat amyotrophic lateral sclerosis model. J Neuropathol Exp Neurol 2007;66(11):1037–44.
[105] Rothstein JD, Patel S, Regan MR, et al. Beta-lactam antibiotics offer neuroprotection by increasing glutamate transporter expression. Nature 2005;433(7021):73–7.
[106] Wang R, Zhang D. Memantine prolongs survival in an amyotrophic lateral sclerosis mouse model. Eur J Neurosci 2005;22(9):2376–80.
[107] Thomas AG, Wozniak KM, Tsukamoto T, et al. Glutamate carboxypeptidase II (NAALADase) inhibition as a novel therapeutic strategy. Adv Exp Med Biol 2006;576:327–37.

[108] Ghadge GD, Slusher BS, Bodner A, et al. Glutamate carboxypeptidase II inhibition protects motor neurons from death in familial amyotrophic lateral sclerosis models. Proc Natl Acad Sci USA 2003;100(16):9554–9.

[109] Nilsson M, Hansson E, Ronnback L. Interactions between valproate, glutamate, aspartate, and GABA with respect to uptake in astroglial primary cultures. Neurochem Res 1992;17: 327–32.

[110] Traynor BJ, Bruijn L, Conwit R, et al. Neuroprotective agents for clinical trials in ALS: a systematic assessment. Neurology 2006;67(1):20–7.

[111] Hu JH, Zhang H, Wagey R, et al. Protein kinase and protein phosphatase expression in amyotrophic lateral sclerosis spinal cord. J Neurochem 2003;85:432–42.

[112] Brooks B, Sanjak M, Roelke K, et al. Phase 2B randomized dose ranging clinical trial of tamoxifen, a selective estrogen receptor modulator[SERM], in ALS: sensitivity analyses of discordance between survival and functional outcomes with long-term follow up. Amyotroph Lateral Scler Other Motor Neuron Disord 2005;6(Suppl 1):118.

[113] Available at: http://www.alsa.org/patient/drug.cfm?id=671. 2008. Ref Type: Internet Communication. Accessed May 24, 2008.

[114] Tikka T, Fiebich BL, Goldsteins G, et al. Minocycline, a tetracycline derivative, is neuroprotective against excitotoxicity by inhibiting activation and proliferation of microglia. J Neurosci 2001;21(8):2580–8.

[115] Zhu S, Stavrovskaya IG, Drozda M, et al. Minocycline inhibits cytochrome c release and delays progression of amyotrophic lateral sclerosis in mice. Nature 2002;417:74–8.

[116] Gordon PH, Moore DH, Miller RG, et al. Western ALS Study Group. Efficacy of minocycline in patients with amyotrophic lateral sclerosis: a phase III randomised trial. Lancet Neurol 2007;6(12):1045–53.

[117] Sagot Y, Toni N, Perrelet D, et al. An orally active anti-apoptotic molecule (CGP 3466B) preserves mitochondria and enhances survival in an animal model of motoneuron disease. Br J Pharmacol 2000;131(4):721–8, 11030721.

[118] Miller R, Bradley W, Cudkowicz M, et al. TCH346 Study Group. Phase II/III randomized trial of TCH346 in patients with ALS. Neurology 2007;69(8):776–84.

[119] Brown IR. Heat shock proteins and protection of the nervous system. Ann N Y Acad Sci 2007;1113:147–58.

[120] Kieran D, Kalmar B, Dick JR, et al. Treatment with arimoclomol, a coinducer of heat shock proteins, delays disease progression in ALS mice. Nat Med 2004;10(4):402–5.

[121] Beal M. Mitochondria and the pathogenesis of ALS. Brain 2000;123:1291–2.

[122] Matthews RT, Yang L, Browne S, et al. Coenzyme Q10 administration increases brain mitochondrial concentrations and exerts neuroprotective effects. Proc Natl Acad Sci USA 1998;95:8892–7.

[123] Ferrante KL, Shefner J, Zhang H, et al. Tolerance of high-dose (3,000 mg/day) coenzyme Q10 in ALS. Neurology 2005;65:1834–6.

[124] Available at: http://www.als-mda.org/research/news/080423coenzyme.html. 2008. Ref Type: Internet Communication. Accessed May 24, 2008.

[125] Yoshino H, Kimura A. Investigation of the therapeutic effects of edaravone, a free radical scavenger, on amyotrophic lateral sclerosis (phase II study). Amyotroph Lateral Scler 2006; 7(4):241–5.

[126] Weishaupt JH, Bartels C, Pölking E, et al. Reduced oxidative damage in ALS by high-dose enteral melatonin treatment. J Pineal Res 2006;41(4):313–23.

[127] Desnuelle C, Dib M, Garrel C, et al. A double-blind, placebo-controlled randomized clinical trial of alpha-tocopherol (vitamin E) in the treatment of amyotrophic lateral sclerosis. ALS Riluzole-Tocopherol Study Group. Amyotroph Lateral Scler Other Motor Neuron Disord 2001;2(1):9–18.

[128] Graf M, Ecker D, Horowski R, et al. German vitamin E/ALS Study Group. High dose vitamin E therapy in amyotrophic lateral sclerosis as add-on therapy to riluzole: results of a placebo-controlled double-blind study. J Neural Transm 2005;112(5):649–60.

[129] Klivenyi P, Ferrante RJ, Matthews RT, et al. Neuroprotective effects of creatine in a transgenic animal model of amyotrophic lateral sclerosis. Nat Med 1999;5(3):347–50.
[130] Lawler JM, Barnes WS, Wu G, et al. Direct antioxidant properties of creatine. Biochem Biophys Res Commun 2002;290(1):47–52.
[131] Angelov DN, Waibel S, Guntinas-Lichius O, et al. Therapeutic vaccine for acute and chronic motor neuron diseases: implications for amyotrophic lateral sclerosis. Proc Natl Acad Sci USA 2003;100(8):4790–5.
[132] Gordon PH, Doorish C, Montes J, et al. Randomized controlled phase II trial of glatiramer acetate in ALS. Neurology 2006;66(7):1117–9.
[133] Kiaei M, Petri S, Kipiani K, et al. Thalidomide and its analogue lenalidomide extend survival in a transgenic mouse model of amyotrophic lateral sclerosis. J Neurosci 2006;26: 2467–73.
[134] Fornai F, Longone P, Cafaro L, et al. Lithium delays progression of amyotrophic lateral sclerosis. Proc Natl Acad Sci USA 2008;105(6):2052–7.
[135] Ochs G, Penn RD, York M, et al. A phase I/II trial of recombinant methionyl human brain derived neurotrophic factor administered by intrathecal infusion to patients with amyotrophic lateral sclerosis. Amyotroph Lateral Scler Other Motor Neuron Disord 2000;1(3): 201–6.
[136] Nagano I, Shiote M, Murakami T, et al. Beneficial effects of intrathecal IGF-1 administration in patients with amyotrophic lateral sclerosis. Neurol Res 2005;27(7):768–72.
[137] Garrity-Moses ME, Teng Q, Liu J, et al. Neuroprotective adeno-associated virus Bcl-xL gene transfer in models of motor neuron disease. Muscle Nerve 2005;32(6):734–44.
[138] Keir SD, Xiao X, Li J, et al. Adeno-associated virus-mediated delivery of glial cell line-derived neurotrophic factor protects motor neuron-like cells from apoptosis. J Neurovirol 2001;7(5):437–46.
[139] Wang LJ, Lu YY, Muramatsu S, et al. Neuroprotective effects of glial cell line-derived neurotrophic factor mediated by an adeno-associated virus vector in a transgenic animal model of amyotrophic lateral sclerosis. J Neurosci 2002;22(16):6920–8.
[140] Kaspar BK, Lladó J, Sherkat N, et al. Retrograde viral delivery of IGF-1 prolongs survival in a mouse ALS model. Science 2003;301(5634):839–42.
[141] Miller TM, Kaspar BK, Kops GJ, et al. Virus-delivered small RNA silencing sustains strength in amyotrophic lateral sclerosis. Ann Neurol 2005;57(5):773–6.
[142] Larsen KE, Benn SC, Ay I, et al. A glial cell line-derived neurotrophic factor [GDNF]: tetanus toxin fragment C protein conjugate improves delivery of GDNF to spinal cord motor neurons in mice. Brain Res 2006;1120(1):1–12.
[143] Zurn AD, Henry H, Schluep M, et al. Evaluation of an intrathecal immune response in amyotrophic lateral sclerosis patients implanted with encapsulated genetically engineered xenogeneic cells. Cell Transplant 2000;9(4):471–84.
[144] Mazzini L, Mareschi K, Ferrero I, et al. Autologous mesenchymal stem cells: clinical applications in amyotrophic lateral sclerosis. Neurol Res 2006;28(5):523–6.
[145] Mazzini L, Mareschi K, Ferrero I, et al. Stem cell treatment in amyotrophic lateral sclerosis. J Neurol Sci 2008;265(1–2):78–83.
[146] Available at: http://www.als-mda.org/research/news/080423coenzyme.html. 2008. Ref Type: Internet Communication. Accessed May 24, 2008.
[147] Zhao P, Ignacio S, Beattie EC, et al. Altered presymptomatic AMPA and cannabinoid receptor trafficking in motor neurons of ALS model mice: implications for excitotoxicity. Eur J Neurosci 2008;27(3):572–9.
[148] Kim K, Moore DH, Makriyannis A, et al. AM1241, a cannabinoid CB2 receptor selective compound, delays disease progression in a mouse model of amyotrophic lateral sclerosis. Eur J Pharmacol 2006;542(1–3):100–5.
[149] Raman C, McAllister SD, Rizvi G, et al. Amyotrophic lateral sclerosis: delayed disease progression in mice by treatment with a cannabinoid. Amyotroph Lateral Scler Other Motor Neuron Disord 2003;5:33–9.

[150] Abood ME, Rizvi G, Sallapudi N, et al. Activation of the CB1 cannabinoid receptor protects cultured mouse spinal neurons against excitotoxicity. Neurosci Lett 2001;309:197–201.

[151] Bilsland LG, Dick JR, Pryce G, et al. Increasing cannabinoid levels by pharmacological and genetic manipulation delays disease progression in SOD1 mice. FASEB J 2006;20:1003–5.

[152] Weydt P, Hong S, Witting A, et al. Cannabinol delays symptom onset in SOD1 transgenic mice without affecting survival. Amyotroph Lateral Scler Other Motor Neuron Disord 2005;6:182–4.

[153] Bello-Haas VD, Florence JM, Kloos AD, et al. A randomized controlled trial of resistance exercise in individuals with ALS. Neurology 2007;68(23):2003–7.

[154] Drory VE, Goltsman E, Reznik JG, et al. The value of muscle exercise in patients with amyotrophic lateral sclerosis. J Neurol Sci 2001;191(1–2):133–7.

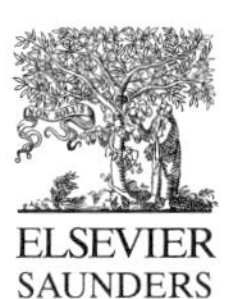

ELSEVIER
SAUNDERS

Phys Med Rehabil Clin N Am
19 (2008) 653–660

PHYSICAL MEDICINE
AND REHABILITATION
CLINICS OF
NORTH AMERICA

Clinical Trials in Spinal Muscular Atrophy

Petra Kaufmann, MD, MSc[a,*],
Susan T. Iannaccone, MD[b]

[a] *The Neurological Institute, Columbia University, 710 West 168th Street, NY 10032, USA*
[b] *Southwestern Medical Center, University of Texas, 2350 Stemmons Freeway, Suite 5074, Dallas, TX 75207, USA*

Spinal muscular atrophy (SMA) is an autosomal recessive disorder characterized by muscle atrophy and weakness due to degeneration of the anterior horn cells in the spinal cord. Hoffmann and Werdnig [1,2] first independently described this disorder in the 1890s, and the genetic defect was localized to 5q11.2-13.3 a century later. The discovery of the underlying mutation in the Survival of Motor Neurons 1 (SMN 1) gene has accelerated preclinical research leading to treatment targets and transgenic mouse models, but there is still no effective treatment. The clinical severity is inversely related to the copy number of SMN 2, a modifying gene producing some full-length SMN transcript. Drugs shown to increase SMN 2 function *in vitro*, therefore, have the potential to benefit SMA patients [3].

As several drugs are approaching clinical investigation, the following elements become important as a basis for successful clinical trials. First, we need recent data on the natural history of SMA. Second, we need sensitive, reliable and clinically meaningful outcome measures. Third, we need an SMA clinical trials infrastructure that allows for adequate patient recruitment and that makes it easy for patients to participate in trials.

Historically, three types are defined clinically but they overlap, so that the classification is often not used in clinical research [4]. SMA 1 is designated as that of patients who have onset before 6 months of age who never achieve the ability to sit. SMA 2 is defined by onset between 6 and 18 months and not reaching the motor milestone of standing. Patients who have SMA 3 by

Funding for this article was provided by the National Institutes of Health, National Institute of Neurological Disorders and Stroke, RO1 NS39327 (STI), National Institutes of Health 1 UL1 RR024156, and the Spinal Muscular Atrophy Foundation (PK).

* Corresponding author.
E-mail address: pk88@columbia.edu (P. Kaufmann).

doi:10.1016/j.pmr.2008.04.006

definition have disease onset after 18 months and gain the ability to walk. In addition, the term SMA 4 is sometimes used to describe patients who have adult-onset SMA and achieve the ability to walk. Children who have SMA 2 typically survive to adulthood. SMA 3 patients have a normal life expectancy.

The natural history of SMA, especially for the more severe phenotypes, is a moving target, as illustrated by several studies conducted in recent decades. Byers and Banker [5] described 25 SMA 1 subjects in 1961 with a mean age at death (n = 23) of 10 months (range 17 days to 52 months), and a mean age of 17 months (range 10–24 months) in those who survived (n = 2). Zerres and Rudnik-Schöneborn [6] reported outcomes in 197 SMA 1 subjects in 1995 and found a survival probability of 32% at 2 years, 18% at 4 years, 8% at 10 years, and 0% at 20 years. Borkowska [7] studied SMA 1 patients who survived past 36 months, and found a mean age at death (n = 18) of 11 years (range 5–24 years). In a recent, United States registry-based study of 150 patients who had SMA 1, among patients born between 1980 and1994, 57 (80.3%) had died with a mean age at death of 17.9 months (range 1.0–193.5) compared to 28 (35.4%) had died with a mean age at death of 22.1 months (range 2.5–112) among those born between 1995 and 2006 [8].

The natural history of SMA 2 and 3 suggests that patients enter a chronic phase with little if any disease progression. Although a cross-sectional study found better performance on timed tasks in younger, compared with older, ambulatory patients who had SMA [9], longitudinal studies suggest that motor function often does not change over time periods that can be readily studied in clinical trials. Over periods of several years, loss of motor function is frequently observed [10]. However, in a prospective study, improved motor function and acquired milestones were documented [11]. The Dallas-Cincinnati-Newington Spinal Muscular Atrophy (DCN-SMA) study group found no change in muscle strength over 8 years in a cohort of patients with SMA 2 or 3. No mortality occurred during the study [12].

Outcome measures

Quantitative muscle testing (QMT) using the Richmond Quantitative Measurement System was used to test grip, knee flexion and extension, and elbow flexion in 12 children aged 2 to 14 who had SMA. QMT showed greater variability among the weakest children than did other measures. The investigators therefore concluded that a motor function measure may be more useful in clinical trials of childhood SMA than QMT [13]. Myometry using a hand-held dynamometer may be less fatiguing than QMT, and it does not require expensive and fixed equipment. Three muscle groups, elbow flexors, knee flexors, and knee extensors, have been reported as showing the feasibility and reproducibility of QMT when tested with a hand-held device in 33 SMA patients [14]. Reference values for maximum isometric muscle force in hand-held dynamometry have been established in 270 children aged 4 to 17 [15]. In addition to issues related to cooperation and variability in children, motor function measures are often considered more inherently clinically meaningful than muscle strength measures.

Several gross motor function measures have been investigated in SMA. The gross motor function measure (GMFM), a proprietary instrument (McMaster University) has been validated in children who have SMA and has shown high interrater reliability. The GMFM contains 88 items in five dimensions: (1) lying and rolling, (2) sitting, (3) crawling, (4) standing, and (5) walking. Patients continue in each dimension to their maximum ability. The American Spinal Muscular Atrophy Randomized Trials (AmSMART) investigators found the GMFM reliable in children older than age 2 and all subjects performed in at least two dimensions [13,16]. An alternative scale, the Hammersmith Functional Motor Scale (HFMS), has been developed specifically for SMA 2 and takes less time to administer than the GMFM [17]. However, the HFMS is specific to non-ambulatory SMA patients so that its use in clinical trials can be limited by a floor or ceiling effect. Recently, an expanded HFMS has been proposed to broaden the range of motor function tested in the original HFMS [18].

Timed tasks, such as time walking, can be considered as outcomes in ambulatory subjects, because they are easily quantifiable, meaningful to patients, and have been successfully used in neuromuscular research [9,19,20].

Pulmonary function measures can be performed in patients aged 5 or older. Potential measures include inspiratory vital capacity, forced expiratory vital capacity (as a percent predicted for age and height) [21], maximal inspiratory and expiratory pressures, and peak expiratory flow [22]. Pulmonary measures have been validated in SMA clinical research [13].

Quality of life can be evaluated in subjects aged 2 to 18 years using the PedsQL Generic Quality of Life Inventory instrument [23,24], which has been validated by the AmSMART investigators for SMA [15]. The development and validation of a neuromuscular module are in progress. In subjects 18 years and older a range of quality of life measures are available, including the 36-Item Short Form Health Survey; it is a generic measure of health-related quality of life designed for self administration that can be completed in less than 30 minutes by most patients [25]. Controlled clinical trials are required by the United States Food and Drug Administration (USFDA) to approve drugs for the treatment of patients. Therefore, clinical trials are associated not only with potential scientific benefit to the community, but also potential benefit to the population of SMA patients. In addition, some patients perceive direct benefit from trial participation, for example in terms of learning more about their disease or in terms of frequent interactions with healthcare professionals [26]. However, recruitment has been difficult in recent US clinical trials for SMA [27].

Drug trials published

Albuterol

Albuterol is thought to have an anabolic effect on muscle, but more recently has also been suggested as an up-regulator of SMN 2 function. An open-label study of albuterol over 6 months in 13 patients with SMA 2 or 3 showed modest benefits in strength [28].

Gabapentin

Two placebo-controlled trials of gabapentin in SMA were negative [29,30]. The initial trial included 84 adult patients with SMA 2 or 3 who were treated over 12 months and evaluated with myometry. A second trial included 120 patients with SMA 2 or 3, aged 5 to 60, who were also treated for 12 months and evaluated with myometry.

Riluzole

Riluzole, a neuroprotective agent with modest benefit in amyotrophic lateral sclerosis, showed possible benefit in seven patients who had SMA 1 compared with three placebo-treated patients, with a targeted follow-up period of 9 months. A subsequent open-label study had insufficient enrollment but pharmacokinetic studies in three subjects showed adequate blood levels after oral administration to infants [10].

Phenylbutyrate

Phenylbutyrate showed promise in an open-label pilot study of 10 patients who had SMA 2 treated for 9 weeks [31], but a placebo-controlled trial of intermittent treatment over 13 weeks in 107 SMA 2 patients aged 2 to 13 was negative [32,33]. Both phenylbutyrate studies were designed to demonstrate functional motor benefit.

Valproic acid

Valproic acid resulted in increased SMN mRNA, and protein levels increased after treatment in 7 of 10 carriers and 7 of 20 patients but remained unchanged or decreased in 13 patients [34]. In a second open-label pilot study in the United States, 7 patients aged 17 to 45 who had SMA 3 or 4 treated with valproic acid for 8 months on average showed improvement in muscle strength and function [35].

Hydroxyurea

Hydroxyurea treatment for 8 weeks in 33 patients with SMA 2 or 3 has shown slight benefit in muscle strength scores [36]. This trial was not placebo-controlled.

Summary

Challenges

Fragility of patients who have spinal muscular atrophy type 1

Trials for SMA 1 infants are challenging because recruitment and retention are affected by the often severe and frequent concurrent illnesses in this population. However, patients who have SMA 1 may be the most appropriate target population for new treatments. Their disability is severe, whereas their nervous systems may be more plastic than those of older patients who have chronic forms of SMA.

Late diagnosis

Most patients who have SMA have entered a stable disease course when they present for trial participation. Therefore, trials are designed to detect an improvement in the treatment group compared with the placebo group in these chronic patients. Treating patients in the initial, potentially more progressive stages of SMA is currently not feasible, because patients typically do not receive a diagnosis and present to an SMA clinical research center until they have entered the chronic phase. Newborn screening for SMA is controversial, but if it ever becomes a reality, it might afford opportunities for presymptomatic treatment or for treatment in the early phase of the disease.

Frequency of visits

For patients who have a disability, but in particular for fragile patients who have SMA 1, frequent visits to a clinical trial site are burdensome and often simply not feasible. Investigators should therefore design the visit schedule around the patient's need, and make sure that the site is as accessible as possible. Research visits to the patient's home or outcome measures that can be ascertained remotely are another solution to this problem.

Lack of standard of care

Current SMA management is through supportive care, ideally using a multidisciplinary approach. The variability in clinical care among centers can modify the clinical course of the disease, which can theoretically create a challenge for clinical trials. However, in randomized trials with stratification by sites, this problem should not occur. To address differences in standard of care, the International Coordinating Committee (ICC) for Spinal Muscular Atrophy has developed a consensus statement document on care issues [37].

Lack of surrogate markers

When testing new treatments in patients who have SMA, researchers are currently evaluating for a motor function benefit, even in early phase II trials. However, this testing typically requires a large sample size and a long observation period. Surrogate markers can accelerate phase II trials because they are associated with a clinical outcome and can thus provide an early result after a short treatment period. This can potentially shorten the follow-up period required in early phase II trials [38,39].

Opportunities

A great need exists for an effective treatment of SMA, a disease that often causes severe disability in patients who are cognitively intact and can have a normal life expectancy. Unlike many other neurologic diseases, SMA can be easily diagnosed through genetic testing. Also, preclinical progress over the last 2 decades has been major, with the discovery of the gene and of a "druggable" modifying gene that provides one of several promising targets for treatment. SMA is rare but is a common orphan disease, so trials should be feasible. Investigators and patient groups are increasingly well organized, nationally and internationally (eg, International Coordinating Committee for SMA [ICC] and Treat Neuromuscular Disease [Treat NMD]). Suitable outcomes have been developed [17,40] and the Food and Drug Administration has already reviewed trials for this indication [41]. These advances provide opportunities for successful trials and raise the hope that we will find effective treatments for SMA.

References

[1] Hoffmann J. Über chronische spinale Muskelatrophie im Kindesalter, auf familiärer Basis. Deutsche Z Nervenheilkunde 1893;3:427–70 [in German].
[2] Werdnig G. Zwei frühinfantile hereditäre Fälle von progressiver Muskelatrophie unter dem Bilde der Dystrophie, aber auf neurotischer Grundlage. Arch Psychiatr Nervenkr 1891;22: 437–80 [in German].
[3] Sumner CJ. Therapeutics development for spinal muscular atrophy. NeuroRx 2006;3(2): 235–45.
[4] Munsat TL, Davies KE. International SMA Consortium meeting. (26–28 June 1992, Bonn, Germany). Neuromuscul Disord 1992;2(5–6):423–8.
[5] Byers RK, Banker BQ. Infantile muscular atrophy. Arch Neurol 1961;5:140–64.
[6] Zerres K, Rudnik-Schöneborn S. Natural history in proximal spinal muscular atrophy. Clinical analysis of 445 patients and suggestions for a modification of existing classifications. Arch Neurol 1995;52(5):518–23.
[7] Borkowska J, Rudnik-Schöneborn S, Hausmanowa-Petrusewicz I, et al. Early infantile form of spinal muscular atrophy (Werdnig-Hoffmann disease) with prolonged survival. Folia Neuropathol 2002;40(1):19–26.
[8] Oskoui M, Levy G, Garland CJ, et al. The changing natural history of spinal muscular atrophy type 1. Neurology 2007;69(20):1931–6.
[9] Merlini L, Bertini E, Minetti C, et al. Motor function-muscle strength relationship in spinal muscular atrophy. Muscle Nerve 2004;29(4):548–52.
[10] Russman BS, Buncher CR, White M, et al. Function changes in spinal muscular atrophy II and III. The DCN/SMA Group. Neurology 1996;47(4):973–6.

[11] Iannaccone ST, Browne RH, Samaha FJ, et al. Prospective study of spinal muscular atrophy before age 6 years. DCN/SMA Group. Pediatr Neurol 1993;9(3):187–93.
[12] Iannaccone ST, Russman BS, Browne RH, et al. Prospective analysis of strength in spinal muscular atrophy. DCN/Spinal Muscular Atrophy Group. J Child Neurol 2000;15(2):97–101.
[13] Iannaccone ST. Outcome measures for pediatric spinal muscular atrophy. Arch Neurol 2002;59(9):1445–50.
[14] Merlini L, Mazzone ES, Solari A, et al. Reliability of hand-held dynamometry in spinal muscular atrophy. Muscle Nerve 2002;26(1):64–70.
[15] Beenakker EA, van der Hoeven JH, Fock JM, et al. Reference values of maximum isometric muscle force obtained in 270 children aged 4-16 years by hand-held dynamometry. Neuromuscul Disord 2001;11(5):441–6.
[16] Nelson L, Owens H, Hynan LS, et al. The gross motor function measure trade mark is a valid and sensitive outcome measure for spinal muscular atrophy. Neuromuscul Disord 2006; 16(6):374–80.
[17] Main M, Kairon H, Mercuri E, et al. The Hammersmith functional motor scale for children with spinal muscular atrophy: a scale to test ability and monitor progress in children with limited ambulation. Eur J Paediatr Neurol 2003;7(4):155–9.
[18] O'Hagen JM, Glanzman AM, McDermott MP, et al. An expanded version of the Hammersmith functional motor scale for SMA II and III patients. Neuromuscul Disord 2007; 17(9–10):693–7.
[19] Beenakker EA, Maurits NM, Fock JM, et al. Functional ability and muscle force in healthy children and ambulant Duchenne muscular dystrophy patients. Eur J Paediatr Neurol 2005; 9(6):387–93.
[20] Nair KP, Vasanth A, Gourie-Devi M, et al. Disabilities in children with Duchenne muscular dystrophy: a profile. J Rehabil Med 2001;33(4):147–9.
[21] Wang X, Dockery DW, Wypij D, et al. Pulmonary function between 6 and 18 years of age. Pediatr Pulmonol 1993;15(2):75–88.
[22] Bach JR, Goncalves MR, Paez S, et al. Expiratory flow maneuvers in patients with neuromuscular diseases. Am J Phys Med Rehabil 2006;85(2):105–11.
[23] Varni JW, Rode CA, Seid M, et al. The pediatric cancer quality of life inventory-32 (PCQL-32). II. Feasibility and range of measurement. J Behav Med 1999;22(4):397–406.
[24] Varni JW, Seid M, Rode CA. The PedsQL: measurement model for the pediatric quality of life inventory. Med Care 1999;37(2):126–39.
[25] Ware J Jr, Kosinski M, Keller SD. A 12-Item Short-Form Health Survey: construction of scales and preliminary tests of reliability and validity. Med Care 1996;34(3):220–33.
[26] Verheggen FW, Nieman FH, Reerink E, et al. Patient satisfaction with clinical trial participation. Int J Qual Health Care 1998;10(4):319–30.
[27] Iannaccone S, Hynan LS, Group A. Challenges of enrollment for SMA type 1 clinical trials [abstract]. Neuromuscul Discord 2007;17:780.
[28] Kinali M, Mercuri E, Main M, et al. Pilot trial of albuterol in spinal muscular atrophy-Neurology 2002;59(4):609–10.
[29] Miller RG, Moore DH, Dronsky V, et al. A placebo-controlled trial of gabapentin in spinal muscular atrophy. J Neurol Sci 2001;191(1–2):127–31.
[30] Merlini L, Solari A, Vita G, et al. Role of gabapentin in spinal muscular atrophy: results of a multicenter, randomized Italian study. J Child Neurol 2003;18(8):537–41.
[31] Mercuri E, Bertini E, Messina S, et al. Pilot trial of phenylbutyrate in spinal muscular atrophy. Neuromuscul Disord 2004;14(2):130–5.
[32] Mercuri E, Bertini E, Messina S, et al. Randomized, double-blind, placebo-controlled trial of phenylbutyrate in spinal muscular atrophy. Neurology 2007;68(1):51–5.
[33] Kaufmann P, Finkel R. Learning to walk: challenges for spinal muscular atrophy clinical trials. Neurology 2007;68(1):11–2.
[34] Brichta L, Holker I, Haug K, et al. In vivo activation of SMN in spinal muscular atrophy carriers and patients treated with valproate. Ann Neurol 2006;59(6):970–5.

[35] Weihl CC, Connolly AM, Pestronk A. Valproate may improve strength and function in patients with type III/IV spinal muscle atrophy. Neurology 2006;67(3):500–1.
[36] Liang WC, Yuo CY, Chang JG, et al. The effect of hydroxyurea in spinal muscular atrophy cells and patients. J Neurol Sci 2008;268(1–2):87–94.
[37] Wang CH, Finkel RS, Bertini ES, et al. Consensus statement for standard of care in spinal muscular atrophy. J Child Neurol 2007;22(8):1027–49.
[38] De Gruttola VG, Clax P, DeMets DL, et al. Considerations in the evaluation of surrogate endpoints in clinical trials. Summary of a National Institutes Of Health workshop. Control Clin Trials 2001;22(5):485–502.
[39] Lesko LJ, Atkinson AJ Jr. Use of biomarkers and surrogate endpoints in drug development and regulatory decision making: criteria, validation, strategies. Annu Rev Pharmacol Toxicol 2001;41:347–66.
[40] Iannaccone ST, Hynan LS. Reliability of 4 outcome measures in pediatric spinal muscular atrophy. Arch Neurol 2003;60(8):1130–6.
[41] NTPUNE. Available at: https://www.clinicalresearchnetworks.org/profile.asp?NetworkID=6420.

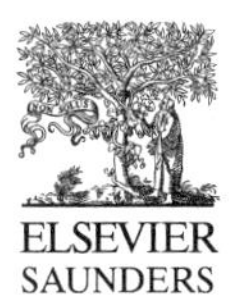
ELSEVIER
SAUNDERS

Phys Med Rehabil Clin N Am
19 (2008) 661–680

PHYSICAL MEDICINE AND REHABILITATION CLINICS OF NORTH AMERICA

Diagnosis and Clinical Management of Spinal Muscular Atrophy

Jay J. Han, MD*, Craig M. McDonald, MD

Department of Physical Medicine and Rehabilitation, University of California–Davis, 4860 Y Street, Suite 3850, Sacramento, CA 95817, USA

Spinal muscular atrophy (SMA) is a term used to describe a varied group of inherited disorders characterized by weakness and muscle wasting secondary to degeneration of motor neurons in the spinal cord and brainstem. In the late 19th century, an early-onset form of SMA presenting in infancy was first described independently by Werdnig [1] and Hoffmann [2]. Oppenheim [3] subsequently described a more benign form presenting in early childhood. Wohlfart and colleagues [4] and Kugelberg and Welander [5] later described a more slowly progressing hereditary form of SMA with survival into adulthood. The wide spectrum of disease severity in childhood SMA was noted by Byers and Banker [6], who divided patients into three categories, depending on age of onset and different life expectancies. Since then, other rare SMA syndromes with childhood and adult onset have been recognized, with varied clinical phenotypes and inheritance pattern. This article focuses on autosomal recessive, predominantly proximal SMA, which is the second most common neuromuscular disease of childhood (after Duchenne muscular dystrophy) estimated to occur in approximately 1:6,000 to 1:10,000 live births [7,8].

Classification, patterns of severity, and survival

SMA is generally divided into clinical subtypes using age of onset, achieved developmental milestones, ability to achieve independent sitting, standing, walking, and survival as classification criteria. The International Consortium on SMA attempted to standardize the classification of SMA to provide a rational basis for linkage studies and therapeutic trials (Table 1)

This work was supported by Grant H133B031118 05 from the National Institute of Disability and Rehabilitation Research (NIDRR).

* Corresponding author.
E-mail address: jay.han@ucdmc.ucdavis.edu (J.J. Han).

1047-9651/08/$ - see front matter
doi:10.1016/j.pmr.2008.02.004 *pmr.theclinics.com*

Table 1
Classification of autosomal recessive predominantly proximal spinal muscular atrophy (International Spinal Muscular Atrophy Consortium classification)

Type	Onset	Achieved milestones	Survival
I	≤6 mo	Never sits without support	Usually less than 2 y
II	≤18 mo	Sits independently but never stands or walks without aids	Usually more than 2 y; often to adulthood
III	>18 mo	Stands or walks without support	Adulthood

[9,10]. SMA type I (SMA I) (Werdnig-Hoffmann, severe form) was defined by the consortium as follows: onset from birth to 6 months, no achievement of sitting without support, and death usually before the age of 2. In SMA type II (SMA II) (intermediate form), onset is before 18 months, sitting is achieved but standing and ambulation are never obtained, and death occurs after the age of 2 years. In SMA type III (SMA III) (Kugelberg-Welander, mild form), onset is after the age of 18 months, patients develop the ability to stand and walk, and death is in adulthood. However, considerable variability in severity and occasionally some overlap exist within each of the three groups [11–15]. Clinically, an adult-onset type of SMA with mild disease phenotype, presenting usually in the second or third decade, has been recognized. These patients are able to ambulate with minor motor impairments. Although the adult-onset type of SMA is not classified formally by the criteria set forth by the consortium, among clinicians, SMA type IV (SMA IV), denoting this adult-onset group of patients who have mild disease features, has been used widely. A modified classification scheme has been proposed by Zerres and Rudnik-Schoneborn [15], as shown in Table 2.

Life expectancy is closely related to SMA type. Pooled data regarding age of onset and survival from the United Kingdom [16] and Finalnd [13] are shown in Table 3. Survival past 2 years is rare for those presenting before 6 months. In a large series, 197 patients classified as type I had the following survival probabilities: 32% at the age of 2, 18% at the age of 4, 8% at the age of 10, and 0% at the age of 20 [15]. For 104 cases classified as SMA II,

Table 2
University of Bonn (Germany) spinal muscular atrophy classification

Type	Definition	Mean age of onset	Range of onset	Survival probability at age 20
I	Never sat alone	1.9 mo	0–10 mo	0
II	Sits alone, never walked	8.6 mo	0–18 mo	77%
IIIa	Walks without support; age of onset <3 y	17.9 mo	3–30 mo	Normal
IIIb	Walks without support; age of onset 3–30 y	10.4 y	3–24 y	Normal
IV	Age of onset >30 y	44.8 y	33–54 y	N/A

Abbreviation: N/A, not applicable.

Table 3
Age at death related to age of onset

Age of onset (mo)	Number of patients	Mean age at death (mo)	Maximum survival (mo)
Birth	29	4.5	12
<1	19	6.1	18
>1–2	24	6.4	12
>2–3	18	13.6	25[a]
>3–6	10	15.2	30

[a] Excluding two patients who never sat unaided and survived to 10 and >18 years, and a third patient who survived 8 years with tracheostomy and mechanical ventilation.

98% survived to the age of 10 and 77% to the age of 20. In a prospective study including SMA II patients younger than 6 years old, no deaths occurred during a 5-year period in those cases whose onset of symptoms occurred at the age of 6 months or later [12]. A 10-year prospective study reported by Carter and colleagues [17] documented seven deaths among 32 SMA II patients (mean age at death, 21 years). Patients who have SMA II have been documented to live to as late as the fifth decade with and without mechanical ventilation [14,17,18]. Although no survival data exist for patients who have SMA III, cases without mechanical ventilation have been followed into the eighth decade [15,17].

Genetics of autosomal recessive, predominantly proximal spinal muscular atrophy

The carrier frequency for SMA in the general population is estimated at about 1 in 40 to 50 individuals [19]. Autosomal recessive inheritance has long been documented in proximal SMA with childhood onset. In 1990, all three forms of SMA were mapped to chromosomal region 5q13, indicating that allelic variants of the same disease locus account for the clinical heterogeneity [20,21]. During the past 2 decades, tremendous advances have been made in our understanding of the genetic basis for SMA [22–27]. A detailed analysis of the 5q13 region revealed that this chromosomal region in humans contained a large inverted duplication, with at least 2 genes present in telomeric and centromeric copies.

Further studies have identified the SMA causative gene as the survival motor neuron (SMN) 1 gene (SMN1, telomeric copy), along with a disease modifying gene (SMN2, centromeric copy) [22–24]. Briefly, the two SMN genes are nearly identical except for a difference of only five nucleotides in their 3′ regions, without any alteration of the amino acid sequence of the protein. However, the critical difference between the SMN1 and SMN2 genes is a C-T transition located within the exon-splicing region of the SMN2 that affects the splicing of exon 7. This change results in frequent exon 7 skipping during the splicing of SMN2 transcripts [28,29]. It is thought that the resulting truncated SMN protein, without its exon 7 contribution, is a less stable form of SMN protein, and therefore, rapidly degraded. In about 95% of SMA patients, both copies of SMN1 exon 7 are absent because of mutations. In the remaining SMA-affected patients, other small or subtle mutations have been identified [22].

Genetic studies have now established that SMA is caused by mutations in the telomeric SMN1 gene, with all patients having at least one copy of the centromeric SMN2 gene. At least one copy of the SMN2 must be present in the setting of homozygous SMN1 mutations; otherwise, embryonic lethality occurs. The copy number of SMN2 varies in the population, and this variation appears to have some important modifying effects on SMA disease severity [30–32]. It appears that a higher number of SMN2 copies in the setting of SMN1 mutations results in a less severe clinical SMA phenotype. However, substantial variations in SMA phenotype and disease severity can exist with a given SMN2 copy number, so it is not recommended that disease severity be predicted based on SMN2 copy numbers. Although we now know that SMN protein is expressed widely in many tissues throughout the body, its function is still not completely understood at this time [33].

Physical examination findings

Spinal muscular atrophy I

In many instances, mothers of SMA I cases report experiencing reduced fetal movements. Most cases present within the first 2 months. Weak suck, dysphagia, labored breathing during feeding, aspiration of food or secretions, and a weak cry are also frequently noted. Examination shows generalized hypotonia and symmetric weakness involving the lower extremities earlier and to a greater extent than the upper extremities. Proximal muscles are weaker than distal muscles. In the supine position, the lower extremities may be abducted and externally rotated in a "frog-leg" position. Volitional movements of fingers and hands persist well past the time when the shoulders and elbows cannot be flexed against gravity. The thorax is flattened anteroposteriorly, and may be described as bell shaped. The diaphragm is usually more preserved relative to the intercostal and abdominal musculature, which results in a diaphragmatic breathing pattern during respiration, with abdominal protrusion, paradoxical thoracic depression, and intercostal retraction. Neck flexor and extensor weakness are noted with head lag during examination. With advanced disease, the mouth may remain open as a result of masticatory muscle weakness. Facial weakness has been noted in as many as 50% of SMA I patients [34]. Tongue fasciculations have been reported in 56% to 61% of patients [12,35]. Deep tendon reflexes have been absent in all four extremities in about 74% of cases [12]. Appendicular muscle fasciculations and distal tremor may be present. Extraocular and myocardial muscles are spared. Contractures are generally not severe, although hip, knee, and elbow flexion contractures may be observed. Wrist contractures with ulnar drift of the fingers may be noted. Varus or valgus deformities of the ankles may also be present. Hip subluxation or frank hip dislocation is occasionally observed. Severe arthrogryposis is not typically observed but can be present.

Spinal muscular atrophy II

The onset of SMA II is usually more insidious than that of SMA I. The findings of generalized hypotonia, symmetric weakness, and delayed motor milestones are hallmarks of SMA II. Weakness involves proximal muscles more than distal muscles, and lower extremity more than upper extremity. A fine tremor of the fingers and hands occurs in some patients. Wasting tends to be more conspicuous in SMA II than in SMA I. The deep tendon reflexes are depressed and usually absent in the lower extremities. Appendicular or thoracic wall muscle fasciculations may be observed. Tongue fasciculations have been observed in 30% to 70% of SMA II patients [9,12,35,36]. Progressive kyphoscoliosis and neuromuscular restrictive lung disease is almost invariably seen in the late first decade. Contractures of the hip flexors, tensor fasciae latae, hamstrings, triceps surae, elbow flexors, and finger flexors are common. Hip subluxation and dislocations have been noted commonly in SMA II patients [35]. Sensory examination is normal. Extraocular, sphincter, and myocardial muscles are spared.

Spinal muscular atrophy III

In SMA III, weakness usually initially occurs between the ages of 18 months and the late teens. Motor milestones may be delayed in infancy. Proximal weakness is observed, with the pelvic girdle being more affected than the shoulder girdle. Lumbar lordosis and anterior pelvic tilt are exaggerated, owing to hip extensor weakness. The patient also usually has a waddling gait pattern with pelvic drop and lateral trunk lean over the stance phase side, secondary to hip abductor weakness. If ankle plantar flexion strength is sufficient, the patient may show primarily forefoot or toe contact during gait without heel strike, which is a compensatory measure to maintain a stabilizing extension moment at the knee. The patient may exhibit a Gower's sign when arising from the floor; stair climbing is also difficult because of hip flexor weakness. Fasciculations in the limb and thoracic wall muscles are common. Fasciculations of the tongue are noted in about one half of the patients and are more common later in the disease course [9]. Deep tendon reflexes are diminished and often become absent over time. Significant scoliosis and contractures are rare in SMA III.

Laboratory findings in spinal muscular atrophy

Serum laboratory studies

Creatine kinase levels have been found to be normal to elevated two to four times in SMA I and II [35]. SMA III patients can also have normal to slightly elevated creatine kinase values [37]. A serum creatine kinase level greater than 10 times the upper limit of normal is generally an exclusionary criterion for SMA [10] and workup for other disorders such as inflammatory or dystrophic myopathies should be pursued. Functional status and disease progression did not correlate with creatine kinase level in a series of SMA III cases [37]. Adolase may also be normal to slightly elevated in SMA.

Electrodiagnosis

Needle electromyography

The predictive value of needle electromyography in the diagnosis of SMA has been established [38,39]. The findings have largely been consistent with motor axonal loss, denervation, and reinnervation. In the infant, spontaneous activity may be more easily determined with the study of muscles that are not as readily recruited (vastus lateralis, gastrocnemius, triceps, and first dorsal interosseous). Recruitment and motor unit characteristics can be assessed in muscles that are readily activated (anterior tibialis, iliopsoas, biceps, and flexor digitorum sublimes) [40]. The paraspinal muscles are usually not studied because of poor relaxation. The tongue muscle can be examined with needle electromyography; however, for practical reasons, it is rarely performed or needed in the evaluation of the hypotonic infant.

Although some investigators [41] have described high-density fibrillation potentials in infants with poorer prognosis, most studies have not demonstrated abundant fibrillation potentials in the infantile form of SMA [35,36,42]. In SMA III, the incidence of fibrillation potentials ranged from 20% to 40% in one series [43], to 64% in another [44]. The incidence of fibrillation potentials in SMA II appears higher than in SMA III. Spontaneous activity has been observed more frequently in the lower than in the upper limbs, and in proximal more than distal muscles [43]. Fasciculations are more common in SMA I than in SMA II or III [35,36,45]. The degree of spontaneous activity has not been found to be independently associated with a worse prognosis [39].

Voluntary motor unit action potentials (MUAPs) frequently fire with an increased frequency, although recruitment frequency may be difficult to determine consistently in infants. Compared with age-matched norms, MUAPs show longer duration and higher amplitude, particularly in older subjects; however, a bimodal distribution may be seen, with some concomitant, low-amplitude, short-duration potentials [42]. Large-amplitude, long-duration MUAPs may be absent in many infants with SMA I but are more commonly observed in SMA II and III [35]. Other signs of reinnervation, such as polyphasic MUAPs, may be observed in more chronic and mild SMA. A reduced recruitment pattern with maximal effort is perhaps the most consistent finding in all SMA types.

Nerve conduction studies

Motor nerve conduction velocities and compound muscle action potential (CMAP) amplitude have been shown to be reduced in many patients who have infantile SMA. The degree of motor conduction slowing tends to be mild and the conduction velocity tends to be greater than 70% of the lower limit of normal [14,36,43,46,47]. Significant reductions in CMAP amplitudes have been frequently reported in SMA I to III [35,39,43]. A tendency toward greater reductions in CMAP amplitude among patients with earlier age of onset and shorter survival has been reported [43]. Sensory nerve conduction studies are essentially normal. Significant abnormalities in sensory studies exclude a diagnosis of SMA, whereas minor abnormalities in sensory conduction velocities have been noted infrequently [47–49].

Pathologic evaluation in spinal muscular atrophy

Histologic changes on muscle biopsy are characterized by sheets of round atrophic fibers (2–8 μM in diameter) intermingled with groups of normal or hypertrophic fibers. Fiber-type grouping is not usually observed in infants but may be observed in older children with SMA. Significant fiber necrosis is usually absent, although occasional muscle fiber changes, such as basophilia, fiber slitting, and internal nuclei, may be observed. Overall, the extent of histologic changes seen within muscle biopsy specimens does not predict the severity or the disease course for children with SMA [50,51]. Histologic evaluation of the spinal cord from postmortem specimens shows loss of anterior horn cells at all cord levels [52]. Residual anterior horn cells may show swelling, chromatolysis, thickened neurofibrils, and increased lipofuscin granules. The ventral roots are atrophic with myelin loss, whereas the dorsal roots are spared.

Clinical issues in spinal muscular atrophy

Diagnostic evaluations

If the diagnosis of SMA is strongly suspected, a SMN gene deletion test can be done to confirm the diagnosis. At this time, a genetic test for SMA is commercially available. The test is based on the homozygous absence of SMN1 exon 7, with or without a concomitant exon 8 deletion. The sensitivity and specificity of the gene deletion test are excellent and approach 95% and 100%, respectively. The test results are usually available in several weeks. The copy number of the SMN2 gene is also typically reported. If the SMN gene test is negative, then the diagnosis of SMA should be seriously questioned, and work up for other potential neuromuscular diagnoses pursued. However, if further workup and electromyography results continue to point to a motor neuron disease in an individual with the clinical features of SMA, then additional testing for more subtle SMN mutations can be undertaken. SMN1 gene copy number testing and sequencing of the SMN1 gene are available through some research laboratories (www.genetests.org).

Family education and genetic counseling

After the diagnosis is established, a meeting with the patient and family is important to explain the disease process, phenotype classification, and prognosis. A geneticist consultation may be necessary for more detailed questions regarding sibling or carrier testing, recurrence risk, and reproductive planning issues. The issues regarding testing of unaffected siblings for presymptomatic diagnosis and prenatal screening for SMA may be discussed with the help of a geneticist. The patients and families should also receive information regarding various support networks or advocacy groups. In addition, information regarding ongoing SMA clinical trials can be obtained through the Web site, www.clinicaltrials.gov.

Clinical management of impairment and disability in spinal muscular atrophy

Strength profiles and exercise

Many studies have performed strength evaluations in SMA patients [53–57]. Manual muscle test across 34 muscle groups showed that proximal weakness was greater than distal weakness in SMA II and III [53]. Strength measurements across a large age span showed increasing proximal muscle weakness with increasing age, whereas distal muscles showed minimal decline in strength with age [53,56,57]. SMA III patients did not show a significant rate of decline in strength when age and disease duration were considered. Extensor muscle groups appear to be weaker than flexor groups at the elbow, wrist, hip, and knee, whereas neck flexors are weaker than neck extensors [53,55]. In SMA patients 5 years or older, markedly reduced muscle strength approximating 20% of that predicted from age- and gender-matched normative data were found [55].

The potential benefits of exercise in neuromuscular disorders such as SMA have been described previously [41,58]. These benefits include increased endurance, greater aerobic capacity, reduction in O_2 cost of locomotion, improved daily functional abilities, improved flexibility, and psychosocial benefits. Limited data exist regarding the effects of strength training in SMA specifically. Strength profile studies have shown no effect of side dominance in SMA [12,53,54]. At this time, little clinical evidence suggests that overuse weakness occurs in SMA. One study of resistive exercises included three subjects with SMA II [59]. Strength and endurance were improved in these subjects and exercise was well tolerated. In addition, recent studies in a mouse model of SMA have provided evidence of potential neuroprotective and survival benefits of exercise [60,61]. A moderate resistance exercise program has been advocated for the postpubertal patient who has a slowly progressive neuromuscular condition such as SMA [41,62,63]. Based on the functional status of the patient, a regular exercise program including swimming, aquatherapy, and adaptive sports should be encouraged.

Bulbar dysfunction and swallowing problems

Bulbar dysfunction is more commonly observed in SMA I, but can also occur in SMA II and III patients, especially during the later stages of the disease. Such bulbar involvement leads to problems in buccal and pharyngeal propulsion activities during eating, and it can also contribute to impaired airway protection [64–66]. The prevalence of self-reported symptoms of swallowing difficulty in 85 SMA II and III patients was 36.5% in one study [66]. Fluoroscopic swallowing evaluations in four SMA I patients revealed involvement of the anterior and posterior phases [65]. Impairment of facial musculature in SMA results in weakened mastication. In addition, SMA patients have been found to have abnormal craniofacial growth patterns. The malocclusion of teeth has been attributed to various factors, including weakness of masticatory muscles, tendency for mouth breathing, and poor head positioning [67,68]. Management of malocclusion in SMA patients may be important for optimal nutrition and respiratory function.

Body composition and nutrition

Patients who have SMA I and II are often of small stature and have greatly diminished muscle bulk [69,70]. MRI of limbs has demonstrated severe muscular atrophy in SMA I and II [71]. In addition, increased subcutaneous fat is observed in these patients. Muscles of SMA III patients, in comparison, showed less atrophy but significant fatty infiltration. In these more chronic cases, the use of skin fold measurements may not accurately reflect percent of lean and fat mass.

Diffuse weakness, bulbar dysfunction, or respiratory distress may affect feeding in SMA patients. Therapeutic modifications may include use of a premature baby nipple with a large opening, use of proper head and jaw position along with a semireclined trunk position, and use of frequent small feedings to minimize fatigue [35,70]. The use of larger bolus feeds may distend the stomach and encroach on the diaphragm. Improved nourishment and nutritional status in individuals with SMA has shown to lead to a feeling of well-being and a better quality of life [70]. Poor nutritional status, labored feeding, or symptoms of dysphagia are indications for the initiation of supplemental enteral feedings by way of nasogastric tube or gastrostomy. Supplemental enteral feedings may be performed by bolus, gravity drip, or continuously during the night by way of a pump. Another common issue facing SMA patients, especially infants, is constipation. Constipation is thought to be caused by a combination of weak abdominal muscles and immobility. Chronic constipation and impaction can further decrease the already impaired lung function, and can decrease oral intake in these patients. Appropriate dietary management and hydration, supplemented with laxatives, are effective in the maintenance of optimal bowel care for these patients.

Cardiac function

Although the myocardium is not primarily involved in SMA, mild nonspecific electrocardiogram changes have been described [52,72,73]. Baseline irregularities in tracings, at times caused by skeletal muscle fibrillations, may be observed [53]. Electrocardiogram findings consistent with atrial and ventricular enlargement may be observed in SMA II [53,72]; however, echocardiograms have not shown concomitant atrial or ventricular dilation [72].

Pulmonary function testing and respiratory management

The restrictive lung disease is the most common and serious complication facing patients who have SMA. In general, the severity of restrictive lung disease is proportional to the weakness and functional class of SMA. It is most severe in infants with SMA I but it may not affect patients who have SMA III [74,75]. Samahu and colleagues [76] showed that absolute forced vital capacity (FVC) was significantly related to height index and functional level in 5- to 18-year-olds who had SMA. Ambulatory patients showed normal or near-normal values, whereas nonsitters showed the lowest values, with absolute FVC of less than 1 to 1.56 L. A need for ventilatory support through intermittent positive pressure breathing was directly related to FVC and functional status. Two thirds of those who could only sit supported used intermittent positive pressure breathing, compared with only 5% of those who walked independently [76]. Carter and colleagues [17] showed significant reductions in FVC over time with increasing disease durations in SMA II, but not in SMA III subjects. In addition, SMA II patients showed more severe declines in maximal expiratory pressure versus maximal inspiratory pressure, suggesting relative diaphragmatic sparing [53,77–79]. Progressive restrictive lung disease in SMA III was shown to be mild and rarely necessitated the institution of ventilatory support [17,37,80–83].

Although no specific spirometry parameters for beginning ventilatory support have been established, it has been found that the institution of mechanical ventilation in SMA II was generally not required until FVC was about 20% of the predicted value [81,84]. This parameter is not absolute and ventilatory support has been initiated at FVC values of mid-30% [80]. Other pulmonary function measurements including maximal inspiratory pressure, maximal expiratory pressure, and peak cough flow are also useful. When these values decline, they can indicate poor airway clearance function, increased risk for infection, and hastened respiratory failure. In most specialty neuromuscular disease clinics, spirometry evaluation is typically performed at least annually for those SMA patients who have impaired lung function (and every 6 months or more frequently for those at higher risk). Children older than 5 years can usually cooperate and follow directions reliably enough to perform spirometry.

Over the last decade, advances in noninvasive ventilation technology, an increased variety of ventilation interface devices, and miniaturization of ventilators leading to better portability have all contributed to improved pulmonary management of patients who have SMA. Treatment of severe respiratory insufficiency in SMA may use noninvasive intermittent positive pressure ventilation (NIPPV) by way of oral or nasal interfaces, nasally applied bi-level positive airway pressure (BiPAP), or positive pressure mechanical ventilation by way of a tracheostomy [5,81,83,85]. In any method, the most important goal is to obtain a good seal around the interface. The noninvasive ventilation method is particularly convenient for nighttime use. In general, nocturnal NIPPV appears to be effective for sleep-disordered breathing and night-time hypoventilation encountered in patients who have various neuromuscular diseases. In most cases, the BiPAP mode of ventilation, rather than the continuous positive airway pressure, is appropriate for most restrictive lung volume processes secondary to progressive neuromuscular diseases. However, continuous positive airway pressure may have a role, particularly in young infants with SMA I who are unable to synchronize effectively with BiPAP. In all cases, frequent monitoring for adequate mask fit and appropriate ventilator pressure level settings is necessary.

Continuous invasive ventilatory support by way of a tracheostomy should be considered when contraindications or patient aversion to noninvasive ventilation are present, or when noninvasive ventilation is not feasible because of severe bulbar weakness or dysfunction. In these cases, discussions allowing careful consideration of the patient/family's desires, the child's prognosis, and the child's quality of life can often lead to a satisfactory resolution. For those SMA patients requiring full-time ventilatory support, portable ventilators can now be easily attached to power wheelchairs, markedly improving the quality of life for these patients in the community.

Secretion management and airway clearance are also important aspects of respiratory care in SMA patients. Manual cough-assist techniques performed by the caregiver/family, or mechanical insufflator-exsufflators (cough-assist machines), can help improve airway clearance and secretion management. In addition, the use of these methods in conjunction with noninvasive ventilation pre- and postoperatively have helped significantly improve the pulmonary care of patients who have SMA and are undergoing surgery. Intrapulmonary percussive devices and ventilators are also available to help mobilize secretions and improve pulmonary hygiene.

Sleep-disordered breathing and nocturnal alveolar hypoventilation are manifestations of worsening restrictive lung disease and respiratory failure in SMA. Sleep-disordered breathing is now recognized as a significant cause of morbidity in SMA [86]. Common signs and symptoms suggesting sleep-disordered breathing are nightmares, morning headache, and daytime drowsiness. A polysomnography with continuous CO_2 monitoring is helpful in determining sleep-related hypoventilation. However, a nocturnal pulse oximetry in the home environment can serve as an acceptable screening tool for sleep-related oxyhemoglobin desaturation and alveolar hypoventilation when polysomnography is unavailable. Other general measures for patients who have restrictive lung disease include yearly influenza and pneumococcal vaccination. For more detail, a recent update regarding the respiratory care of patients and a consensus statement for standard of care in SMA are available [87,88].

Spine deformity

Scoliosis has been estimated to occur in 78% to nearly 100% of SMA II patients [53,89,90]. Scoliosis almost always begins in the first decade of life as a result of severe truncal weakness. The curves are collapsing in nature and are thoracolumbar (62%), thoracic (12%), or lumbar (10%), or are double curves involving thoracic with lumbar or thoracic with thoracolumbar (16%) [89,91–96]. The average deformity observed over 10 studies was 90°, with a reported range of from 20° to 164° [97]. Severe kyphosis may be a common associated deformity [90] and virtually all patients who have severe scoliosis have significant pelvic obliquity [92]. In contrast, SMA III patients who are ambulatory have less scoliosis, with a reported prevalence of 8% to 63% [72,89,90]. Spinal bracing is generally used in SMA patients who are unable to walk, or to improve sitting balance. However, bracing has been repeatedly shown to be ineffective in preventing eventual progression of the scoliosis [90,91,93,94]. In addition, a concern with bracing is that it may compress the rib cage and further impair the pulmonary function by lowering the vital capacity [98,99].

Spinal fusion surgery is the only effective treatment for scoliosis in SMA [89–96,99,100]. For children over the age of 10 years with curves exceeding 60°, instrumentation with posterior fusion is the definitive choice [92]. Most consider improved cosmesis, balance, and comfort in the sitting position to be the primary goals of surgery. Segmental sublaminar wiring with Harrington rods or, more recently, Luque instrumentation, has resulted in an average correction of approximately 50%, with maintenance of the correction years after surgery [92]. Anterior surgical approaches in SMA patients can result in significant respiratory difficulty postoperatively and diminished pulmonary function over the long term. Nocturnal pulse oximetry can provide valuable information about potential postoperative ventilation need. In those patients at risk, preoperative mask-fitting and initiation of NIPPV can improve postoperative respiratory recovery [101]. Postoperative management after scoliosis surgery includes early involvement of physical and occupational therapies, mobilization out of bed when clinically stable, pain control, ventilatory support as needed, and appropriate pulmonary toilet. As in other neuromuscular diseases, spinal arthrodesis does not significantly improve the restrictive lung disease component of SMA by increasing the FVC.

Decline in some functional activities can occur after spinal arthrodesis. The most common include decreased gross motor skills, transfer ability, self-feeding, hygiene, dressing, independent toileting, and ambulation [96,102,103]. Spinal fixation may impair compensatory lumbar lordosis and lateral trunk sway, which are used by ambulatory patients to compensate for proximal weakness. Therefore, surgery is best deferred until ambulatory function loss is imminent or already lost. Patients and care providers should be adequately informed about possible short-term and long term functional consequences of spinal arthrodesis.

Hip dislocations and contractures

Nonambulatory SMA patients have a high incidence of coxa valga of the proximal femur and hip subluxation. Frank hip dislocation associated with pelvic obliquity is commonly noted. Significant pain associated with hip subluxation or dislocation is rare [104,105]. Operative treatment of hip subluxation or dislocation in SMA appears to be poor, with a high recurrence rate [105,106]. The current consensus is for nonoperative conservative management. Contractures are problematic in SMA II and SMA III patients who have lost ambulatory function. Reductions in range of motion by greater than 20° were found among 22% to 50% of SMA II subjects [53]. Hip, knee, and wrist contractures are the most common. Patients who have SMA perceive their elbow flexion contractures to hinder one or more daily functions and the contractures have been reported to be associated with greater discomfort [107]. Occupational and physical therapy referral, and a daily home stretching program with caregivers, should continue to prevent formation of significant joint contractures. Serial casting for contractures can be used, but a clear and practical goal of improved range of motion should be kept in mind.

Osteopenia and fractures

Osteopenia is a common finding among SMA patients. Fractures at birth may occur in SMA [108]. Falls may also lead to fractures in SMA after seemingly trivial trauma [109,110]. In one series, fractures occurred in 15% of SMA II cases and 12% of SMA III subjects [111]. Bone mineral density is significantly reduced in SMA, and the nature of bone mineralization at the epiphysis as compared with the diaphysis may be different. A recent study of bone density in SMA patients by dual energy x-ray absorptiometry (DEXA) scan suggests that osteopenia may be secondary to factors other than immobility [112]. Studies now suggest a possible SMN protein role in bone remodeling [113,114]. Rigid cast immobilization of fractures should be avoided to prevent a cycle of worsening osteopenia and further fractures. Calcium and vitamin D supplementation is reasonable, based on DEXA results.

Functional status evaluation in spinal muscular atrophy

Functional status evaluation, including gross motor milestone acquisition, independence in mobility, hand function, activities of daily living, and timed motor performance, have all been shown to be correlated with strength in SMA II and SMA III [14,53,54]. Patients have been documented to lose motor function over time without loss in absolute muscle strength [14,115]. Especially in severely weak patients who have SMA, traditional strength measurements are not as useful or clinically meaningful as functional measures. More recently, in evaluating clinical outcome measures in SMA patients, gross motor function measurements showed high reliability compared with quantitative muscle testing [115]. Other evaluation methods are now used, such as the Hammersmith and modified-Hammersmith Functional Motor Scale (HFMS), and a recently developed expanded version of HFMS available for SMA patients [116–120].

A detailed functional status evaluation of SMA patients shows that for self-care activities, 100% SMA I and 73% SMA II patients require assistance, whereas 45% and 37% of SMA IIIa and IIIb patients require assistance [57]. Bathing and dressing were the most difficult tasks. For the mobility function, assistance was needed in more than 90% of SMA I, II, and IIIa, whereas 63% of SMA IIIb patients required assistance. Stair management was the major obstacle for independence in achieving mobility for all types of SMA [57].

Interventions to improve the function of SMA patients depend on each patient's disease severity, level of weakness, comorbidity, and patient/family goal. For nonambulatory children who have SMA, early referral to a pediatric occupational and physical therapist for evaluation of appropriate adaptive equipment for self-care, seating system, and mobility devices is important. In general, evaluation for power wheelchair mobility can be explored as early as 18 to 20 months of age. Evaluations for adaptive equipment for dressing, feeding, and self-care should take place as appropriate, but frequently enough to challenge the patient's functional skills and improve independence. For those patients who have adequate truncal control but not enough strength for functional ambulation, reciprocal gait orthoses or a light-weight knee ankle-foot orthosis can be considered for standing and therapeutic exercises. Standing frame and mobile stander with ankle-foot orthosis may be additional options for those children who do not have sufficient strength to participate in standing activities. For ambulatory SMA patients, based on an individual's functional level, judicious use of an ankle-foot orthosis, a walker, a scooter, and a power wheelchair can improve community mobility function and independence.

Psychosocial evaluation

Normal intellectual function has been documented among SMA patients [17,121]. In regards to comorbid behavioral problems, a recent study found that 12.5% of SMA patients fulfilled the criteria for a *Diagnostic and Statistical Manual of Mental Disorders* (Fourth Edition) diagnosis, with separation anxiety disorder being the most common diagnosis [122]. The investigators concluded that children and adolescents who have SMA are characterized by a low psychiatric comorbidity and are not significantly different from control individuals. A study looking into the stress level of parents caring for a child who has SMA found that parental stress is lower in the SMA families with good coping skills, and lower than in families caring for a child with severe mental retardation [123]. Good social support was found to be an important factor in reducing emotional strain and stressors for families. During the care of patients who have SMA, providers should also be attuned to the needs of the caregivers. Keeping the family well informed of medical issues and treatment decisions, and being responsive to their needs, will improve the overall quality of life and care for the SMA patients.

Summary

Although many advances have been made regarding our understanding of SMA, unfortunately, no cure is yet available. However, neuromuscular medicine specialists have an important role in the care of patients who have SMA to maximize their functional capacities, prolong or maintain independent locomotion, prevent physical deformity and medical complications, and improve the quality of life. Many complex medical issues are associated with SMA that can be managed effectively by medical providers. The comprehensive management of clinical and rehabilitative issues associated with the care of patients who have SMA requires a coordinated multidisciplinary approach.

References

[1] Werding G. Zwei fruhinfantuile heriditaren falle von progressiver muskelatrophie unter bilde der dystrophie, aber auf neurotischer grundlage. Arch Psychiatr Nervenkr 1891;22:437–80 [in German].

[2] Hoffman J. Uber chronische spinal muskelatrophie in kindestalter auf familiarer basis. Dtsch Z Nervenheilkd 1893;3:427–70 [in German].

[3] Oppenheim H. Gber allgemeine und localisierte atonie der muskulatur (myatonie) im frGhen kindesalter. Mschr Psychiat Neurol 1990;8:232–3 [in German].

[4] Wohlfart G, Fex J, Eliasson S. Hereditary proximal spinal muscular atrophy—a clinical entity simulating progressive muscular dystrophy. Acta Psychiatr Scand 1955;30:395–406.

[5] Kugelberg E, Welander L. Heredofamilial juvenile muscular atrophy simulating muscular dystrophy. Arch Neurol Psychiatry 1956;75:500–9.

[6] Byers RK, Banker BQ. Infantile muscular atrophy. Arch Neurol 1961;5:140–64.

[7] Ogino S, Leonard DG, Rennert H, et al. Genetic risk assessment in carrier testing for spinal muscular atrophy. Am J Med Genet 2002;110(4):301–7.

[8] Pearn J. Incidence, prevalence, and gene frequency studies of chronic childhood spinal muscular atrophy. J Med Genet 1978;15(6):409–13.

[9] Munsat TL, Davies KE. Meeting report: International SMA consortium meeting. Neuromuscul Disord 1992;2:423–8.
[10] Munsat TL. Workshop report: International SMA collaboration. Neuromuscul Disord 1991;1:81.
[11] Dubowitz V. Chaos in the classification of SMA: a possible resolution. Neuromuscul Disord 1995;5(1):3–5.
[12] Iannaccone ST, Browne RH, Samaha FJ, et al. Prospective study of spinal muscular atrophy before age 6 years. Pediatr Neurol 1993;9:187–93.
[13] Ignatius J. The natural history of severe spinal muscular atrophy—further evidence for clinical subtypes. Neuromuscul Disord 1994;4(5–6)):527–8.
[14] Russman BS, Iannoccone ST, Buncher CR, et al. Spinal muscular atrophy: new thoughts on the pathogenesis and classification schema. J Child Neurol 1992;7(4):347–53.
[15] Zerres K, Rudnik-Schoneborn S. Natural history in proximal spinal muscular atrophy. Arch Neurol 1995;52:518–23.
[16] Thomas NH, Dubowitz V. The natural history of type I (severe) spinal muscular atrophy. Neuromuscul Disord 1994;4(5–6)):497–502.
[17] Carter GT, Abresch RT, Fowler WM Jr, et al. Profiles of neuromuscular diseases: spinal muscular atrophy. Am J Phys Med Rehabil 1995;74(Suppl):S150–9.
[18] Munsat TL, Skerry L, Korf B, et al. Phenotypic heterogeneity of spinal muscular atrophy mapping to chromosome 5q11-13.3 (SMA 5q). Neurology 1990;40:1831–6.
[19] Pearn J. Classification of spinal muscular atrophies. Lancet 1980;1(8174):919–22.
[20] Brzustowicz LM, Lehner T, Castilla LH, et al. Genetic mapping of chronic childhood-onset spinal muscular atrophy to chromosomes 5q11.2-13.3. Nature 1990;334:540–1.
[21] Gillium TC, Brzustowicz LM, Castilla LH, et al. Genetic homogeneity between acute and chronic forms of spinal atrophy. Nature 1990;345:823–5.
[22] Lefebvre S, Bürglen L, Reboullet S, et al. Identification and characterization of a spinal muscular atrophy-determining gene. Cell 1995;80(1):155–65.
[23] Scheffer H, Cobben JM, Mensink RG, et al. SMA carrier testing–validation of hemizygous SMN exon 7 deletion test for the identification of proximal spinal muscular atrophy carriers and patients with a single allele deletion. Eur J Hum Genet 2000;8(2):79–86.
[24] Feldkötter M, Schwarzer V, Wirth R, et al. Quantitative analyses of SMN1 and SMN2 based on real-time lightCycler PCR: fast and highly reliable carrier testing and prediction of severity of spinal muscular atrophy. Am J Hum Genet 2002;70(2):358–68.
[25] Battaglia G, Princivalle A, Forti F, et al. Expression of the SMN gene, the spinal muscular atrophy determining gene, in the mammalian central nervous system. Hum Mol Genet 1997;6(11):1961–71.
[26] Boda B, Mas C, Giudicelli C, et al. Survival motor neuron SMN1 and SMN2 gene promoters: identical sequences and differential expression in neurons and non-neuronal cells. Eur J Hum Genet 2004;12(9):729–37.
[27] Wirth B, Brichta L, Schrank B, et al. Mildly affected patients with spinal muscular atrophy are partially protected by an increased SMN2 copy number. Hum Genet 2006;119(4):422–8.
[28] Lorson CL, Hahnen E, Androphy EJ, et al. A single nucleotide in the SMN gene regulates splicing and is responsible for spinal muscular atrophy. Proc Natl Acad Sci U S A 1999;96(11):6307–11.
[29] Monani UR, Lorson CL, Parsons DW, et al. A single nucleotide difference that alters splicing patterns distinguishes the SMA gene SMN1 from the copy gene SMN2. Hum Mol Genet 1999;8(7):1177–83.
[30] Parsons DW, McAndrew PE, Iannaccone ST, et al. Intragenic telSMN mutations: frequency, distribution, evidence of a founder effect, and modification of the spinal muscular atrophy phenotype by cenSMN copy number. Am J Hum Genet 1998;63(6):1712–23.
[31] Zerres K, Wirth B, Rudnik-Schöneborn S. Spinal muscular atrophy–clinical and genetic correlations. Neuromuscul Disord 1997;7(3):202–7.

[32] Swoboda KJ, Prior TW, Scott CB, et al. Natural history of denervation in SMA: relation to age, SMN2 copy number, and function. Ann Neurol 2005;57(5):704–12.

[33] Hausmanowa-Petrusewicz I, Vrbová G. Spinal muscular atrophy: a delayed development hypothesis. Neuroreport 2005;16(7):657–61.

[34] Moosa A, Dawood A. Spinal muscular atrophy in African children. Neuropediatrics 1990; 21(1):27–31.

[35] Eng GB, Binder H, Koch B. Spinal muscular atrophy: experience in diagnosis and rehabilitation in management of 60 patients. Arch Phys Med Rehabil 1984;65:549–53.

[36] Parano E, Fiumara A, Falsaperla R, et al. A clinical study of childhood spinal muscular atrophy in Sicily: a review of 75 cases. Brain Dev 1994;16(2):104–7.

[37] Dorsher PT, Sinaki M, Mulder DW, et al. Wohlfart-Kugelberg-Welander syndrome: serum creatine kinase and functional outcome. Arch Phys Med Rehabil 1991;72:587–91.

[38] Packer RJ, Brown MJ, Berman PH. The diagnostic value of electromyography in infantile hypotonia. Am J Dis Child 1982;136:1057–9.

[39] Russell JW, Afifi AK, Ross MA. Predictive value of electromyography in diagnosis and prognosis of the hypotonic infant. J Child Neurol 1992;7:387–91.

[40] Jones HR. EMG evaluation of the floppy infant: differential diagnosis and technical aspects. Muscle Nerve 1990;13:338–47.

[41] Kilmer DD, McDonald CM. Exercise in childhood progressive neuromuscular disease. In: Goldberg B, editor. Sports, exercise, and childhood chronic disease. Champaign (IL): Human Kinetics; 1995. p. 109–21.

[42] Hausmanowa-Petrusewicz I, Karwanska A. Electromyographic findings in different forms of infantile and juvenile proximal spinal muscular atrophy. Muscle Nerve 1986; 9:37–46.

[43] Hausmanowa-Petrusewicz I, Fidzianska A, Dobosz I, et al. Is Kugelberg-Welander spinal muscular atrophy a fetal defect? Muscle Nerve 1980;3:389–402.

[44] Kuntz NL, Daube JR. Electrophysiological profile of childhood spinal muscular atrophy. Muscle Nerve 1982;5:S106.

[45] Buchthal F, Olsen PZ. Electromyography and muscle biopsy in infantile spinal muscular atrophy. Brain 1970;93:15–30.

[46] Imai T, Minami R, Nagaoka M, et al. Proximal and distal motor nerve conduction velocities in Werdnig-Hoffmann disease. Pediatr Neurol 1990;6(2):82–6.

[47] Moosa A, Dubowitz V. Motor nerve conduction velocity in spinal muscular atrophy of childhood. Arch Dis Child 1976;51:974–7.

[48] Raimbault J, Laget P. Electromyography in the diagnosis of infantile spinal amyotrophy of Werdnig-Hoffman type. Pathol Biol 1972;20:287–96.

[49] Schwartz MS, Moosa A. Sensory nerve conduction in the spinal muscular atrophies. Dev Med Child Neurol 1977;19:50–3.

[50] Dubowitz V. Muscle biopsy: a practical approach. London: BailliereTindall; 1985.

[51] Zalneraitis EL, Halperin JJ, Grunnet ML, et al. Muscle biopsy and the clinical course of infantile spinal muscular atrophy. J Child Neurol 1991;6:324–8.

[52] Malamud W. Infantile progressive muscular atrophy. In: Minckler J, editor. Pathology of the nervous system, vol. 1New York: McGraw-Hill; 1968.

[53] Carter GT, Abresch RT, Fowler WM Jr, et al. Profiles of neuromuscular diseases: hereditary motor and sensory neuropathy, types I and II. Am J Phys Med Rehabil 1995; 74(Suppl):S140–9.

[54] Koch BM, Simerson RL. Upper extremity strength and function in children with spinal muscular atrophy type II. Arch Phys Med Rehabil 1992;73:241–5.

[55] Merlini L, Bertini E, Minetti C, et al. Motor function-muscle strength relationship in spinal muscular atrophy. Muscle Nerve 2004;29(4):548–52.

[56] Kroksmark AK, Beckung E, Tulinius M. Muscle strength and motor function in children and adolescents with spinal muscular atrophy II and III. Eur J Paediatr Neurol 2001;5(5): 191–8.

[57] Chung BH, Wong VC, Ip P. Spinal muscular atrophy: survival pattern and functional status. Pediatrics 2004;114(5):e548–53.
[58] Bar-Or O. Role of exercise in the assessment and management of neuromuscular disease in children. Med Sci Sports Exerc 1996;28(4):421–7.
[59] McCartney N, Moroz D, Gamer SH, et al. The effects of strength training in patients with selected neuromuscular disorders. Med Sci Sports Exerc 1988;20:362–8.
[60] Charbonnier F. Exercise-induced neuroprotection in SMA model mice: a means for determining new therapeutic strategies. Mol Neurobiol 2007;35(3):217–23.
[61] Grondard C, Biondi O, Armand AS, et al. Regular exercise prolongs survival in a type 2 spinal muscular atrophy model mouse. J Neurosci 2005;25(33):7615–22, Erratum in: J Neurosci. 2005 14;25(37):8587.
[62] Aitkens SG, McCrory MA, Kilmer DD, et al. Moderate resistance exercise program: its effect in slowly progressive neuromuscular disease. Arch Phys Med Rehabil 1993;74:711–5.
[63] Kilmer DD, McCrory MA, Wright MC, et al. The effect of a high resistance exercise program in slowly progressive neuromuscular disease. Arch Phys Med Rehabil 1994;75:560–3.
[64] Barois A, Estournet B, Duval-Beaupere G, et al. Amyotrophic spinale infantile. Rev Neurol (Paris) 1989;145:299–304.
[65] Nutman J, Nitzan M, Grunebaum M. Swallowing disturbances in Werdnig-Hoffmann disease. Harefuah 1981;101:301–3.
[66] Willig TN, Paulus J, Lacau Saint Guily J, et al. Swallowing problems in neuromuscular disorders. Arch Phys Med Rehabil 1994;75:1175–81.
[67] Houston K, Buschang PH, Iannaccone ST, et al. Craniofacial morphology of spinal muscular atrophy. Pediatr Res 1994;36:265–9.
[68] Houston K, Bushang PH, Duffy D, et al. Occlusal characteristics of children with spinal muscular atrophy. Pediatr Dent 1994;16(1):59–61.
[69] Ballestrazzi A, Ballardini D, Battistini N, et al. Growth pattern and body composition in spinal muscular atrophy. In: Merlini L, Granata C, Dubowitz V, editors. Current concepts in childhood spinal muscular atrophy. New York: Springer-Verlag; 1989. p. 221–6.
[70] Bindfer H. New ideas in the rehabilitation of children with spinal muscular atrophy. In: Merlini L, Granata C, Dubowitz V, editors. Current concepts in childhood spinal muscular atrophy. New York: Springer-Verlag; 1989. p. 117–25.
[71] Liu GC, Jong YJ, Chiang CH, et al. Spinal muscular atrophy: MR evaluation. Pediatr Radiol 1992;22(8):584–6.
[72] Coletta C, Carboni P, Carunchio A, et al. Electrocardiographic abnormalities in childhood spinal muscular atrophy. Int J Cardiol 1989;24:283–8.
[73] Tanaka H, Uemera N, Toyama Y, et al. Cardiac involvement in the Kugelberg-Welander syndrome. Am J Cardiol 1976;38:528–32.
[74] Balantic Z, Zupan A. Measurements of respiratory capacity in patients with neuromuscular diseases. Exp Lung Res 2003;29(8):537–48.
[75] Iannaccone ST, Hynan LS, , American Spinal Muscular Atrophy Randomized Trials (AmSMART) Group. Reliability of 4 outcome measures in pediatric spinal muscular atrophy. Arch Neurol 2003;60(8):1130–6.
[76] Samahu FJ, Buncher CR, Russman BS, et al. Pulmonary function in spinal muscular atrophy. J Child Neurol 1994;9(3):326–9.
[77] Johnson ER, Abresch RT, Carter GT, et al. Profiles of neuromuscular diseases: myotonic muscular dystrophy. Am J Phys Med Rehabil 1995;74(Suppl):S104–16.
[78] McDonald CM, Abresch RT, Carter GT, et al. Profiles of neuromuscular diseases: Becker's muscular dystrophy. Am J Phys Med Rehabil 1995;74(Suppl):S93–103.
[79] McDonald CM, Abresch RT, Carter GT, et al. Profiles of neuromuscular diseases: Duchenne muscular dystrophy. Am J Phys Med Rehabil 1995;74(Suppl):S70–92.
[80] Bach JR, Wang TG. Noninvasive long-term ventilatory support for individuals with spinal muscular atrophy and functional bulbar musculature. Arch Phys Med Rehabil 1995;76: 213–7.

[81] Gilgoff IS, Kahlstrom E, MacLaughlin E, et al. Long-term ventilatory support in spinal muscular atrophy. J Pediatr 1989;115:904–9.
[82] Haas H, Johnson JR, Gill TH, et al. Diaphragm paralysis and ventilatory failure in chronic proximal spinal muscular atrophy. Am Rev Respir Dis 1981;123:465–7.
[83] Want TG, Bach JR, Avilla C, et al. Survival of individuals with spinal muscular atrophy on ventilatory support. Am J Phys Med Rehabil 1994;73:207–11.
[84] Lyager S, Steffensen B, Juhl B. Indicators of need for mechanical ventilation in Duchenne muscular dystrophy and spinal muscular atrophy. Chest 1995;108(3):779–85.
[85] Padman R, Lawless S, Von Nessen S. Use of BiPAP by nasal mask in the treatment of respiratory insufficiency in pediatric patients: preliminary investigation. Pediatr Pulmonol 1994;17:119–23
[86] Mellies U, Dohna-Schwake C, Stehling F, et al. Sleep disordered breathing in spinal muscular atrophy. Neuromuscul Disord 2004;14(12):797–803.
[87] Iannaccone ST. Modern management of spinal muscular atrophy. J Child Neurol 2007; 22(8):974–8.
[88] Wang CH, Finkel RS, Bertini ES, et al, Participants of the International Conference on SMA Standard of Care. Consensus statement for standard of care in spinal muscular atrophy. J Child Neurol 2007;22(8):1027–49.
[89] Evans GA, Drennan JR, Russman BS. Functional classification and orthopedic management of spinal muscular atrophy. J Bone Joint Surg Br 1981;63(4):516–22.
[90] Granata C, Merlini L, Magni E, et al. Spinal muscular atrophy: natural history and orthopedic treatment of scoliosis. Spine 1989;14:760–2.
[91] Aprin H, Bowen JR, MacEwen GD, et al. Spine arthrodesis in patients with spinal muscular atrophy. J Bone Joint Surg Am 1982;65:1179–87.
[92] Granata C, Cervellati S, Ballestrazzi A, et al. Spine surgery in spinal muscular atrophy. Long term results. Neuromuscul Disord 1993;3:207–15.
[93] Hensinger RN, MacEwen GD. Spinal deformity associated with heritable neurological conditions: spinal muscular atrophy. Friedreich's ataxia, familial dysautonomia, and Charcot-Marie-Tooth disease. J Bone Joint Surg Am 1976;58:13–24.
[94] Merlini L, Granata C, Bonfiglioti S, et al. Scoliosis in spinal muscular atrophy: natural history and management. Dev Med Child Neurol 1989;31:501–8.
[95] Piasecki JO, Mahinpour S, Levine DB. Long-term follow-up of spinal fusion in spinal muscular atrophy population. Clin Orthop 1986;207:44–54.
[96] Schwentker EP, Gibson DA. The orthopedic aspects of spinal muscular atrophy. J Bone Joint Surg Am 1976;58:32–8.
[97] Shapiro F, Specht L. The diagnosis and orthopedic treatment of childhood spinal muscular atrophy, peripheral neuropathy, Friedreich's ataxia, and arthrogryposis. J Bone Joint Surg Am 1993;75:1699–714.
[98] Noble-Jamieson C, Heckmatt JZ, Dubowitz V, et al. Effects of posture and spinal bracing on respiratory function in neuromuscular disease. Arch Dis Child 1986;61: 178–81.
[99] Riddick MF, Winter RB, Lutter LD. Spinal deformities in patients with spinal muscle atrophy: a review of 36 patients. Spine 1982;7:476–83.
[100] Daher YH, Lonstein JE, Winter RB, et al. Spinal surgery in spinal muscular atrophy. J Pediatr Orthop 1985;5:391–5.
[101] Bach JR, Sabharwal S. High pulmonary risk scoliosis surgery: role of noninvasive ventilation and related techniques. J Spinal Disord Tech 2005;18(6):527–30.
[102] Brown JC, Zeller JL, Swant SM, et al. Surgical and functional results of spine fusion in spinal muscular atrophy. Spine 1989;14:763–70.
[103] Furumasu J, Swank SM, Brown JC, et al. Functional activities in spinal muscular atrophy patients after spinal fusion. Spine 1989;14:771–5.
[104] Sporer SM, Smith BG. Hip dislocation in patients with spinal muscular atrophy. J Pediatr Orthop 2003;23(1):10–4.

[105] Zenios M, Sampath J, Cole C, et al. Operative treatment for hip subluxation in spinal muscular atrophy. J Bone Joint Surg Br 2005;87(11):1541–4.
[106] Thompson CE, Larsen LJ. Recurrent hip dislocation in intermediate spine atrophy. J Pediatr Orthop 1990;10:638–41.
[107] Willilg TN, Bach JR, Rouffet MJ, et al. Correlation of flexion contractures with upper extremity function and pain for spinal muscular atrophy and congenital myopathy patients. Am J Phys Med Rehabil 1995;74:33–8.
[108] Burke SW, Jameson VP, Roberts JM, et al. Birth fractures in spinal muscular atrophy. J Pediatr Orthop 1986;6:34–6.
[109] Gray B, Hsu JD, Furumasu J. Fractures caused by falling from a wheelchair in patients with neuromuscular disease. Dev Med Child Neurol 1992;34:589–92.
[110] Vestergaard P, Glerup H, Steffensen BF, et al. Fracture risk in patients with muscular dystrophy and spinal muscular atrophy. J Rehabil Med 2001;33(4):150–5.
[111] Hsu JD. Skeletal changes in children with neuromuscular disorders. Prog Clin Biol Res 1982;101:553–7.
[112] Kinali M, Banks LM, Mercuri E, et al. Bone mineral density in a pediatric spinal muscular atrophy population. Neuropediatrics 2004;35(6):325–8.
[113] Shanmugarajan S, Swoboda KJ, Iannaccone ST, et al. Congenital bone fractures in spinal muscular atrophy: functional role for SMN protein in bone remodeling. J Child Neurol 2007;22(8):967–73.
[114] Kurihara N, Menaa C, Maeda H, et al. Osteoclast-stimulating factor interacts with the spinal muscular atrophy gene product to stimulate osteoclast formation. J Biol Chem 2001; 276(44):41035–9.
[115] Iannaccone ST, American Spinal Muscular Atrophy Randomized Trials (AmSMART) Group. Outcome measures for pediatric spinal muscular atrophy. Arch Neurol 2002; 59(9):1445–50.
[116] Main M, Kairon H, Mercuri E, et al. The Hammersmith functional motor scale for children with spinal muscular atrophy: a scale to test ability and monitor progress in children with limited ambulation. Eur J Paediatr Neurol 2003;7(4):155–9.
[117] Mercuri E, Messina S, Battini R, et al. Reliability of the Hammersmith functional motor scale for spinal muscular atrophy in a multicentric study. Neuromuscul Disord 2006; 16(2):93–8.
[118] Krosschell KJ, Maczulski JA, Crawford TO, et al. A modified Hammersmith functional motor scale for use in multi-center research on spinal muscular atrophy. Neuromuscul Disord 2006;16(7):417–26.
[119] Nelson L, Owens H, Hynan LS, et al. The gross motor function measure is a valid and sensitive outcome measure for spinal muscular atrophy. Neuromuscul Disord 2006;16(6): 374–80.
[120] O'Hagen JM, Glanzman AM, McDermott MP, et al. An expanded version of the Hammersmith functional motor scale for SMA II and III patients. Neuromuscul Disord 2007; 17(9–10):693–7.
[121] Billard C, Gillett P, Signoret JL, et al. Cognitive function in Duchenne muscular dystrophy: a reappraisal and comparison with spinal muscular atrophy. Neuromuscul Disord 1992;2: 371–8.
[122] Laufersweiler-Plass C, Rudnik-Schöneborn S, Zerres K, et al. Behavioral problems in children and adolescents with spinal muscular atrophy and their siblings. Dev Med Child Neurol 2003;45(1):44–9.
[123] von Gontard A, Backes M, Laufersweiler-Plass C, et al. Psychopathology and familial stress—comparison of boys with Fragile X syndrome and spinal muscular atrophy. J Child Psychol Psychiatry 2002;43(7):949–57.

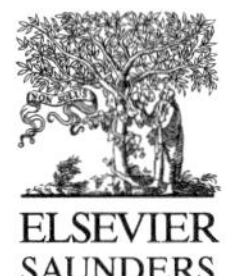

ELSEVIER
SAUNDERS

Phys Med Rehabil Clin N Am
19 (2008) 681–690

PHYSICAL MEDICINE
AND REHABILITATION
CLINICS OF
NORTH AMERICA

Index

Note: Page numbers of article titles are in **boldface** type.

A

doi:10.1016/S1047-9651(08)00054-5

B

N

O

P

Q

R

S

T

Moving?

Make sure your subscription moves with you!

To notify us of your new address, find your **Clinics Account Number** (located on your mailing label above your name), and contact customer service at:

E-mail: elspcs@elsevier.com

800-654-2452 (subscribers in the U.S. & Canada)
1-407-563-6020 (subscribers outside of the U.S. & Canada)

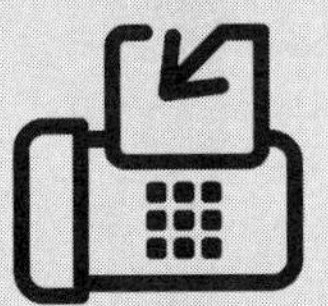

Fax number: 407-363-9661

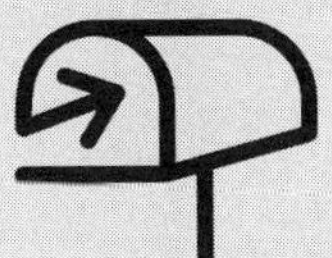

Elsevier Periodicals Customer Service
6277 Sea Harbor Drive
Orlando, FL 32887-4800

*To ensure uninterrupted delivery of your subscription, please notify us at least 4 weeks in advance of move.

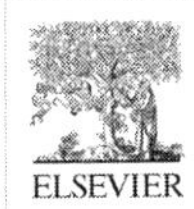